D1289517

ATTACHMENT FROM INFANCY TO ADULTHOOD

ATTACHMENT
from
INFANCY to ADULTHOOD
The Major Longitudinal Studies

Edited by
KLAUS E. GROSSMANN
KARIN GROSSMANN
EVERETT WATERS

THE GUILFORD PRESS
New York   London

© 2005 The Guilford Press
A Division of Guilford Publications, Inc.
72 Spring Street, New York, NY 10012

All rights reserved

No part of this book may be reproduced, translated, stored in a retrieval
system, or transmitted, in any form or by any means, electronic,
mechanical, photocopying, microfilming, recording, or otherwise, without
written permission from the Publisher.

Printed in the United States of America

This book is printed on acid-free paper.

Last digit is print number: 9 8 7 6 5 4 3 2 1

Library of Congress Cataloging-in-Publication Data

Attachment from infancy to adulthood : the major longitudinal studies /
edited by Klaus E. Grossmann, Karin Grossmann, Everett Waters.
     p. cm.
  Includes bibliographical references and index.
  ISBN 1-59385-145-6 (hardcover)
  1. Attachment behavior—Longitudinal studies. I. Grossmann, Klaus E.,
1935– II. Grossmann, Karin. III. Waters, Everett.
  BF575.A86A78 2005
  155.2—dc22

                                                    2004023994

About the Editors

Klaus E. Grossmann (PhD, University of Arkansas, 1965; Hab., University of Freiburg, 1970) first discovered the work of John Bowlby and Mary Ainsworth while conducting ethological and experimental research at the University of Freiburg's Institute for Biology after receiving his doctoral degree. He was appointed Full Professor at Bielefeld University, Germany, in 1970, and began the Bielefeld Longitudinal Study in 1973. In 1977, he moved his laboratory to the University of Regensburg and started a second long-term longitudinal attachment study. Professor Grossmann's numerous publications include, most recently, a collection of John Bowlby's and Mary Ainsworth's key papers in German translation with commentary (coedited with Karin Grossmann).

Karin Grossmann (PhD, University of Regensburg, 1984) is a Senior Scientist in Psychology at the University of Regensburg, Germany. Her research focuses on longitudinal and cross-cultural research in attachment. Widely published, Dr. Grossmann recently coauthored (with Klaus Grossmann) a book based on the Bielefeld and Regensburg longitudinal studies. She also teaches and publishes on the applications of attachment theory and research in family matters.

Everett Waters (PhD, University of Minnesota, 1977) is Professor of Psychology at the State University of New York at Stony Brook and a founding member of the New York Attachment Consortium. At the University of Minnesota's Institute of Child Development, Dr. Waters studied ethology and evolution with William Charlesworth and the concept of development and emotional development with L. Alan Sroufe. His extensive publications include the classic volume *Patterns of Attachment* (coauthored with Mary Ainsworth and colleagues) and two *Monographs of the Society for Research in Child Development* on attachment.

Contributors

Ora Aviezer, PhD, Center for the Study of Child Development, University of Haifa, Haifa, Israel

Jay Belsky, PhD, Institute for the Study of Children, Families, and Social Issues, Birkbeck University of London, London, United Kingdom

Inge Bretherton, PhD, Department of Human Development and Family Studies, University of Wisconsin, Madison, Wisconsin

Elizabeth Carlson, PhD, Institute of Child Development, University of Minnesota, Minneapolis, Minnesota

W. Andrew Collins, PhD, Institute of Child Development, University of Minnesota, Minneapolis, Minnesota

Judith Crowell, MD, Department of Child and Adolescent Psychiatry, State University of New York, Stony Brook, New York

Mary Dozier, PhD, Department of Psychology, University of Delaware, Newark, Delaware

Byron Egeland, PhD, Institute of Child Development, University of Minnesota, Minneapolis, Minnesota

Karin Grossmann, PhD, Department of Psychology, University of Regensburg, Regensburg, Germany

Klaus E. Grossmann, PhD, Department of Psychology, University of Regensburg, Regensburg, Germany

Erik Hesse, PhD, Department of Psychology, University of California, Berkeley, California

Robert A. Hinde, PhD, Department of Zoology, Sub-Department of Animal Behavior, St. John's College, University of Cambridge, Cambridge, United Kingdom

Nancy Kaplan, PhD, Department of Psychology, University of California, Berkeley, California

Heinz Kindler, PhD, Deutsches Jugendinstitut, München, Germany

Oliver Lindhiem, BA, Department of Psychology, University of Delaware, Newark, Delaware

Mary Main, PhD, Department of Psychology, University of California, Berkeley, California

Melissa Manni, MA, Department of Psychology, University of Delaware, Newark, Delaware

Avi Sagi-Schwartz, PhD, Center for the Study of Child Development, University of Haifa, Haifa, Israel

L. Alan Sroufe, PhD, Institute of Child Development, University of Minnesota, Minneapolis, Minnesota

Howard Steele, PhD, Graduate Faculty of Political and Social Science, New School University, New York, New York

Miriam Steele, PhD, Graduate Faculty of Political and Social Science, New School University, New York, New York

Joan Stevenson-Hinde, PhD, Department of Zoology, Sub-Department of Animal Behavior, St. John's College, University of Cambridge, Cambridge, United Kingdom

Everett Waters, PhD, Department of Psychology, State University of New York, Stony Brook, New York

Preface

Life courses or individual development can only be adequately understood longitudinally. Cross-sectional studies provide valuable comparisons among individuals at certain points in their lives. But the actual trajectories of individuals' lives are only accessible when the same people are studied at different ages. Longitudinal studies therefore have a long history in developmental research. And yet, because they are always designed and interpreted in the context of prevailing theory, methods, and culture, they are never entirely satisfactory. The coherence and impact of a longitudinal study depend on a productive back-and-forth movement between meaning, provided by a rich theoretical framework, and methods for translating theory into age-appropriate assessment. Ultimately, coherence and meaning also depend on the context provided by other studies, and certainly on future developments regarding the value of close bonds between children and parents.

No area in developmental psychology has a richer legacy of truly long-term longitudinal studies than attachment research in the Bowlby–Ainsworth tradition. The major longitudinal studies of attachment and its role in individual development are masterpieces of methodological problem solving and monuments to developmental analysis. Their key results are well known and widely cited. But each study touches on a wide range of topics, and results are necessarily reported in diverse venues and over the span of many years. Consequently, key results often stand out more clearly than the overall design of the studies. Solutions to difficult problems in age-appropriate assessment, research design, and theoretical work are rarely or only occasionally at center stage. These insights into the art of longitudinal research are as satisfying as specific empirical results, and as important to pass on to the next generation of longitudinal researchers.

In organizing this volume, we have invited the principal investigators from three decades of longitudinal attachment studies to reflect on how their projects originated, on the shape they eventually took, and on how their perspectives changed as the projects went forward. We also asked them to think about the lessons they learned that can be useful to a new generation of longitudinal researchers.

Attachment from Infancy to Adulthood: The Major Longitudinal Studies presents the first collection of original contributions on the major longitudinal attachment research projects. Each project sheds some light on central developmental questions: What actually develops in attachment development? What role does attachment play in the coherence of individual development from infancy to adulthood? And how do we attach meaning to change?

Robert A. Hinde (Chapter 1) shows how important evolutionary theory in general, and ethological observations in particular, were for John Bowlby when he formulated attachment theory. Inge Bretherton (Chapter 2) deepens our understanding of internal working models and the role this concept has played in attachment theory and research.

In this vein, L. Alan Sroufe, Byron Egeland, Elizabeth Carlson, and W. Andrew Collins give the first overview of their unique study of individual, social, and family development in difficult circumstances and across three generations (Chapter 3). Jay Belsky (Chapter 4) has also investigated attachment development in the family context and beyond. Karin and Klaus E. Grossmann and Heinz Kindler (Chapter 5), as well as Howard and Miriam Steele (Chapter 6), point to the distinctive influence of fathers as compared to mothers. Avi Sagi-Schwartz and Ora Aviezer (Chapter 7) have studied the impact of nonparental care.

Beyond specific relationships, Joan Stevenson-Hinde analyzes the interplay of attachment and temperament (Chapter 8). Judith Crowell and Everett Waters focus on secure-base behavior and attachment representations during the development of marriages (Chapter 9). And Mary Main, Erik Hesse, and Nancy Kaplan (Chapter 10) summarize for the first time the longitudinal project that has contributed so much to their thinking on attachment assessment. In the concluding chapter, Mary Dozier, Melissa Manni, and Oliver Lindhiem reflect on the implications of the work assembled here—great improvements in our understanding of developmental trajectories under a range of circumstances, but also issues that remain unresolved.

In the late 1960s and early 1970s, Mary Ainsworth's reports of her observations in Uganda and her Baltimore Longitudinal Study set the course for several generations of attachment study. Scholars in earlier periods had made extensive observations of mother–infant interactions (see Grossmann, 1995). But John Bowlby's attachment theory, and his and Ainsworth's commitment to ethological-observational methods, were new. As Hinde (Chapter 1) points out, it was part of Bowlby's genius to realize that behavioral biology provided both a theoretical and an empirical frame for developmental psychology. Infants are equipped with behaviors and expressions of emotions that are—under normal circumstances—intuitively understood and responded to by their caregivers, ensuring the survival of the infants. Bowlby knew about René Spitz's observations about maternal deprivation in orphanages, and he saw with his own eyes the devastating effects of maternal deprivation, depression, and "psychological death" in the infant rhesus monkeys studied by Harry Harlow (Blum, 2002).

Thus Bowlby recognized that an evolutionary ethological perspective must include the environment in which life-history strategies have evolved, and must take into account the "ordinary expectable caregiving environment" in which development occurs. Bowlby had also learned from Konrad Lorenz about the implicit cultural nature of human beings. The question for developmentalists, therefore, is this: What are the limits to adaptability if rearing conditions diverge too much from the "environment of evolutionary adaptedness"?

Bowlby's emphasis on real experience and his lifespan perspective were comfortably integrated with sophisticated ideas about mental representations drawn from cognitive psychology. The wide range of imaginative solutions to research design and age-appropriate assessment studies in this volume drew heavily upon these diverse influences. Here, perhaps more than in any other aspect, we see the critical role of Bowlby's and Ainsworth's theoretical, descriptive, and methodological insights as a "secure base from which to explore close relationships" and an unfailing framework for integrating new and unexpected findings (Waters & Cummings, 2000). These have been central to keeping assessment close to key theoretical constructs.

After more than three decades of attachment study, we are just beginning to realize Bowlby's goals of integrating empirical research on typical and atypical developmental trajectories and applying this research in significant ways to prevention and clinical practice. This is in line with Bowlby's original interest in clinical aspects of attachment development guided by well-posed questions from psychoanalysis. Like Freud, Bowlby considered typical and atypical development to be reflections of the same principles. Understanding attachment and its place in development requires "two stout pillars of evidence—individual development and developmental psychopathology—and a crosspiece of theory" (Bowlby, 1988, p. 2).

The contributors to this volume have integrated many different approaches to the study of attachment and its psychological implications across the lifespan. These pioneering researchers all view attachment development as an open-ended process of discovery from infancy to adulthood. As the reader will see, longitudinal research is a rather uncertain but still intense investment. We like to believe that the lifetime investment of these researchers has been a successful enterprise in helping to establish attachment theory and research as a major branch of developmental psychology.

In July 2003, Klaus and Karin Grossmann invited the contributors to this volume to Regensburg, Germany, to reflect on their careers in longitudinal attachment research. The rest of us (Everett Waters, the contributors, and the discussants) thank them for going beyond the usual "scientific" reports to share their very personal reflections on their own work.

We editors and contributors also thank the colleagues who, along with the editors, have commented on each chapter. These include especially Marinus van IJzendoorn, Peter Zimmermann, Gottfried Spangler, Lieselotte Ahnert, Isabel Soares, and Gabriele Gloger-Tippelt, whose knowledge and research greatly enriched the Regensburg discussions and this volume. The contributions collected here are reflections on attachment study and a foundation on which to continue building.

The meeting of the contributors and the discussants in Regensburg was generously supported by the Lotte Koehler Stiftung, München. We appreciate the unfailing assistance of Margit Frimberger, Anika Keppler, Ludwig Kreuzpointner, and Kerstin Stöcker in preparing and executing this meeting.

KLAUS E. GROSSMANN
KARIN GROSSMANN
EVERETT WATERS

REFERENCES

Blum, D. (2002). *Love at Goon Park: Harry Harlow and the science of affection.* Cambridge, MA: Perseus.

Bowlby, J. (1988). Developmental psychiatry comes of age. *American Journal of Psychiatry, 145,* 1–10.

Grossmann, K. E. (1995). The evolution and history of attachment research and theory. In S. Goldberg, R. Muir, & J. Kerr (Eds.), *Attachment theory: Social, developmental, and clinical perspectives* (pp. 85–102). Hillsdale, NJ: Analytic Press.

Waters, E., & Cummings, E. M. (2000). A secure base from which to explore close relationships. *Child Development, 71,* 164–172.

Contents

ATTACHMENT FROM INFANCY
TO ADULTHOOD

CHAPTER 1

Ethology and Attachment Theory

ROBERT A. HINDE

This chapter is about the role of ethology in John Bowlby's thinking when he was formulating attachment theory. *Ethology* is an approach to animal behavior initiated by Konrad Lorenz and Niko Tinbergen in the 1930s. It flowered between the 1950s and the 1970s, and has now been largely assimilated into other disciplines. It is best regarded not as a theory about behavior, but in terms of three basic attitudes:

1. The description and classification of behavior are essential preliminaries to its understanding.
2. Behavior cannot be studied without some knowledge of the environment to which the species has become adapted through evolution.
3. Questions about the evolution and function of behavior are as important as those about its development and causation.

These attitudes lead to the four questions that have been basic to the ethological approach: causation, development, function, and evolution (Tinbergen, 1963). They are perhaps most easily illustrated by a structural example. Suppose you are asked, "Why does your thumb move in a different way from the four other fingers?" You could answer in terms of *causation*: the bones and muscles of the thumb articulate in a way different from those of the other fingers. You could give a *developmental* answer: as the finger rudiments developed, one came to have a structure different from those of the others. A *functional* answer would refer to the fact that an opposable thumb makes it easier to grasp objects, climb trees, and so on. And finally, you might give an *evolutionary* answer: we are descended from

1

monkey-like ancestors, and have inherited this characteristic from them. All of these answers would be correct, but no one of them would be complete.

Originally ethology was built around a few basic concepts; these concepts were developed, modified, and in some cases discarded by ethologists over the years. But we are concerned here with the ethology of the 1950s, the period during which John Bowlby was forming his ideas. We shall see later that he examined every concept critically for validity and relevance before assimilating it. In addition, it must be emphasized that the fact that concepts basic to the development of a new discipline were subsequently found to be flawed is no reflection on their creators but part of the creative process: one has only to think of how much the same is true of Freud, Piaget, and even Darwin—though interestingly not very true of John Bowlby.

My task here is to survey the influence of these attitudes and 1950s' concepts on the development of attachment theory. I confess to some misgivings about this task because the essence of John Bowlby's approach was broad-minded eclecticism, and to emphasize one strand seems not only a betrayal of the discussions we had when he was formulating his ideas, but necessitates the omission of many other aspects of attachment theory. He made great efforts to present his theory as rooted in the work of Freud, and it is not unfair to describe the 1950s as a period of conflictful synthesis with ethology and other approaches. However, in his writings he made abundant references to the influence that ethology had on him (e.g., Bowlby, 1969, 1991), and in 1962 his closest colleague, Mary Ainsworth, pointed out that one of Bowlby's most significant contributions was to grasp the relevance of ethological concepts and methods for the study of human social development, to reformulate psychoanalytic theory in the light of these concepts, and thus to provide a testable framework.

I shall try to avoid personal bias, but some consequences of selective memory are inevitable.

John Bowlby was first introduced to Konrad Lorenz's writings by a friend in 1951, and the evolutionary biologist Julian Huxley helped him to find his way into the literature (Bowlby, 1980). He resonated to Lorenz's work on the formation of the parent–offspring relationship in geese (see below), and they met at a meeting sponsored by the World Health Organization in London in 1954 (Bowlby, 1991), and possibly earlier. Bowlby was already regarded as somewhat of a renegade by the community of British psychoanalysts. This was primarily because of his views on object relations and defense, which were somewhat discordant with the various schools of psychoanalytic theorizing. In the early chapters of *Attachment and Loss* (1969), he described some of the influences that had led him to depart from traditional psychoanalytic thinking.

I first met John Bowlby at a meeting at the Royal College of Psychiatry in 1954. This was one of my many good fortunes, because the organizers had tried to get Konrad Lorenz and Niko Tinbergen, and fell back on John and me when they declined. Soon afterward John invited me to join a regular seminar that he was starting at the Tavistock Clinic. This seminar was a formative experience for me. It was made possible by one of John's qualities that is too rarely mentioned, his eclecticism. This was demonstrated by the composition of the group, which included a Freudian analyst, a Kleinian analyst, a Hullian learning theorist, a Skinnerian learning theorist, a Piagetian, psychiatric social workers, sometimes an anti-psychiatrist, and myself as an ethologist. We had nothing—repeat nothing—theoretically in common, but we all had an interest in parent–offspring relationships. We met in what I remember as a dingy basement in the old Tavistock Clinic, but the discussions were inspiring. We mostly talked about case histories introduced by a psychiatric social worker or drafts of John's early papers. He was picking from each of us what he thought would be useful.

John's pre-World War II clinical work, epitomized by his study of "44 thieves" (Bowlby, 1944), led John to want to explore the mother–child relationship. Although the importance of a continuing relationship with another figure seemed clear, it was based on retrospective evidence. It was crucial to John to know what *really* went on between mother and child. Chapter 1 of *Attachment and Loss* (Vol. 1) starts with an exposition of the importance of direct observation, and he takes issue with psychoanalysis for starting with a clinical symptom or syndrome and making "hypotheses about events and processes which are thought to have contributed to its development" (1969, p. 4).

Two main factors influenced John to lay emphasis on an observational approach. First, in the postwar years in Great Britain parental visiting to children in hospitals was often limited to a single visit each week. The careful observations of children undergoing separation experiences in the hospital by James Robertson (e.g., 1952) showed that children could suffer a great deal from the separation. Second, John Bowlby was also much influenced by Mary Ainsworth's observations in Uganda (published in detail only in 1967 but carried out much earlier) which gave his theorizing an early impetus. He was thus entirely open to the ethological emphasis on description and classification. This aspect of his work is perhaps the more remarkable in that he was not an observer himself, and it was Ainsworth (Ainsworth, Blehar, Waters, & Wall, 1978) who developed the link between observational data and theory.

During the 1950s (see below) John became completely wedded to the two other basic attitudes of ethology. First, he embraced its emphasis on function. Many aspects of infant and child behavior and of mother–child interaction seem irrelevant to the modern world, and can only be understood in terms of the evolution of humans in an environment very different from the modern city. For instance, the fear of darkness, of strange situations, and of falling, and especially of separation from the mother, generally regarded then as "the irrational fears of childhood," make sense only when seen as *functional* in the environments in which humans evolved. John came to see proximity-seeking behavior as biologically adaptive: maternal protection would have been crucial in preventing starvation, exposure, and the attacks of predators.

John tied such observations together with the concept of the "environment of evolutionary adaptedness" (EEA) in which humans probably evolved as hunter-gatherers. In the EEA these apparently irrational aspects of behavior would have been essential for an infant primate dependent on its mother for care and protection.[1] The concept of function thus became central to ethological theory, giving rise to such questions as "Why do babies cry?" and "Why do babies direct their smiles preferentially at their mothers?" More recently, a number of authors have written about the possible functions not only of the "ideal" caregiver–child relationship, but also of "insecure" relationships (e.g., Belsky, 1999; Main & Hesse, 1990).

In association with the importance of the question of function, John realized the importance of recognizing humans' evolutionary origins. He frequently quoted comparative data to substantiate his theorizing, was delighted by the early publications from Harlow's laboratory on mother–infant interaction, and encouraged work on animals in others (see below). The evolutionary origins of human behavior became very much part of John's thinking, and he advocated an extensive use of the comparative approach.

I now turn from consideration of ethological *attitudes* to the influence of some of the *early concepts* of ethology on John's formulation of attachment theory.

Since John Bowlby first met ethology through the writings of Konrad Lorenz, but was later influenced more by the rather different approach epitomized by Niko Tinbergen, it is necessary first to say something about the early ethological concepts used by these two men. Although they were both basically naturalists and shared (with Karl von Frisch) a Nobel Prize, there were many differences between their approaches to ethology—differences that stemmed from differences in their personalities and increased with time (Baerends, 1991; Hinde, 1995). Two concepts developed by Konrad Lorenz in the early days of ethology must be mentioned first: the fixed action pattern (FAP) (Lorenz, 1935) and the innate releasing mechanism (IRM) (von Uexküll, 1934). Observing that much species-characteristic behavior was elicited by highly specific stimuli, Lorenz postulated the presence in the animal of an IRM that supposedly fitted the stimulus as a lock fits a key. For instance, the begging response of the herring gull chick was seen as elicited and directed by a red spot on the parent's bill (Tinbergen, 1948). And noting that many movements were as characteristic of a species as their anatomical structures, Lorenz referred to them as FAPs. He supposed that each IRM was specific to one FAP. In part because he occasionally observed that FAPs appeared spontaneously, he used an "energy reservoir" model of motivation: each FAP was seen as motivated by reaction-specific energy (RSE) stored in a reservoir that was fed from an endogenous source (Lorenz, 1950). The RSE could be released either by an external stimulus via the IRM or by the hydrostatic pressure of the RSE on a spring valve at the base (Lorenz, 1950).

Lorenz had emphasized that FAPs were often shared between related species, and could be used as taxonomic characters. This had provided a basis for comparative studies of a number of species groups, with shared FAPs being used as an indication of relations between species, and differences between species known to be related on other grounds to indicate the course of behavioral evolution (e.g., Lorenz, 1941; Tinbergen, 1959). (Ethologists were aware of the danger of circularity here.) Although the concept of FAP was later modified as it became apparent that FAPs were not fixed but had some variability (Barlow, 1977), John was impressed by the species-characteristic actions shown even by newborns, and incorporated the concept into his scheme. According to Bowlby (1969), "Rooting, grasping, crying, and smiling when they first appear are probably all examples of fixed action patterns and all play an important part in the early phases of social interaction" (p. 66). But in using the concept of FAP he pointed out that in humans they were limited primarily to facial expressions and infant behavior, that FAPs differ in their variability, and that most human behavior was much more variable than the classic examples of FAPs.

Work by Niko Tinbergen and his students and colleagues also necessitated modification of the concept of the IRM. Since one stimulus could influence a number of responses, it became necessary to reject the specificity of IRMs to FAPs postulated by Lorenz. It also became apparent that IRMs were neither necessarily "innate" nor single "mechanisms," and that specific stimuli could have consequences other than releasing FAPs. Most importantly, while some specific stimuli were important for the initiation of behavior, others could turn behavior off when a goal was achieved, implying that an internal correlate of the goal stimulus (the consummatory stimulus, CS) was involved (Bastock, Morris, & Moynihan, 1953). This meshed precisely with John's view that much of toddler and child behavior is "goal-corrected" toward the maintenance of proximity to the mother as a secure base. John preferred the term "terminating stimuli," which he linked to the idea of the "set-goal" of a given behavior or group of behaviors.[2] Of course, one response can also lead to the stimulus situation for another. For instance, Gunther (1955) showed that infant sucking involved successive responses of seeking, finding the nipple, latching on to it, and sucking.

Related to the concept of the CS was that of feedback. Although this had earlier roots (e.g., Craik, 1943), it was introduced into ethology by von Holst and Mittelstaedt (1950) and, as it incorporated the idea of CS, became an accepted part of the ethological approach, at least by Tinbergen and others whom Lorenz later described disparagingly as "English-speaking ethologists."

As might be expected, an issue frequently discussed in the Tavistock seminars was that of motivation. The Freudian concept of libido implied an energy model of motivation, with libido accumulating and being discharged in action. This had much in common with Lorenz's model of RSE released in action when RSE accumulated or the appropriate IRM was encountered. The idea that behavior could cease because of the inhibitory influence of goal stimuli (CS) showed how misleading such energy models could be, and critiques of the Lorenzian reservoir hypothesis (Hinde, 1960) led John to adopt instead references to set-goals, feedback, and behavior systems. Here he married the ethological approach to the test–operate–test–exit (TOTE) model of three American psychologists: Miller, Galanter, and Pribram (1960).

Rejection of the specific connection between IRM and FAP, with recognition that one stimulus could influence a number of behavior patterns, led also to the postulation of a hierarchy of mutually interconnected "nervous centers" (Tinbergen, 1951). Whereas Lorenz had written about his model of a reservoir containing RSE as an "as if" model, Tinbergen incorporated the idea by describing the "nervous centers" as "loaded with motivational impulses." In my view, this was one of the very rare occasions on which Tinbergen was less strict than Lorenz, since Tinbergen's model involved unnecessary speculative physiologizing, and energy models of motivation and the concept of RSE were seen as gross oversimplifications (Hinde, 1956). An even more useful concept proved to be that of the behavioral system.

This behavioral system concept was applied to the motivation and control of a group of behavior patterns that are more or less closely causally (and often also functionally) related to each other (Baerends, 1941, 1976). The concepts of CS ("terminating stimulus," as John called it) and feedback were naturally part of this concept of a behavioral system. This behavior system approach was incorporated into his theory by John as the "attachment behaviour system" with a corresponding "care-giving behaviour system" in the mother. On this view, the development of the child's attachment to the mother depended on a number of apparently pancultural responses (rooting and sucking, clinging, following, crying, etc.) with the biological function of maintaining physical contact, or later proximity, with the mother, and becoming increasingly focused on her as an individual during the first year. Reciprocally, the caregiving behavior system involved sensitivity and appropriate responsiveness to the infant's needs. The component responses were seen as "goal-directed." The infant's attachment behavior system was seen as also interacting with other behavior systems, notably the fear and exploratory systems. Activation of the fear behavior system usually leads to increased, and activation of the exploratory behavior system to decreased, activation of the attachment behavior system.

So far I have focused on the more elemental concepts that John used in developing attachment theory. But of overriding importance is the way in which he saw these as contributing to mother–child relationships. I mentioned earlier that his first contact with ethology was with Lorenz's work on imprinting. Lorenz had shown that young goslings, and the young of other nidifiguous birds, approach and follow the parent as soon as they can walk. However, they will also follow other moving objects. This response is associated with learning the characteristics of the object (normally the mother) and forming a relationship with it that is independent of conventional reinforcement (Lorenz, 1935). This "showed that in some animal species at least a strong bond to an individual mother-figure could develop without the intermediary of food, that it could develop rapidly during a sensitive phase early in life and that it tended to endure" (Bowlby, 1980, p. 650). At that time the current psychoanalytic view held that the infant was primarily motivated to seek food and (in the Freudian sense) sex from the mother, and that it was from these that the mother–infant bond emerged. Bowlby was empowered to reject this "dependency" hypothesis by Lorenz's goose data. When Harlow and Zimmermann (1959) demonstrated the importance of "contact comfort" in the formation of the mother–infant relationship in rhesus monkeys and the relative unimportance of nutrition, it was, of course, strong support for his view that the formation of a monotropic relationship with the caregiver was of central importance, and not the provision of material comforts. He also followed with interest the later work of Harlow, Mason, and colleagues on the formation of "affectional bonds" in nonhuman primates, with the reservation that their experiments were carried out in unnatural and impoverished laboratory situations (for a review, see Blum, 2003).

In the late 1950s John was trying to persuade hospitals to relax their restrictions on parental visiting hours, and needed experimental evidence to support his clinical or retrospective arguments. Such experiments would, of course, be ethically impossible with human children, but were considered acceptable with monkeys. He therefore helped me to find funds to establish a colony of group-living rhesus monkeys, partly in order to study the mother–infant relationship in detail in a more natural social context, and partly to obtain experimental evidence that maternal separation could have long-term effects. The social situation used, with a male, several females, and their young living together in a fairly large cage, seemed an acceptable compromise between nature and a small laboratory cage.

I cite one result as an example of the way in which attachment theory influenced ethological research.

In the short term, the response of the infant monkeys to separation could be characterized as "protest" and "despair," very similar to those demonstrated by Robertson (1952) in human infants during a stay in the hospital with very limited parental visiting. To simulate the types of separation in humans, we used four procedures, in each of which the infants were 30–32 weeks old and the procedure lasted 13 days (Hinde & McGinnis, 1977):

1. *M/R*. Mother removed, infant remains in familiar surroundings ("Mother goes to the hospital").
2. *I/R*. Infant removed, mother remains in the group ("Infant goes to the hospital").
3. *M-I/R*. Mother and infant removed and separated ("Mother and infant go to different hospitals").
4. *(MI)/R* Mother and infant removed but not separated ("Mother and infant go to the same hospital").

Although the group sizes were small (n = 6 or 7), the results were of some interest in throwing light on the importance of the precise circumstances of the separation. The nonseparated infants were less affected by the procedure than any of the other groups (I/R and M-I/R groups showed greatest frequency of distress calling and activity). The "protest" period lasted longer in the infants in a strange environment (I/R, M-I/R) than in those left in the home group (M/R), the latter lapsing into profound "despair" sooner. After reunion, the infants that had remained in their social group (M/R) showed more prolonged depression than those in the other separated groups and were less effective in getting the mother's attention on reunion than infants who were still protesting vigorously. The nature of the separation also affected the mother's responsiveness. If she had been left in the home pen (I/R), she was responsive to the infant when it was returned, but if she had been removed, then on reunion she was less tolerant of the demands of her infant. The latter result, which differed from that which might be expected in the human case, appeared to be due to the social context, for the removed mothers had to reestablish their relationships with other group members and were therefore less responsive to their demanding infants (Hinde & McGinnis, 1977). Some effects of the procedures on the mother–infant relationship and on behavior in anxiety-provoking situations appeared to be present 6 months later (Hinde, Leighton-Shapiro, & McGinnis, 1978).

In what was probably the last paper that John wrote, he listed 12 "basic features of attachment theory as they contrast with the previously most widely held theory, that postulating a 'dependency need'" (Bowlby, 1991, p. 305). Although it must be said that the paper was entitled "Ethological Light on Psychoanalytical Problems," it is noteworthy that ethological concepts are relevant to at least nine of those points (see also Simpson, 1999).

What is particularly impressive is the meticulous care with which John carefully examined every concept that he used. "Attachment and loss" was not a mere stitching together of instinct theory, control systems, and psychoanalysis: he analyzed every ethological concept that he used, even "instinct" itself. He recognized that little if any human behavior could be labeled as "instinctive" in the classical sense of the term, but adopted instead a distinction between "environmentally stable" and "labile" behavior (Hinde, 1970), recognizing that children had the potential to develop certain patterns of behavior, but that the course of development depended on environmental input. The result was real integration. In our discussions I sometimes said that I thought he spent too much space on aligning his views with Freudian ones. I was wrong: he was not just defending his back against psychoanalytic criticism, he was producing a true amalgam.

What of the future? Two points are worth emphasizing in the present context. First, and here I certainly betray my bias as an erstwhile primatologist/ethologist, some lessons from the monkey work seem to have been underexploited. For instance, the importance and implications of parent–infant conflict emphasized so brilliantly by Trivers (1974) and illustrated by the rhesus data (Hinde, 1969) have been cited in theoretical papers concerned with attachment, but seem to have had little effect on attachment research. In essence, Trivers argued that, as the infant developed, its demands on its mother would increase and the mother's willingness to accede to those demands would decrease because (in an evolutionary sense) the resulting diminution in her resources would diminish her chances of rearing further young successfully. Eventually, the latter effect would predominate. A variety of predictions concerning especially the relative amount of maternal care likely to be bestowed on successive infants follow from this. For instance, a last-born is likely to receive excellent care since any effect on the mother's later reproductive success will be unaffected. This surely is a matter worth consideration in research on maternal sensitivity, and also in research concerned with the differential effects of the age of separation on the nature of the mother–infant relationship.

Similarly, the relations between further maternal conception and infant behavior at weaning must involve differences in the maternal care received

(Berman, Rasmussen, & Suomi, 1993; Simpson, Hooley, & Zunz, 1981). This should surely have relevance to attachment theorists.

And second, to reiterate yet again a point made earlier, attachment theorists must never lose sight of the importance of eclecticism. For a number of years John's eclecticism was neglected and attachment research was limited to a rather small group of workers who paid little attention to the work of others—probably a necessary phase as the necessary but difficult techniques were established. But already attachment theorists are beginning to incorporate other approaches and to exploit advances in other disciplines (e.g., cognitive science, neuroscience; see Hesse & Main, 1999; Main, 1999) and the way seems open for a wider integration.

NOTES

1. The concept of the EEA has been criticized by authors insensitive to its relevance at the time, principally on the grounds that the environments in which humans evolved were probably more heterogeneous than was formerly supposed (see Laland & Brown, 2002). However, this criticism does not apply to those aspects of the environment with which John Bowlby was concerned.
2. John has written that Lorenz introduced him to the concept of "consummatory stimulus" in 1954, and that this was a factor influencing him to become interested in ethology. This is historically interesting since the concept had been clearly formulated only in 1953, and Lorenz, unhappy with it because it conflicted with his view of RSE, had difficulty in accepting it.

REFERENCES

Ainsworth, M. D. (1962). The effects of maternal deprivation: A review of findings and controversy in the context of research strategy. In *Deprivation of maternal care* (pp. 97–165). Geneva: World Health Organization.

Ainsworth, M. D. (1967). *Infancy in Uganda: infant care and the growth of attachment*. Baltimore: Johns Hopkins University Press.

Ainsworth, M. D. S., Blehar, M. C., Waters, E., & Wall, S. (1978). *Patterns of attachment*. Hillsdale, NJ: Erlbaum.

Baerends, G. P (1941). Fortpflanzungsverhalten und Orientierung der Grabwespe Ammophila campestris. *Tijdschrift Voor Entomologie, 84,* 68–275.

Baerends, G. P. (1976). The functional organisation of behaviour. *Animal Behaviour, 24,* 726–38.

Baerends, G. P. (1991). Early ethology: Growing from Dutch roots. In M. S. Dawkins, T. R. Hallliday, R. Dankins (Eds.), *The Tinbergen legacy* (pp. 1–15. London: Chapman & Hall.

Barlow, G. W. (1977). Modal action patterns. In T. A. Sebeok (Ed.), *How animals communicate* (pp. 98–136). Bloomington: Indiana University Press.

Bastock, M., Morris, D., & Moynihan, M. (1953). Some comments on conflict and thwarting in animals. *Behaviour, 6,* 66–84.

Belsky, J. A. (1999). Modern evolutionary theory and patterns of attachment. In J. Cassidy & P. R. Shaver (Eds.), *Handbook of attachment: Theory, research, and clinical applications* (pp. 141–161). New York: Guilford Press.

Berman, C. M., Rasmussen, K. L. R., & Suomi, S. J. (1993). Reproductive consequences of maternal care patterns during estrus among free-ranging rhesus monkeys. *Behavioral Ecology and Sociobiology, 32*, 391–399.

Blum, D. (2003). *Love at Goon Park*. Chichester, UK: Wiley.

Bowlby, J. (1944). Forty-four juvenile thieves: Their characters and home life. *International Journal of Psycho-analysis*, pp. 25–52, 107–127.

Bowlby, J. (1969). *Attachment and loss: Vol. 1. Attachment*. London: Hogarth Press.

Bowlby, J. (1980). By ethology out of psychoanalysis: An experiment in interbreeding. *Animal Behaviour, 28*, 649–65.

Bowlby, J. (1991). Ethological light on psychoanalytical problems. In P. Bateson (Ed.), *The development and integration of behaviour* (pp. 301–314). Cambridge, UK: Cambridge University Press.

Craik, K. J. W. (1943). *The nature of explanation*. London: Cambridge University Press.

Gunther, M. (1955). Instinct and the nursing couple. *Lancet, 268*, 575–78.

Harlow, H. F., & Zimmermann, R. R. (1959). Affectional responses in the infant monkey. *Science, 130*, 421–432.

Hesse, E., & Main, M. (1999). Psychoanalytic theory and attachment research: Theoretical considerations. *Psychoanalytic Inquiry, 19*.

Hinde, R. A. (1956). Ethological models and the concept of "drive." *British Journal for the Philosophy of Science, 6*, 321–331.

Hinde, R. A. (1960). Energy models of motivation. *Symposia of the Society for Experimental Biology, 14*, 199–213.

Hinde, R. A. (1969). Assessing the roles of the partners in a behavioural interaction. *Annals of the New York Academy of Sciences, 159*, 651–667.

Hinde, R. A, (1970). *Animal behavior* (2nd ed.). New York: McGraw-Hill. (First edition published 1966)

Hinde, R. A. (1995). Lorenz and Tinbergen. In R. Fuller (Ed.), *Seven pioneers of psychology* (pp. 75–106). London: Routledge.

Hinde, R. A., Leighton-Shapiro, M., & McGinnis, L. (1978). Effects of various types of separation experience on rhesus monkeys 5 months later. *Journal of Child Psychology and Psychiatry, 19*, 199–211.

Hinde, R. A., & McGinnis, L. (1977). Some factors influencing the effects of temporary mother–infant separation: Some experiments with rhesus monkeys. *Psychological Medicine, 7*, 197–222.

Laland, K., & Brown, G. (2002). *Sense and nonsense*. Oxford, UK: Oxford University Press.

Lorenz, K. (1935). Der Kumpan in des Umwelt des Vogels. *Journal für Ornithologie, 83*, 137–213, 289–413.

Lorenz, K. (1941). Vergleichende Bewegungsstudien an Anatinen. *Journal für Ornithologie 89*(Suppl.), 194–294.

Lorenz, K. (1950). The comparative method in studying innate behaviour patterns. *Symposia of the Society for Experimental Biology, 4*, 221–268.

Main, M. (1999). Epilogue. In J. Cassidy & P. R. Shaver (Eds.), *Handbook of attach-*

ment: Theory, research, and clinical applications (pp. 845–887). New York: Guilford Press.

Main, M., & Hesse, E. (1990). Parents' unresolved traumatic experiences are related to attachment status: Is frightened and/or frightening behaviour the linking mechanism? In M. Greenberg, D. Cicchetti, & E. M. Cummings (Eds.), *Attachment in the preschool years* (pp. 161–182). Chicago: University of Chicago Press.

Miller, G. A., Galanter, E., & Pribram, K.H. (1960). *Plans and the structure of behavior.* New York: Holt, Rinehart & Winston.

Simpson, J. A. (1999). Attachment theory in modern evolutionary perspective. In J. Cassidy & P. R. Shaver (Eds.), *Handbook of attachment: Theory, research, and clinical applications* (pp. 115–140). New York: Guilford Press.

Simpson, M. J. A., Simpson, A. E., Hooley, J., & Zunz, M. (1981). Daytime rest and activity in socially living rhesus monkey infants. *Nature, 290,* 49–51.

Robertson, J. (1952). *A two-year-old goes to hospital* [Film]. London: Tavistock Child Development Research Unit.

Tinbergen, N. (1948). Social releasers and the experimental method required for their study. *Wilson Bulletin, 60,* 6–51.

Tinbergen, N. (1951). *The study of instinct.* Oxford, UK: Clarendon Press.

Tinbergen, N. (1959). Comparative studies of the behaviour of gulls (*Laridae*): A progress report. *Behaviour, 15,* 1–70.

Tinbergen, N. (1963). On aims and methods of ethology. *Zeitschrift für Tierpsychologie, 20,* 410–433.

Trivers, R. (1974). Parent–infant conflict. *American Zoologist, 14,* 249–264.

Uexküll, J. von. (1934). *Streifzüge durch die Umwelten von Tieren und Menschen.* Berlin: Springer. [Translated in 1957 as *Instinctive Behaviour* (C. H. Schiller, Ed.). London: Methuen]

Von Holst, E., & Mittelstaedt, H. (1950). Das Reafferenzprinzip. *Naturwissenschaften, 37,* 464–476.

CHAPTER 2

In Pursuit of the Internal Working Model Construct and Its Relevance to Attachment Relationships

INGE BRETHERTON

PERSONAL RECOLLECTIONS

After my admission to the psychology program at Johns Hopkins University as an upper-level undergraduate in 1969, one of the first courses in which I enrolled was Mary Ainsworth's introductory class on developmental psychology. Three books were assigned: Bowlby's just published *Attachment* (1969), Freud's *The Ego and the Id* (1923/1960), and Piaget's *The Origin of Intelligence in Children* (1952). As a mother of three young children, I found Mary Ainsworth's observational studies of babies and mothers in their natural environments in Uganda and Baltimore particularly appealing and persuasive, especially as taught in the context of Bowlby's ethological and evolutionary framework. I also resonated to Piaget's view of the development of representation as "interiorized action" that—as I saw it—fit well with Bowlby's notion that infants construct internal working models of themselves in their physical and social environment, and that these models guide their behavior and anticipations, an idea that seemed revolutionary at the time. In 1970, when I became one of Mary Ainsworth's many doctoral advisees, she asked me to play the sometimes stressful role of stranger in a Strange Situation study. This experience led to a joint paper (Bretherton & Ainsworth, 1974) and to my dissertation (see Bretherton, 1978) on the interplay of wariness and affiliation in infants'

13

interaction with unfamiliar people. However, I also continued to be fascinated by Bowlby's "internal working model" approach to representation, and scoured Mary Ainsworth's copy of the prepublication manuscript of *Separation* (Bowlby, 1973) for additional insights.

In 1974, after a position for which I had applied at the University of Colorado–Boulder was offered to Elizabeth (Liz) Bates, I became her research associate. Our collaborative work on the transition from gestural to verbal communication led to my growing interest in young children's understanding of intersubjectivity (Bretherton, 1988; Bretherton & Bates, 1979) and their developing ability to talk about mental states (Bretherton & Beeghly, 1982; Bretherton, McNew, & Beeghly-Smith, 1981; Dunn, Bretherton, & Munn, 1987). Influenced by these findings and emerging research on event schemas and storytelling, I began to interpret symbolic play as evidence for children's early developing ability to mentally represent and manipulate social situations and relationships and to engage in rudimentary hypothetical thinking (Bretherton, 1984).

Another important influence was Robert (Bob) Emde, who invited me to join the Denver Psychobiology Research Group that held bimonthly meetings to discuss and critique members' research. During the Infant Conference in Austin, Texas, in 1980, Bob and I noticed several exciting new trends in attachment research (the Adult Attachment Interview, or AAI; international attachment studies in Germany, Israel, and Japan; the Waters Q-set for assessing secure base behavior; and longitudinal studies with atypical children). In his role as editor of the Monographs for the Society for Research in Child Development, Bob suggested that I might recruit the authors of these studies for a collaborative submission to the monograph series. In the resulting "Growing Points of Attachment Theory and Research" (1985), coedited with Everett Waters, I decided to make a concerted, and I believe successful, effort to interest a broader audience in the "internal working model" construct. I had received much encouragement from Bowlby for an earlier paper I had written on this topic (Bretherton, 1980), but it did not seem to resonate with other colleagues in the attachment field. By the mid-1980s, however, the time seemed ripe for a new attempt. Not only had mental representation become a "hot" topic, but Main, Kaplan, and Cassidy's (1985) empirical findings with the AAI and the Separation Anxiety Test (SAT) had made internal working models more obviously relevant to attachment researchers and clinicians. After my move to Colorado State University, further opportunities to explore the working model construct resulted from Bob's invitation to join the MacArthur Network on the Transition from Infancy to Early Childhood. As a member of the network's Attachment Work Group (headed by Mark Greenberg) and in line with the group's focus on attachment beyond the preschool years, I decided to create an attachment-based story completion task (ASCT) in collaboration with Doreen Ridgeway (Bretherton & Ridgeway, 1990), and in parallel with Helen Buchsbaum and Bob Emde who adopted our technique to examine young children's understanding of moral conflict (Buchsbaum & Emde, 1990). During the second phase of the MacArthur Transition Network, David Oppenheim and I, with input from other members of the Narrative Work Group, created and pilot-tested a "communal" collection of story stems that included attachment and moral conflict themes from the earlier collaborative work, as well as a series of new story stems about moral dilemmas in triadic relationships. This collection, now known as the MacArthur Story Stem Battery, or MSSB, has been in use since 1990 but has only recently been published (Bretherton, Oppenheim, Buchsbaum, Emde, & the MacArthur Narrative Group. 2003).

While pursuing empirical research on story completion tasks for pre-schoolers, I also continued with efforts to flesh out theoretical aspects of the internal working model construct in several integrative papers given at various symposia (Bretherton, 1990, 1991, 1993, 1996). Following in Bowlby's interdisciplinary footsteps, I drew on insights from adjacent fields (object relations psychoanalytic thinking, social cognition and the social self, storytelling, event schemas, memory, trauma) as well as empirical attachment research.

My chapter differs from those by other contributors to this volume because I discuss the origins and development of an idea rather than find-ings from a longitudinal study. I begin by highlighting aspects of Bowlby's (1969, 1973, 1980) working model construct that are frequently misunder-stood. I then switch to empirical work on working models, but with a selec-tive focus on studies of preschool children that have used the ASCT (Bretherton & Ridgeway, 1990) as a window into young children's work-ing model of self and attachment figure(s). In the third section I integrate ASCT findings with recent research on mother–child talk about memories of everyday life and traumatic experiences. I also consider developmental research on implanted memories that is relevant to Bowlby's (1980) pro-posals about defensive processes in the construction of working models.

INTERNAL WORKING MODELS: A CLARIFICATION OF BOWLBY'S PERSPECTIVE

It is *not* surprising that Bowlby, a psychoanalyst trained in the object rela-tions tradition, concerned himself with the function of mental representa-tion in attachment relationships. Undeterred by the still dominating influ-ence of behaviorism, his aim was to bring a new perspective to "the internal worlds of traditional psychoanalysis" (Bowlby, 1969, p. 82). What *is* surprising, however, is that he adopted the notion of representation as mental models before empirical support for this speculative idea became available. Bowlby had discovered the notion of internal working models in the writings of an eminent zoologist who studied the behavior of octopi (Young, 1964), but its origin was an influential book by Kenneth Craik, titled *The Nature of Explanation* (1943). Commenting that the idea might seem fanciful to researchers "steeped in extreme behaviorism," Bowlby (1969, p. 81) maintained that the human capacity for foresightful and insightful human behavior was difficult to understand *without* making the assumption that the brain builds up mentally manipulable models of the environment and the self in it.

Internal Working Models:
A General Approach to Representation

Since 1969, when Bowlby first used Craik's term "internal working model," it has been independently adopted by cognitive psychologists (e.g., Johnson-Laird, 1983), philosophers of mind (Metzinger, 2003), and neuroscientists (Gallese, in press). Yet few attachment researchers realize or acknowledge that mental model building constitutes a *general* approach to representation that applies to the physical as well as to the interpersonal world and that is by no means limited to attachment relationships. As Bowlby explained later:

> Every situation we meet with in life is construed in terms of the representa-
> tional models we have of the world about us and of ourselves. Information
> reaching us through our sense organs is selected and interpreted in terms of
> those models, its significance for us and those we care for is evaluated in
> terms of them, and plans of action executed with those models in mind. On
> how we interpret and evaluate each situation, moreover, turns also how we
> feel. (1980, p. 229)

Bowlby held that "in the working model of the world that anyone builds, a key feature is his notion of who his attachment figures are, where they may be found, and how they may be expected to respond" (1973, p. 208). Children with sensitive and responsive attachment figures, he posited, would learn to approach the world with confidence or seek help if they could not manage on their own. They would, hence, develop working models of a secure self, caring parents, and a reasonably benign world. In contrast, children who could not count on an available and responsive attachment figure would come to see the world as unreliable and unpredictable, leading them to either retreat from it or to fight it. From outside attachment theory, Nelson (1996) recently made a related claim, namely, that the specific bond with a primary caregiver is a key early ingredient in the individuality or uniqueness of the infant's model of the world.

Working Models in Attachment Relationships

In the remainder of this section I narrow my focus to working models of self and attachment figure (more briefly, attachment working models) and attempt to address four frequently asked questions: (1) whether attachment working models should be regarded as relationship-specific or as representations of general strategies of relating; (2) in what sense we can talk about stability of security in the context of developmental change of attachment working models; (3) the degree to which attachment working models are consciously accessible or rendered inaccessible by defensive processes; and (4) whether "fantasies" have a place in theorizing about attachment.

The first question, whether attachment working models should be seen as relationship-specific or as representing general strategies of relating, has a straightforward answer as long as we limit the discussion to one attachment figure. Bowlby conceived of attachment working models as a translation of actual relationship patterns into interdependent representations of self and attachment figure (e.g., parent as loving-protecting, self as loved-secure), that is, as relationship-specific. He also assumed, however, that early relationship patterns influenced how a child might enter into relationships with other caregiving adults and peers, as well as with future mates and offspring in adulthood (Bowlby, 1988).

Unfortunately, this explanation becomes problematic when a child's relationship with one attachment figure is secure but that with another insecure. A number of studies comparing child–mother and child–father attachments have revealed that attachment security with the mother more consistently and strongly predicts later patterns of relating to peers than attachment security with the father (for a meta-analysis, see van IJzendoorn & Bakermans-Kranenburg, 1996). In other studies, however, two secure relationships predicted better child outcomes than two insecure relationships, with intermediate results when one parent–child relationship is secure and the other insecure. Much, therefore, remains to be discovered about whether, when, and how a child constructs an integrated self-model while participating in two (or more) qualitatively different attachment relationships (for a discussion of this topic in light of sociocognitive development, see Bretherton, 1991). In view of Bowlby's (1969) proposal that one attachment figure tends to play the primary role, one might hypothesize that the primary figure would have the greatest influence on personality and relational development, but studies tend not to identify which of a child's several attachment figures should be considered primary (those that do so tend to find that this role is more often played by the mother). In addition, the degree to which individuals develop relationship-specific working models with teachers and peers, and whether and how these in turn feed into a generalized working model of relating to others, deserves much further thought and study.

Regarding the second question, how to conceptualize stability of security in the face of developmental change, Bowlby's explanation is again straightforward if we restrict ourselves to one secure attachment relationship. In such a relationship, gradual changes in a child's behavioral, cognitive, and emotional competencies result in similarly gradual revisions of the child's working models (Bowlby, 1969, p. 82) and, I would add, the parent's working model of the child. However, over time a profound change takes place as children gain a greater understanding of their attachment figure's feelings and motives. Young children who have reached this level of psychological insight, Bowlby claimed, become able to develop *shared* working models of attachment relationships in which there is give-and-take on both sides, and in which conflicting goals can more easily be aligned through reciprocal negotiation. His label for this more sophisticated level of relating was "goal-corrected partnership" (Bowlby, 1969, p. 355). In terms of trust and security, such a relationship has remained secure from infancy to childhood, but, developmentally speaking, the security offered by a goal-corrected partnership is more sophisticated than that experienced by an infant (Bretherton & Munholland, 1999).

The third question, conscious accessibility versus inaccessibility of attachment working models, arises most often when severe family or environmental stresses adversely affect an attachment figure's ability to respond sensitively to a child's attachment needs. The revision of attachment working models under these circumstances becomes problematic because defensive processes tend to interfere with adaptive model reconstruction. Attempting to replace Freud's ideas on defence mechanisms with a more current perspective, Bowlby (1980) availed himself of the growing literature on information processing and memory. It is important to point out, however, that he regarded his theorizing in this area as tentative, cautioning that "there is clearly a long way to go before the theory sketched is within sight of doing justice to the wide range of defensive phenomena met with clinically" (1980, p. 44).

Bowlby (1980) proposed two major defensive strategies: "defensive exclusion" and "segregation of principal systems." As I understand his exposition, both have the effect of shutting available, but potentially anxiety-provoking, information out of awareness, with the second (involving a "split" in the ego) being more severe. Bowlby speaks of "defensive exclusion" when an individual has developed two inconsistent working models of the same relationship, but only one of dominant in consciousness while the other is repressed or suppressed. In contrast, "segregation of principal systems" occurs when two or more selves or egos are segregated from each other, each having "access to its own sectionalized memory store" or working model. What Bowlby seems to have had in mind are dissociative processes, including dissociative identity disorder or fugues (1980, p. 59; see also Bowlby, 1988, pp. 113–115). The distinction between defensive exclusion and segregation of principal systems can perhaps be clarified with the help of William James's (1890/1950) constructs of the "I" (self as agent and knower) and the "Me" (self as object or representation). Within this terminology, defensive exclusion would involve a unified principal system or "I" operating with one or more "Me's" that are differentially accessible to consciousness. Segregation of principal systems, in contrast, would involve two or more distinct but conflicting "I's," each with its own internally consistent IWM, but with no communication between the two "I's" and their respective "Me's." In a later publication, however, Bowlby (1988, p. 113) referred to defensive processes as "a spectrum of related syndromes with commoner and more severe forms," perhaps hinting that the distinction between repression and dissociative processes is not always easy to make.

Bowlby believed that young children before 3 years of age were especially vulnerable to conditions instigating defensive processes (1980, p. 72), but he also held that adolescents and adults continued to remain at risk. Relying on clinical case studies, he contended that when parents reject, ignore, or ridicule their children's attachment behavior in highly stressful or traumatic situations, the children may respond by repressing these experiences, especially if parents also insist that their rejecting behavior be seen as caring and the child him- or herself as incompetent or bad (1973, p. 315). Although not all children in such situations adopt their parents' (false) views, some may develop contradictory working models of self and attachment figure, one based on his or her own memories, and another based on parental (mis)interpretations. Often, the latter working model will dominate the child's awareness while the former is likely to be wholly or partially repressed. Moreover because it is based on the level of understanding available at the time it was formed, it may never have been translated into language, and hence never have been revised. Updating and reprocessing of such early models would—according to Bowlby—require conscious reworking:

> In individuals suffering from emotional disturbance, the model that has the greatest influence may have been developed during the early years on fairly simple lines, yet one of which the individual is not aware, in contrast to a later, much more sophisticated model of which the individual is more aware and that he believes to be dominant. During therapy a model of doubtful validity may become intelligible when the patient's history is explored during years of immaturity. (1973, p. 205; see also p. 23)

In previous discussions, I have described defensive exclusion (Bowlby, 1973, 1980) as an all-or-nothing process, but this was an oversimplification of what Bowlby actually claimed. Rather, he proposed that the dominance of the more readily accessible (conscious) working models over the defensively excluded models should not be considered as absolute. Fragments of contradictory nonconscious or partially conscious subordinate model(s) may leak into awareness, and activate fragments of attachment behavior, and associated moods, or dreams. Alternatively, two or more contradictory working models may oscillate in becoming conscious, explaining the activation of erratic interpersonal behavior. Sometimes what is defensively excluded is not the memory of a traumatic event, but emotions become cognitively disconnected from the person who aroused them. Thus, a distressing situation primarily caused by the self may erroneously be blamed on another person, or the self may falsely take responsibility for a situation caused by someone else (especially to absolve a parent from blame). Another possibility is that a person may become so preoccupied with the details of his or her own suffering that he or she is unable to reflect on the reasons for a painful interpersonal situation (Bowlby, 1980, p. 68). Such defensive misattributions render the revision of contradictory working models of self and attachment figure very difficult.

Taking his cue from the emerging notion that humans may operate with several distinct memory systems Bowlby (1980, citing Tulving, 1972) speculated that defensive exclusion and misattribution may be facilitated when information from different sources (personal experience vs. what parents or others tell the child about these experiences) is stored in separate systems. For example, the original memory of how a child experienced an event might be stored in what Tulving (1972) termed the "episodic" (autobiographical) memory system, whereas representations of what parents or others (misleadingly) told the child might come to be stored in the "semantic" memory system or general knowledge base. In support of these proposals, Bowlby pointed out that some patients provide general descriptions that portray their parents as highly admirable while their detailed accounts of how the parents had actually behaved or what they actually said throw doubt upon these idealized general descriptions. In other cases, "uniformly adverse" generalizations about parents are contradicted by detailed memories suggesting a more favorable image. It is in this context that Bowlby remarked that "the generalizations of mother, father, and self enshrined in what I am terming working models or representational models will be stored semantically" (1980, p. 62). It is not clear, however, why he regarded semantic, but not episodic, memory as involved in the construction of internal working models.

While not quarreling with the defensive phenomena Bowlby described, I suggest that his proposals based on Tulving's (1972) memory research should be revisited in light of current thinking. Memory theorists are not unanimous over how to differentiate between episodic and semantic memory because semantic memory seems to be necessary to generate and store episodic memories. In addition, some researchers tend to contrast semantic and episodic memory (both accessible to consciousness) with procedural memory (not accessible to deliberate recall). It is unclear to me why Bowlby failed to include procedural memory in his discussion of memory systems even though it too was proposed in Tulving's 1972 chapter. Bowlby did, however, point out that habitual interaction patterns can become so automated that they operate outside awareness, having become what some call "proceduralized." Several attachment researchers have begun to use the construct of procedural memory in their theorizing (see Crittenden, 1989; Spangler & Zimmermann, 1999; Zimmermann, 1999), but without clarifying what aspect of procedural memory they have in mind. Such clarifications seem called for, in view of Wheeler, Stuss, and Tulving's (1997) definition of procedural memory as a collection of multiple systems that include motor skill memory, conditioning, and priming. Finally, some memory theorists employ the newer terms *explicit* and *implicit* to refer to memory systems, an approach rejected by Schacter and Tulving (1994) who protest that the adjectives *explicit* and *implicit* memory describe types of processing, not types of storage. According to this approach, a child could use attachment working models implicitly (without conscious awareness) to guide ongoing interactions with a caregiver, and explicitly to reflect on what might happen in the more distant future. I will return to this issue in the third section of this chapter.

Finally, I would like to address the topic of fantasies whose relevance to attachment theory and working models is often denied. Bowlby was extremely wary of this term because he strongly disagreed with those of his psychoanalytic colleagues who viewed fantasies as the product of instincts and as unrelated to actual experiences in the family (Bowlby & Parkes, 1970, p. 215). Instead of using the label "fantasy," he preferred to talk about a "belief that X will occur," or a "hope that Y will still be possible," even if what was expressed seemed totally impossible to outside observers unacquainted with a patient's history. In a paper on mourning, Bowlby (1960) described a boy who left his bedroom door open every night "in the hope that a large dog would come to him, be very kind to him, and fulfill all his wishes." Bowlby interpreted this "fantasy" as an expression of the boy's longing for his dead mother whom he had not been allowed to mourn, let alone talk about. In another example, Bowlby (1988) mentioned a 6-year-old girl who had developed a terror that creatures looking like chairs and other pieces of furniture—she called them "daleks"—would fly across the room to strike her. It turned out that the child's father had repeatedly broken furniture and thrown it at the child when she was 2 years old, and had also beaten and thrown the child herself across the room. Based on these and similar cases, Bowlby (1980) maintained that seemingly unrealistic wishes or fears can seem reasonable when a person's history is taken into account. These notions are important in the interpretation of children's responses to representational attachment measures that I consider in the next section. If taken in Bowlby's sense, I see a place for "fantasies" within attachment theory.

RESEARCH ON CHILDREN'S
ATTACHMENT REPRESENTATIONS

Empirical studies of attachment up to the mid-1980s focused almost exclusively on infant–parent attachment patterns assessed in the Strange Situation, either to predict later developmental outcomes or to examine precursors of secure and insecure attachment classifications. During this period, Bowlby's theorizing about working models had little impact, but in the course of the 1980s, Main and her collaborators (1985) began to study attachment relationships at the level of representation. They examined adults', especially parents', attachment histories via the Adult Attachment Interview (AAI; George, Kaplan, & Main, 1984/1996), and accessed children's representations of attachment experiences using pictures of parent–child separation. In this section I reflect on the development and meaning of instruments designed to access children's attachment working models with particular emphasis on findings obtained with the Attachment Story Completion Task (Bretherton & Ridgeway, 1990).

Beginnings: The Separation Anxiety Test

The first representational attachment measure for children was the Separation Anxiety Test (SAT), adapted by Kaplan (1987; Main et al., 1985) from Klagsbrun and Bowlby's (1976) earlier version, itself derived from Hansburg's (1972) SAT for adolescents. The SAT is based on the assumption that children draw on their working models of actual attachment experiences in responding to the task.

Kaplan's version of the test consisted of six drawings depicting mild and severe parent–child separation experiences (e.g., the parents say goodnight at bedtime; the parents leave for a 2-week vacation). After providing a standard description of each picture, an interviewer asked the 6-year-old participants to say how the child in the picture was feeling and what he or she was going to do next. Kaplan (1987) identified four distinct patterns of responses to this separation test. "Resourceful" 6-year-olds were able to talk about the pictured separations with emotional openness, producing coherent explanations of how the child in the picture would feel and behave. Many spontaneously mentioned their own separation experiences. "Inactive" children labeled the pictured child as sad, but had little or nothing to say about what the child might do in response to the separation. "Ambivalent" children described contradictory parental behaviors in response to the pictures. Finally, "fearful" children either remained completely silent or ascribed overwhelming fears to the pictured child. There was significant concordance between resourceful, inactive, ambivalent, and fearful classifications of separation pictures and children's secure, avoidant, ambivalent, and disorganized infant–mother attachment patterns observed in the Strange Situation in infancy. Coherence, constructive resolutions, and emotional openness versus incoherence, bizarre resolutions, and emotional constriction in children's picture responses turned out to be excellent predictors of observed reunion behaviors in these and a number of subsequent studies (for a review, see Solomon & George, 1999). These findings are consonant with Bowlby's proposal that working models of self and attachment figure in secure relationships are easily retrievable from memory because they are not subject to extensive defensive processes, and, conversely, that the interference of defensive processes in working model construction and access would make it more difficult for insecure children to create coherent and constructive story resolutions. Interestingly, even though they were developed independently (N. Kaplan, personal communication, June 2004), both Main and Goldwyn' (1984/1998) classification system for the AAI and Kaplan's (1987) classification system for children's responses to separation pictures corroborated the theoretically expected link between attachment security and a coherent well-organized attachment working model, including the ability to "operate" this model without defensiveness during discussions with a nonjudgmental interviewer.

Development of an Enactive Attachment Story Completion Task

The discovery that classifications of mothers' AAIs and of children's responses to the SAT could be predicted from infant–mother attachment patterns in the Strange Situation (Kaplan, 1987; Main, 1995) inspired researchers to create additional representational attachment measures. These included interviews designed to capture parental perceptions of the relationship with a specific child (e.g., the Parent Development Interview by Aber, Slade, Berger, Bresgi, & Kaplan [1985]; the Parent Attachment Interview by Bretherton, Biringen, & Ridgeway [1989]; the Experiences of Caregiving Interview by George & Solomon [1994/97]; and the Working Model of the Child Interview by Zeahnah [1989]). Additional child measures consisted either of new versions of the Separation Anxiety Test

(Slough & Greenberg, 1990) or enactive story completion tasks (e.g., Bretherton & Ridgeway, 1990; Cassidy, 1988; Mueller & Tingley, 1990; Oppenheim, 1997).

My own attempt to develop an assessment capable of revealing aspects of attachment working models in even younger children than those studied by Main and colleagues (1985) was prompted by emerging studies of toddlers' and preschoolers' understanding of social relationships. Particularly relevant were findings about the development of pretend play (e.g., Bretherton, 1984; Nelson & Seidman, 1984; Wolf, Rygh, & Altshuler, 1984), the ability to talk meaningfully about inner states (Bretherton et al., 1981; Bretherton & Beeghly, 1982; Dunn & Bretherton, 1987), and to produce coherent event representations or scripts (Nelson, 1986; Nelson & Gruendel, 1981). Also influential was Erikson's (1950) proposition that "play is the child's expression of the human capacity to deal with experience by *creating model situations* and to master reality by experiment and planning" (p. 214).

Judging that the purely verbal responses called for by the picture-based SAT might underestimate the complexity of young preschoolers' attachment working models, I wondered whether the introduction of manipulable figures and props, similar to those used by play therapists, might help children as young as 36 months of age generate attachment story completions. There are a number of reasons why "mimetic," or physically enacted, representations might support a young child's ability to both understand and complete a story beginning (Donald's [1991] notion of mimetic representation was introduced to developmental psychology by Nelson [1996]). Spatial and temporal relations can be portrayed (and understood) without language through sequencing of actions and placement of figures. Actions do not have to be described verbally, but can be acted out, though clarifications are sometimes needed. Proper use of pronouns and conventions such as "he said" and "she said" are not necessary because figures can be activated or touched while making them talk. Emotions can be conveyed by tone of voice, even facial expressions, or the way in which figures are moved. In short, the presence of the figures and props both lessens the required memory load and the extent to which narrative devices must be used to tell the story.

With my colleague Doreen Ridgeway, I devised and pilot-tested a number of story beginnings that depicted a greater variety of attachment scenarios than the SAT, including situations in which a child protagonist caused an accidental mishap (spilled juice at the dinner table), felt pain (fell off a rock in the park), was afraid (a monster in the bedroom), and experienced a separation from and reunion with parents (the parents leave for an overnight trip while the grandmother looks after the children).

To make it easier for the children to understand and complete the story stems, we used Mandler and Johnson's (1977; see also Stein & Glenn,

1979) findings about story grammars (well-structured stories include a set-ting, initiating event, attempt, and resolution). We saw to it that the spatial layout of the family figures and props facilitated children's understanding of the initial "setting" and that the story beginnings (or "initiating situa-tion") portrayed common events with which any young child might be familiar. We used props that were suggestive without being so elaborate as to distract children from the task. After presenting each story beginning or stem, the interviewer was to invite the child to produce a resolution of the story problem with: "Show me and tell me what happens next" (for fur-ther details on techniques on story stem presentation, see Bretherton & Oppenheim, 2003).

Our criteria for coding children's responses to the ASCT were based on detailed analyses of story transcriptions, but also relied heavily on Main and colleagues' (1985) summary of Kaplan's coding for the SAT. We began by creating individualized criteria for evaluating each story, with particular attention to the constructiveness of story resolutions, the degree to which story completions were coherent versus avoidant or bizarre/chaotic, and assessed the spontaneity/emotional openness of the child's responses. Based on these criteria, considered jointly, we devised a 4-point security scale for the story task. Story security scores turned out to be significantly correlated with mother–child reunion behavior at the same age (rated by Cassidy), security scores from the Waters and Deane (1985) Attachment Q-sort per-formed by mothers at 25 months, and (though more modestly) the Strange Situation with mother at 18 months (Bretherton, Ridgeway, & Cassidy, 1990). In addition, story security was predicted by maternal insight/sensi-tivity as rated from the Parent Attachment Interview as well as family cohe-sion/ adaptability and marital quality rated by the mother at 37 months (Bretherton, Biringen, Ridgeway, Maslin, & Sherman, 1989). An independ-ent analysis of longitudinal data from the study developed by Waters, Rodrigues, and Ridgeway (1998) ranked children's story responses in terms of their resemblance to an ideal secure script. This reanalysis not only cor-roborated the earlier findings, but also revealed significant correlations between children's story completions performed at 3 and 4.5 years, as well as moderate but significant correlations of the 4.5-year story productions with the earlier observational attachment measures. As would be expected, however, the story completions of the 4.5-year-olds were more complex (Bretherton, Prentiss, & Ridgeway, 1990; Waters et al., 1998).

Findings obtained with the ASCT have been validated in several subse-quent studies with older preschoolers and school-age children as well as in one replication with 3-year-olds. These support our assumption that story completions reflect the child's attachment working models. Some of these studies devised new or more elaborate coding systems and/or classification procedures. Solomon, George, and DeJong (1995) adapted the attachment stories for use with 6-year-old children, but published findings only for

the separation–reunion story. They identified four patterns of responding (confident-secure, casual-avoidant, busy-ambivalent, and frightened-
disorganized) that overlapped significantly with secure, avoidant, resistant,
and controlling classifications during an actual separation–reunion with the
mother at age 6, using the classification system by Main and Cassidy
(1988).

Gloger-Tippelt, Gomille, König, and Vetter (2002) administered the
attachment stories (in a German translation with slight adaptations) to 29
children ages 5–7 years who had been seen with their mothers in the
Strange Situation at 13 months. In addition, the mothers had taken part in
the AAI when the children were 4–5 years old. The Gloger-Tippelt and
König (2000) story coding manual provides detailed instructions, supple-
menting the ASCT criteria suggested by Bretherton, Ridgeway, and Cassidy
(1990), complemented by adaptations of criteria for classifying the AAI
(Main & Goldwyn, 1984/1998). For each story the authors established
necessary, possible, and excluding criteria (i.e., what must be, can be, and
may not be present) and rated the stories as very secure, secure, insecure,
and very insecure. Their overall security rating, based on the number of
secure story completions a child had produced, showed excellent concordance with infant–mother Strange Situation and mothers' AAI classifications. The authors used ratings rather than classifications to evaluate the
ASCT because, like Bretherton and colleagues and Cassidy (1988), they
found it difficult to unambiguously identify an ambivalent pattern of
responding, perhaps due to the small sample size.

Miljkovitch, Pierrehumbert, Bretherton, and Halfon (2004) administered a French translation of the ASCT, supplemented by one story from
Oppenheim (1997), to 31 children ages 36–39 months. Instead of security
ratings to evaluate the children's responses, they developed a Q-set com-
posed of 65 items derived from several extant coding systems and their
own observations. They then created Q-set mega-items that captured
secure, deactivating, hyperactivating, and disorganized story responses.
These mega-items were based on the notion that insecure-avoidant children defensively deactivate attachment feelings, thoughts, and behaviors,
whereas insecure-ambivalent children engage in hyperactivation of the
attachment behavioral system, and insecure-disorganized children have no
consistent attachment strategy. Scores based on these mega-items were
meaningfully related to maternal, but not paternal, AAI classifications
(secure-autonomous, dismissing, preoccupied, and unresolved).

In a methodologically important study, Ongari, Tomasi, and Zoccatelli
(2003) administered an Italian translation of the ASCT to 71 preschoolers
ages 3–7 years. Comparing the efficacy of several existing coding systems,
they reported significant intercorrelations among the Gloger–Tippelt and
König system, the Miljkovitch Q-set, and a system developed for the Mac-
Arthur Story Stem Battery by Robinson, Mantz-Simmons, MacFie, and the

MacArthur Narrative Working Group (1992). The Robinson et al. manual included theme codes for supportive parental representations as well as ratings of narrative coherence. Particularly interesting was the finding that for each of the five story stems, children with insecure stories (assessed with the Gloger-Tippelt & König system) scored lower on narrative coherence (Robinson et al. system) than the secure children, but that the divergence was greatest for the separation-reunion story.

In a study with older children, Granot and Mayseless (2001) showed that the ASCT—translated into Hebrew with slight adaptations—could yield useful findings even with 9-year-olds who were unlikely to need family figures and props to support their verbal storytelling. Based on a coding system adapted from Main and Goldwyn's (1984/1998) AAI classification criteria, the authors were able to predict the children's concurrent social competence at school. Finally, in the first study using physiological measures, Bar-Haim, Fox, VanMeenen, and Marshall (2004) found that 7-year-olds' responses to the separation-reunion story stems and an additional story stem about a child's first day at school elicited increases in heart rate, during both the "presentation" and the "production" phases of the task. They also found that suppression of vagal tone was related to coherent story productions.

The ASCT has also begun to yield interesting insights in studies of children experiencing various types of stress. Among these are children of incarcerated mothers (Poehlmann, 2004), divorced families (Bretherton & Page, 2004; Gloger-Tippelt & König, 2000; Page & Bretherton, 2001), and maltreated children (e.g., MacFie, Cicchetti, & Toth, 2001; Toth, Cicchetti, MacFie, Maughan, & VanMeenen, 2000; Toth, Cicchetti, MacFie, Rogosch, Robinson, & Maughan, 2000).

Finally, correlational findings similar to those described for the ASCT have been obtained with alternative versions of the SAT (e.g., Slough & Greenberg, 1990; Shouldice Stevenson-Hinde, 1992), and with subsets of the MacArthur Story Stem Battery (e.g., Steele et al., 2003). In addition, Verschueren, Marcoen, and Schoefs (1996) reported correlations between the separation picture responses and scores based on a selection of story stems from the Bretherton and Ridgeway (1990) ASCT and Cassidy's (1988) stems about the self. The Manchester Child Attachment Story Task (Green, Stanley, Smith, & Goldwyn, 2000), based on five distress stories for children ages 5–7.5 years, revealed correlations between children's disorganized story productions and their mothers' unresolved AAI classifications.

That attachment story- and picture-based representational assessments evaluated with a variety of coding systems yielded similar predictions of children's observed relations with parents and/or peers supports the original assumption that children draw on their internal working models of actual relationships to address the story problems. Meaningful correlations have been obtained both with coding systems that capture children's regulatory strategies during story production (narrative coherence and emotional openness vs. avoidance or emotional dysregulation) and coding systems that assess constructive story themes and story resolutions. This contrasts with results obtained with the AAI where coherence turns out to be a stronger predictor of how a parent relates to his or her own infant than positive portrayals of the parents' childhood attachments in the family of origin (Main et al., 1985). The reason for the discrepancy may be that some adults, classified as "autonomous-secure," give highly coherent accounts of adverse attachment experiences in childhood that they have later been able to work through (Main et al., 1985). This type of "earned security" is, however, unlikely to be seen in young children who are still living with their parents.

In summary, there is now fairly consistent *correlational* evidence that attachment security as expressed in story completions is associated with security assessed in the Strange Situation and related procedures, and with maternal representations conveyed in the AAI. In a global sense, this allows us to conclude that the ASCT as well as the SAT and related measures can provide insight into children's attachment working models. I nevertheless have strong reservations about treating ASCT ratings and classifications as equivalent to observational attachment measures. First, concordances or correlations of the two types of assessment, though significant, are not sufficiently high to justify this. Second, unlike interviews about remembered relationship experiences, attachment story completion tasks do not require the child to represent actual life events. Whereas children's responses to the ASCT *do* include memories of actual experiences, they also contain accounts of what seem to be feared and hoped-for episodes that are quite unrealistic. In addition, they may incorporate fragments of family or picture book stories, and (perhaps) depict emotions in metaphorical form. This raises important questions about exactly in what sense children's attachment story productions can be said to offer a window into their working models of attachment to parents, a topic that I discuss next.

Story Meaning and the Working Model Construct

In a review of representational attachment measures, Oppenheim and Waters (1995, p. 203) suggested that "it may be useful to think of narrative assessments of attachment as measuring children's ability to construct narratives about emotionally laden, personal topics and to share these narratives with others." They draw a causal link between this ability and children's history of emotional communication and narrative co-construction of stories with parents. In line with this explanation, they attribute incoherent, bizarre stories to difficulties in communication, preferring not to invoke working models and defensive processes. I partially disagree with their approach. Under attachment theory, the influences of communication and representation have always been regarded as reciprocal. Well-organized, consciously accessible, well-adapted working models are believed to develop in the context of responsive parent–child interaction and emotionally open parent–child dialogue, while avoidant or ambivalent parent–child interaction and communication are thought to lead to ill-organized working models that are difficult to update adaptively (Bowlby, 1973; see also Bretherton, 1990, 1993). Oppenheim and Waters have, however, performed a useful service by placing emphasis on the creative, communicative, and co-constructive aspects of storytelling, and by underscoring the need to state more clearly in what sense attachment story completions reflect attachment working models.

Some children draw parallels between their ASCT stories and actual attachment, socialization, and mastery experiences, suggesting that they are tapping into aspects of their attachment working models. An example is a child saying "This is what my mommy does when I fall down," after making the mother figure pick up and comfort the child figure in the Hurt-Knee story. Along similar lines, Kaplan (1987) noted that children whose responses to separation pictures were classified as secure tended to share memories of actual separation experiences with the interviewer. The adoption of adult forms of speech is another indicator that story stems evoke material derived from the child's experience. An example is a mother figure telling a father figure to "settle down" during a quarrel, an expression that this child may have overheard at home. Third, some children identify the story mother as "my mommy" (not just "the mommy") and/or call the child protagonist by the participant's first name, instead of using the name supplied by the interviewer. More detailed examination of these phenomena is needed.

Children also enact positive and negative story events, however, that are highly *unlikely* to have occurred or to occur in the future. This became especially evident in our study of 4.5–5-year-old children of divorced parents with an expanded version of the ASCT in which mother and father were represented as living in different houses, symbolized by pieces of felt (Bretherton & Page, 2004). Although the story stems themselves had no divorce content, a very high percentage of the children enacted family reunifications, often accompanied by explicit comments that the parents were not divorced anymore. I suggest that these children were revealing working models of a hoped-for restored and harmonious family life. Other children enacted what looked like a wish that could not be sustained and became emotionally dysregulating. Thus, some reunifications were followed by severe family discord, even death (e.g., the father figure throws the mother and child on a garbage heap; the child becomes a ghost trapped under the couch). Here the child may be revealing working models of the self as affectively "thrown away" or rejected by the father. Similarly, depictions of a toy wagon that goes berserk, hitting all family figures, or of a tornado that scatters and kills the story family, may metaphorically represent the child's working model of out-of-control family relationships (Bretherton & Page, 2004). Finally, in response to a story stem by Zahn-Waxler and colleagues (1994), in which the mother figure cries "because Uncle Fred has died," a considerable number of children in the divorce study created stories in which it was the father figure who died (Herman & Bretherton, 2001). I suspect that these enactments reflected the children's fear of father loss or loss of access to the father, which is a working model of a feared future without the actual father. Following Bowlby (1980), who encouraged us to search for the reality behind seemingly unrealistic "fantasies," I contend that some of the extreme or unlikely events in children's stories are most plausibly interpreted as reflecting wishes, hopes, and fears related to experiences that are or have been anxiety-provoking to the child. Some enactments, normally classified as bizarre, make sense when interpreted metaphorically.

In some cases, children enact neither remembered interactions nor unrealistically positive or chaotic sequences, but engage in a variety of avoidant responses, such as saying "I don't know," denying that the problematic event occurred ("No, he didn't spill" or "No, she didn't get hurt"), inventing a completely unrelated story, or talking about the physical appearance of characters or props instead of attending to attachment issues (e.g., saying "This car is made of wood and paint" when the parent figures return home from their overnight trip). In this case, we can make inferences about the affective organization of the child's working model of self and attachment figure(s), based on the correlational findings presented earlier, but recent studies of mother–child reminiscing may shed more light on these avoidant narratives. New insights from the literature on memory development and narrative competence are also relevant given that story coherence and elaboration increases with age, and that story content in some studies reveals gender differences and even statistical interactions with child gender (Bretherton & Page, 2004; Page & Bretherton, 2001; Steele et al., 2003). In the next section I offer selected findings from this literature.

MEMORY AND REMINISCING RESEARCH

As I have already mentioned, research during the past two to three decades has revealed that preschoolers' narrative ability and understanding of relationships are far more advanced than had been assumed by Piaget (1951,

1954). These findings contributed to my work on story completion tasks and my attempts to flesh out the working model construct (Bretherton, 1985, 1987, 1990, 1991, 1993, 1995; Bretherton & Munholland, 1999). In this section I reflect on new findings on memory development and mother–child reminiscing that parallel and converge with discoveries independently made by attachment researchers.

Particularly relevant is Nelson's (1996) theorizing about distinct memory systems in relation to Bowlby's (1980) notions about episodic and semantic memory. Also revealing are studies documenting differences in mother–child reminiscing styles during talk about positive and highly stressful experiences. Findings about implanted memories are relevant to Bowlby's (1973, 1980) notions about defensive processes.

Memory Systems

Nelson's view of memory, like Bowlby's (1969, 1980), is a functional one: Memory conserves information, supports action in the present, and predicts future outcomes on the basis of past probabilities. Also consonant with Bowlby, Nelson (1996) proposes that event memory is the basic "experiential" memory system that develops first, and provides the initial building blocks for the child's "world model." She considers semantic memory ("general knowledge, undated and unlocalized," p. 154) as derived from reprocessing of the constituents of generic event memory, and in this differs from Schacter and Tulving (1994), who subsume event memory under the semantic system.

Several studies show that, already in the second year, toddlers can recall both generic and unique events by reenacting them as external (mimetic) representations after delays of weeks to months (e.g., Bauer & Wewerka, 1995). Later in the second year, they begin to translate their increasingly sophisticated mimetic and procedural event representations into language and gain rudimentary mastery of the process in the reverse direction by learning to translate narratives produced by others back into meaningful mental representations. The mastery of this process is lengthy and extends over the preschool years (Nelson, 1996).

By 2–2.5 years of age, children who are asked to talk about what happened at supper last night tend to describe generic routines, not a unique event (Fivush & Hamond, 1990). The authors speculate that children of this age may need to embed specific events in familiar routines or that scripts provide the necessary structure to hold new memories. However, if the event is sufficiently novel, and if prompted and supported, children of this age *can* narrate memories of unique events after delays of weeks and months, and this delay can be lengthened if the memories are intermittently "reinstated" (Fivush & Hamond, 1990). Nevertheless, although some autobiographical memories for significant events during this early age can be recalled for some time, few endure into later childhood (Pillemer, 1998). Nelson (1996) speculates that these memories do not disappear but are overwritten by similar episodes (i.e., they become aspects of internal working models). Only autobiographical memories formed after 3–4 years of age tend to be consciously retained into adulthood, and form the basis for creating a life story and a sense of identity. As research on mother–child reminiscing shows, attachment figures appear to be vitally involved in the development of the autobiographical memory system, but these important aspects of the working model of self and relationships have so far been neglected by attachment theorists.

Styles of Mother–Child Reminiscing

In discussing the role of verbal communication in the creation of shared working models, Bowlby (1973, p. 322) highlighted the importance of "frank communication by parents of working models—of themselves, of child, and of others—that are not only tolerably valid but are open to be questioned and revised." Relevant to these proposals, Pillemer and White (1989) contended that an initial memory system, present at birth, allows infants to store memories as images, emotions, or behaviors that can only be evoked by situational or affective cues. A second "intentionally addressable" personal memory system develops during the preschool years through parent–child conversation about past events (e.g., "Do you remember when .. . ?"). This system comes to coexist with (but does not replace) the initial system, and enables children to actively reflect and perhaps reevaluate remembered events and discuss them with others.

Fivush and Fromhoff (1988; see also Engel, 1986) discovered that mothers have different ways of fostering the development of children's autobiographical memory through joint reminiscing, beginning at the end of the second year. "Elaborative" mothers provide a coherent story line accompanied by rich detail. They welcome their child's contributions, even if they are minimal. "Repetitive mothers," in contrast, seem more interested in obtaining a correct answer than in co-constructing a memory, and tend to repeatedly ask the same or similar questions.

Subsequent longitudinal studies of reminiscing have demonstrated that children adopt their mothers' elaborative or repetitive style of reminiscing, whether conversing with their mothers or with experimenters (Reese, Haden, & Fivush, 1993). One might assume that these findings are due the influence of children's verbal skills, but this is unlikely because a mother's elaborative style is evident even before the child can contribute much to the conversation him- or herself. Moreover, the elaborative style is highly compatible with maternal sensitivity as described by Ainsworth, Bell, and

Stayton (1974), whereas the repetitive style, with its disavowal of the child's contributions to the conversation, seems much less sensitive and supportive. To examine the role of attachment in learning to reminisce, Reese and Farrant (2003) assessed child–mother attachment security with version 3.0 of the Attachment Q-set (Waters, 1995) in a group of 56 19-month-olds and mother–child memory talk at 25, 32, and 40 months. Attachment security turned out to be significantly correlated with elaborative reminiscing by mother and child at all three ages. In an extension of that study, Newcombe and Reese (2004) found that evaluative statements in particular (e.g., internal state words, intensifiers, affect modifiers, and emphasis) distinguished the reminiscing of secure from that of insecure dyads at 19, 25, 32, 40, and 51 months. In secure, but in not insecure dyads, the use of evaluative language by mothers and children was systematically intercorrelated and increased systematically with child age. Along similar lines, Fivush and Vasudeva (2002) discovered that 4-year-olds' attachment security scores (also based on the Waters Attachment Behavior Q-set, sorted by mothers) predicted more elaborative reminiscing, with results holding for both mothers and children, and equally for boys and girls.

Coming at the same topic from an attachment story perspective, Heller (2000) used a selection of nine story stems from the ASCT and the MacArthur Story Stem Battery in a study of middle-class preschoolers and disadvantaged children participating in Headstart programs. In children from both groups, story-derived security scores were significantly related to maternal sensitivity/elaborative style assessed during mother–child talk about the past (modeled on Kuebli, Butler, & Fivush, 1995) and mother–child co-construction of a separation–reunion story (modeled on Oppenheim, Nir, Warren, & Emde, 1997). Additionally, children's secure and coherent attachment story resolutions were predicted by security scores from the Waters (1995) Attachment Behavior Q-set, sorted by observers.

Memory, Stress, and Defensive Exclusion

The mother–child reminiscing studies cited above suggest that autobiographical memory develops differently in secure and insecure dyads. A drawback of these studies, however, is that memory talk in this research focused mostly on positive events. Conversations about traumatic experiences might heighten such differences because defensive biases are more likely to come into play if children cannot count on a parent's willingness to help them comprehend such experiences. Bowlby (1973, p. 322) noted that children in such circumstances may be pressured "to adopt and thereby to confirm, a parent's false models—of self, of child, and of their relationship." Elaborating on the role of language in the building of working models, Grossmann (1999) points out that parents who provide misleading explanations, and who either ridicule or taboo discussions about events that have been stressful and traumatic, do not make the world meaningful to their children, leaving them without any corresponding reality or interpretation of their private feelings.

Several researchers interested in children as reliable witnesses (of sexual abuse) and traumatic memory (as in posttraumatic stress disorder) have investigated children's ability to talk about natural disasters and injuries. These are relevant to the issues raised by Bowlby (1980) and Grossmann (1999).

Reminiscing about Stressful Experiences

During interviews of 5- to 12-year-olds from violent neighborhoods, Fivush, Hazzard, Sales, Sarfati, and Brown (2003) unexpectedly found that the children's accounts of negative events were more coherent and involved greater disclosure of feelings and thoughts than discussions of positive past experiences. Bahrick, Parker, Merritt, and Fivush (1998) interviewed younger children who were 3–4 years of age when they lived through a devastating hurricane. Six months after the event, children from families most affected by the disaster reported slightly fewer details than the others, but 6 years later all of the children who could be tracked down (now 9–10 years of age) provided more detailed narratives about the disaster than at the earlier interview. Those who had been most highly stressed recalled most but required somewhat more prompting from the interviewers. Peterson (1999), who studied children with injuries that required treatment in a hospital emergency room, observed less recall of detail after a 2-year delay, but only with respect to hospital-related stress, not the prior injury (Peterson & Bell, 1996). Finally, in the only study of mother–child reminiscing about traumatic events, Ackil, Van Abbema, and Bauer (2003) found that 29 mothers and their children ages 2.6 to 11.8 produced considerably more detailed and narratively coherent talk about a tornado that had caused great destruction in their neighborhood than about two nontraumatic events, both 4 and 6 months after the storm. The study did not distinguish the child's from the mother's contribution, however.

Variations in these findings may be due to differences in how the data were obtained and how traumatic the experiences were perceived by the children, but overall these studies did not reveal striking defensive processes. If anything, the children participating in these studies talked with greater elaboration and coherence about highly negative events. Perhaps the disasters and injuries investigated were not the kinds of situations (e.g., sexual abuse, parental suicide) that are particularly likely to be "falsified" or "silenced" by parents. It is possible, however, that more detailed examination of the transcripts might have revealed such effects for some of the dyads, especially given that the parents themselves were stressed by the natural disasters or their children's injuries. In two studies, maternal attachment style was linked to children's accuracy of in the recall of medical procedures (Eisen & Goodman, 1998; Quas et al., 1999). Children of parents with higher avoidance scores produced somewhat less accurate memories. However, the questions asked in these two studies were mostly factual, rather than probing feelings.

Defensive (distorting) responses *were*, however, observed in two studies using clinical interviews. In both, parents had failed to explain stressful situations to their children. Steward (1993) observed young hospitalized children diagnosed with cancer. She found that when parents kept the diagnosis secret to protect the children's feelings, children invented their own horrific explanations for medical procedures (e.g., that nurses were stealing their blood). Silence, in this case, was not security-promoting, but rather left the children alone with their fears (or as Grossmann [1999] put it, without narrative correspondence). Terr (1983; see also Terr, 1991) interviewed 5- to 14-year-old children who had been abducted and trapped in a trailer-truck that was buried underground for 24 hours before they were able to escape. During a clinical interview 4 years later the children's accounts of the original event were unusually clear, detailed, and vivid. Unlike adults suffering from posttraumatic stress disorder, they remembered the abduction itself quite well, but had suppressed/repressed memories of panic attacks and nightmares that they had mentioned during a first interview, held immediately after the kidnapping. Most notably, however, in terms of their internal working model of self, the children had acquired a frighteningly pessimistic outlook on life. Many felt that they would die young or that the world might soon come to an end. Furthermore, many had reinterpreted events prior to the kidnapping as omens that ought to have warned them or their parents of the impending disaster (defensively opting for guilt and anxiety over helplessness). Although these children seemed to have repressed/suppressed their own emotional reactions to the kidnapping, they had created a malignant working model of the external world and a model of the self as helpless.

Research on Implanted Memories

In his discussion of defensive processes, Bowlby (1980) claimed that some children repress their memories of traumatic situations in favor of false explanations supplied by parents. Citing clinical cases, he noted that parents may do so under two kinds of circumstances: (1) when they have behaved abusively toward the child and (2) when the child has witnessed an event that the parent does not want the child to know about. Researchers interested in eyewitness testimony who have attempted to implant false autobiographical "memories" in young children's minds have shown that this can be quite effective, especially if the untrue episode (in this case, getting lost in a mall at a young age) is made more plausible by placing it in a familiar location (Loftus & Ketcham, 1994). After experimenters repeatedly insisted that the children had experienced the fictitious event, some children began to produce detailed autobiographical "memories" of the false episode. In another study, 3- to 6-year-old children were invited to narrate their "memories" of untrue positive and negative events, with two additional twists. They were told that the experimenters had learned about the event from their mothers and were asked "to make a picture of the event" in their heads (Ceci, Loftus, Leichtman, & Bruck, 1994, p. 216). Over 12 repeated sessions during which the children were pressured to remember true and untrue events, the percentage reporting false memories increased markedly from around 30% to over 50% for positive and from about 15% to about 30% for negative events. Loftus, Coan, and Pickrell (1996) suggest that merely asking individuals to imagine a scene increases the likelihood of falsely remembering it at a subsequent session.

Whereas this research is consonant with Bowlby's claim that some children can develop working models on the basis of what they are (deceptively) told by parents, it also demonstrates that what they can begin to "remember" under such pressure are not merely semantic facts, as Bowlby proposed, but detailed, yet false autobiographical episodes. Unfortunately, the false memory studies did not collect information about the quality of parent–child relations or reminiscing style. However, Hyman and Billings (1996) report that in a study with adults the tendency to accept false memories as true was related to scores on a dissociative experiences scale and a creative imagination scale. The inclusion of child–parent observational attachment measures and attachment stories into such studies might provide insight into why some of the children were able to resist the researchers' efforts to create false memories.

CONCLUDING REMARKS

The assumed function of internal working models—to make the relational world more predictable, shareable, and meaningful—seems to function well in secure relationships, but story completion studies suggest that this is less true for insecure children, even when their attachment experiences have not been as adverse as the clinical cases of loss and severe trauma on which Bowlby (1980, 1988) based his expositions about defensive processes.

Secure children (assessed observationally) were able to attend to the attachment issues posed in story stems and to produce constructive solutions. They did not become emotionally dysregulated by the story problems, their narratives had a coherent storyline, and they required little prompting. That coherence and emotional openness characterized attachment story production may be the result of having a history of co-constructing memories in a supportive attachment relationship with elaborative mothers. Such joint reminiscing not only offers reassurance after distressing experiences, but also seems to have a more long-term effect on children's autobiographical memory organization. In particular, it may foster the child's capacity for "mentalizing," or understanding others at the psychological level, as required for a well-functioning goal-corrected partnership. In support of this notion, Fonagy and Target (1997) have shown that the degree of coherence of adult attachment narratives goes hand-in-hand with reflective self-awareness. Similarly, Main (1991) found that children classified as securely attached in infancy later had an advantage in mastering a "theory of mind" task, and Grossmann, Grossmann, and Zimmermann (1999) reported that children who were secure as infants were able to display clarity of motives and an orientation to solutions in their discussions of separations. Relatedly, Delius (2004) discovered that preschool children with secure story classifications have a more differentiated knowledge of attachment relationships than children with avoidant classifications.

In contrast, insecure children (classified observationally) had difficulties in responding to attachment story stems, but in different ways. Some avoided or denied the story problems altogether, while others sidestepped them. Were these the children of mothers who had introduced them to a repetitive style of reminiscing and who had adopted this style themselves? I regard this assumption as plausible because the repetitive style is not only relatively unsupportive of the child, but it does not reveal or elicit much about the partner's inner experience. Unfortunately, studies attempting to detect reminiscing styles associated with the different insecure classifications (avoidant, ambivalent, disorganized) have not yet been attempted. One might speculate, for example, that children whose ambivalent attachment stories are elaborated, but conflicted and difficult to follow (Gullon-Rivera & Bretherton, 2003; Page & Bretherton, 2001) may have an elaborative reminiscing style that is accompanied by vacillating interpretations, and perhaps exaggerations of negative and positive affect. Children whose attachment story completions become disrupted by sudden chaos and disaster (akin to the lapses in discourse monitoring that Main [1995] describes for unresolved adult attachment interviews) might have mothers whose reminiscing, especially about negative events, introduces topics of fear and helplessness that are not coherently connected to the narrative. Because many attachment researchers are primarily interested in translating story completions into scores or classifications rather than examining in detail how children convey story meanings, these and similar questions have not yet been asked or studied.

Additional questions remain about the interpretation of the narratives themselves. For example, Solomon and George (1999) equate two types of disorganized responses to attachment stories: (1) being flooded by chaotic material and (2) being intensely inhibited and constricted. Both patterns were related to controlling/disorganized reunion classifications with mothers in a pilot sample. However, this leaves the question as to why defenses break down in the flooded but not in the emotionally constricted children. Also at issue is whether a child with five disorganized story completions should receive the same classification as a child who produces one such story, that is whether sporadic disorganization has the same meaning as pervasive disorganization. In addition, age changes in story responses need greater consideration. Several researchers have reported increasing coherence between the ages of 3 and 6 or 7 years (e.g., Green et al., 2000; Waters et al., 1998). Studies in which age ranges are relatively large may have to create adaptations of the coding scheme for different age levels, but such decisions should be based on research. Aside from coherence, story completions also tend to become more elaborate, in terms of character speech and greater differentiation of adult roles (Bretherton, Prentiss, & Ridgeway, 1990). These and similar issues could be addressed if detailed analyses of the story transcripts were made in conjunction with systematic post hoc analyses of observational attachment and narrative measures and if different coding systems were applied to the same data, following in the footsteps of Ongari and colleagues (2003).

Collaborative studies in which mothers and children reminisce about traumatic situations, together and separately, and in which attachment story completions are also administered, might help us understand why there seems to be so little evidence of bias or defense in the studies of memory talk about injuries and natural disasters. It is possible that group analyses of the data obscured such findings because a majority of the children are likely to have had secure attachment relationships. It is also possible, however, that a more clinical interviewing style and/or the use of story tasks rather than interviews would produce different results because what appear to be defensive phenomena are quite frequently observed in attachment stories about current everyday problems, not traumatic situations. Finally, given the relative ease with which researchers were able to implant false memories in a considerable proportion of children, studies in which children are interviewed about how they experience this pressure would be helpful, especially if attachment observations and stories were also collected.

Continuing our studies of how children construct working models through interaction and how they learn to share their working models with parents and others through dialogue is important, I suggest, not only because such shared meanings make for the smoother operation of secure relationships as well as the growth of self-reliance (Bowlby, 1973), but because working models not only *reflect* but also *create* relational realities. Secure and supportive parent–child relationships in which there is open communication not only encourage the construction of well-organized working models so that memories of emotional experiences can be retrieved and openly discussed with relative ease, but they also help to *generate* relational environments that are optimizing and enhancing for both children and parents. Working models of a secure self seem to set up initial expectations (i.e., a generalized working model) in other relationships with caregiving adults and peers. A trusting attitude is likely to elicit reciprocal trust, though it may sometimes be maladaptive when answered by deceit. A distrustful stance, in contrast, predisposes an individual to interpret others' neutral and even positive behaviors as ill-intentioned, and may indeed elicit negative behavior from them, thus creating a reality that engenders difficulties and anxieties (e.g., Cassidy, Kirsh, Scolton, & Parke, 1996; Dodge, Bates, & Pettit, 1990; Suess, Grossmann, & Sroufe, 1992). In short, meaning- and attribution-making, representational processes and the resulting working models of self, close relationships, and the world are important, not only because they are reality-reflecting, but because they *create* different realities for self and relationship partners.

REFERENCES

Aber, L., Slade, A., Berger, B., Bresgi, I., & Kaplan, M. (1985). *The Parent Development Interview*. Unpublished manuscript, Barnard College, Columbia University, New York, NY.

Ackil, J. K., Van Abbema, D. L., & Bauer, P. J. (2003). After the storm: Enduring differences in mother–child recollections of traumatic and nontraumatic events. *Journal of Experimental Child Psychology, 84*, 286–309.

Ainsworth, M. D. A., Bell, S. V., & Stayton, D. (1974). Infant–mother attachment and social development: "Socialization" as a product of reciprocal responsiveness to signals. In P. M. Richards (Ed.), *The integration of a child into a social world* (pp. 99–135). Cambridge, UK: Cambridge University Press.

Bahrick, L., Parker, J., Merritt, K., & Fivush, R. (1998). Children's memory for Hurricane Andrew. *Journal of Experimental Psychology: Applied, 4*, 308–331.

Bar-Haim, Y. B., Fox, N. A., VanMeenen, K. M., & Marshall, P. J. (2004). Children's narratives and patterns of cardiac reactivity. *Developmental Psychobiology, 44*, 238–249.

Bauer, P. J., & Wewerka, S. S. (1995). One- to two-year-olds' recall of events: The more impressed, the more expressed. *Journal of Experimental Child Psychology, 59*, 475–496.

Bowlby, J. (1960). Grief and mourning in infancy and early childhood. *Psychoanalytic Study of the Child, 15*, 9–52.

Bowlby, J. (1969). *Attachment and loss: Vol. 1. Attachment*. New York: Basic Books.

Bowlby, J. (1973). *Attachment and loss: Vol. 2. Separation.* New York: Basic Books.

Bowlby, J. (1980). *Attachment and loss: Vol. 3. Loss, sadness and depression.* New York: Basic Books.

Bowlby, J. (1988). *A secure base: Parent–child attachment and healthy human development.* New York: Basic Books.

Bowlby, J., & Parkes, C. M. (1970). Separation and loss within the family. In E. J. Anthony & C. Koupernik (Eds.), *The child in his family* (pp. 197–216). New York: Wiley.

Bretherton, I. (1978). Making friends with one-year-olds: An experimental study of infant-stranger interaction. *Merrill-Palmer Quarterly, 24,* 29–51.

Bretherton, I. (1980). Young children in stressful situations: The supporting role of attachment figures and unfamiliar caregivers. In G.V. Coelho & P. Ahmed (Eds.), *Uprooting and development* (pp. 179–210). New York: Plenum Press.

Bretherton, I. (1984). Representing the social world in symbolic play: Reality and fantasy. In I. Bretherton (Ed.), *Symbolic play: The development of social understanding* (pp. 3–41). Orlando, FL: Academic Press.

Bretherton, I. (1985). Attachment theory: Retrospect and prospect. In I. Bretherton & E. Waters (Eds.), Growing points of attachment theory and research. *Monographs of the Society for Research in Child Development, 50*(1–2, Serial No. 209), 3–35.

Bretherton, I. (1987). New perspectives on attachment relations: Security, communication and internal working models. In J. Osofsky (Ed.), *Handbook of infant development* (2nd ed., pp. 1061–1100). New York: Wiley.

Bretherton, I. (1988). How to do things with one word: The ontogenesis of intentional message-making in infancy. In J. Lock & M. Smith (Eds.), *The emergent lexicon* (pp. 225–260). New York: Academic Press.

Bretherton, I. (1990). Open communication and internal working models: Their role in the development of attachment relationships. In R. A. Thompson (Ed.), *Nebraska Symposium on Motivation: Vol. 36. Socioemotional development* (pp. 59–113). Lincoln: University of Nebraska Press.

Bretherton, I. (1991). Pouring new wine into old bottles: The social self as internal working model. In M. Gunnar & L. A. Sroufe (Eds.), *The Minnesota Symposia on Child Psychology: Vol. 23. Self processes in development* (pp. 1–41). Hillsdale, NJ: Erlbaum.

Bretherton, I. (1993). From dialogue to representation: The intergenerational construction of self in relationships. In C. A. Nelson (Ed.), *Minnesota Symposia on Child Psychology: Vol. 26. Memory and affect in development* (pp. 237–263). Hillsdale, NJ: Erlbaum.

Bretherton, I. (1995). Commentary: A communication perspective on attachment relationships and internal working models. In E. Waters, B. Vaughn, G. Posada, & K. Kondo-Ikemura (Eds.), Caregiving, cultural and cognitive perspectives on secure-base behavior and working models. *Monographs of the Society for Research in Child Developmen , 60*(2–3, Serial No. 244), 310–329.

Bretherton, I., & Ainsworth, M. D. S. (1974). The responses of one-year-olds to a stranger in a Strange Situation. In M. Lewis & L. A. Rosenblum (Eds.), *The origins of fear* (pp. 131–164). New York: Wiley.

Bretherton, I., & Bates, E. (1979). The emergence of intentional communication. In I.

C. Uzgiris (Ed.), *Social interaction and communication during infancy* (pp. 81–100). San Francisco: Jossey-Bass.

Bretherton, I., & Beeghly, M. (1982). Talking about internal states: The acquisition of an explicit theory of mind. *Developmental Psychology, 18,* 906–921.

Bretherton, I., Biringen, Z., & Ridgeway, D. (1989). *Parent Attachment Interview.* Unpublished manuscript, University of Wisconsin–Madison.

Bretherton, I., Biringen, Z., Ridgeway, D., Maslin, C. & Sherman, M. (1989). Attachment: The parental perspective. *Infant Mental Health Journal, 10,* 203–221.

Bretherton, I., McNew, S., & Beeghly-Smith, M. (1981). Early person knowledge as expressed in gestural and verbal communication: When do infants acquire a "theory of mind?" In M. Lamb & L. Sherrod (Eds.), *Infant social cognition* (pp. 333–373). Hillsdale, NJ: Erlbaum.

Bretherton, I., & Munholland, K. A. (1999). Internal working models in attachment relationships: A construct revisited. In J. Cassidy & P. R. Shaver (Eds.), *Handbook of attachment: Theory, research, and clinical applications* (pp. 89–111). New York: Guilford Press.

Bretherton, I., & Oppenheim, D. (2003). The MacArthur Story Stem Battery: development, directions for administration, reliability, validity and reflections about meaning. In R. N. Emde, D. P. Wolf, & D. Oppenheim (Eds.), *Revealing the inner world of young children: The MacArthur Story Stem Battery* (pp. 55–80). New York: Oxford University Press.

Bretherton, I., Oppenheim, D., Buchsbaum, H., Emde, R. N., & the MacArthur Narrative Group. (2003). *The MacArthur Story Stem Battery.* In R. N. Emde, D. P. Wolf, & D. Oppenheim (Eds.), *Revealing the inner worlds of young children: The MacArthur Story Stem Battery and parent–child narratives* (pp. 381–396). New York: Oxford University Press.

Bretherton, I., & Page, T. (2004). Shared or conflicting working models?: Relationships in postdivorce families seen through the eyes of mothers and their preschool children. *Development and Psychopathology, 16,* 551–575.

Bretherton, I., Prentiss, C., & Ridgeway, D. (1990). Children's representations of family relationships in a story completion task at 37 and 54 months. In I. Bretherton & M. Watson (Eds.), *Children's perspectives on the family* (pp. 85–105). San Francisco: Jossey-Bass.

Bretherton, I., & Ridgeway, D. (1990). Story completion task to assess young children's internal working models of child and parents in the attachment relationship. In M.T. Greenberg, D. Cicchetti, & E.M. Cummings (Eds.), *Attachment in the preschool years: Theory, research, and intervention* (pp. 300–308). Chicago: University of Chicago Press.

Bretherton, I., Ridgeway, D., & Cassidy, J. (1990). Assessing internal working models of the attachment relationship: An attachment story completion task for 3-year-olds. In M. Greenberg, D. Cicchetti, & M. Cummings (Eds.), *Attachment in the preschool years: Theory, research and intervention* (pp. 273–308). Chicago: University of Chicago Press.

Buchsbaum, H., & Emde, R. N. (1990). Play narratives in 36-month-old children: Early moral development and family relationships. *Psychoanalytic Study of the Child, 40,* 129–155.

Cassidy, J. (1988). Child–mother attachment and the self in six-year-olds. *Child Development, 59,* 121–134.

Cassidy, J., Kirsh, S. J., Scolton, K. L., & Parke, R. D. (1996). Attachment and representations of peer relationships. *Developmental Psychology, 32,* 892–904.

Ceci, S. J., Loftus, E. S., Leichtman, M. D., & Bruck, M. (1994). The possible role of source misattribution in the creation of false beliefs in preschoolers. *International Journal of Clinical and Experimental Hypnosis, 42,* 304–320.

Craik, K. (1943). *The nature of explanation.* Cambridge, UK: Cambridge University Press.

Crittenden, P. (1989). Internal representational models of attachment relationships. *Infant Mental Health Journal, 11,* 259–277.

Delius, A. C. (2004). *"Theory of attachment": Allgemeine Entwicklung und individuelle Unterschiede [General development and individual differences].* Unpublished doctoral dissertation, Justus Liebig University of Giessen, Germany.

Dodge, K., Bates, J. E., & Pettit, G. D. (1990). Mechanisms in the cycle of violence. *Science, 250,* 1678–1683.

Donald, M. (1991). *Origins of the modern mind.* Cambridge, MA: Harvard University Press.

Dunn, J., Bretherton, I., & Munn, P. (1987). Conversations about feeling states between mothers and their young children. *Developmental Psychology, 23,* 132–139.

Eisen, M. L., & Goodman, G. S. (1998). Trauma, memory and suggestibility in children. *Development and Psychopathology, 10,* 717–738.

Engel, S. (1986). *Learning to reminisce: A developmental study of how young children talk about the past.* Unpublished doctoral dissertation, City University of New York Graduate Center, New York, NY.

Erikson, E. H. (1950). *Childhood and society.* New York: Norton.

Fivush, R., & Fromhoff, F. (1988). Style and structure in mother–child conversations about the past. *Discourse Processes, 11,* 337–355.

Fivush, R., & Hamond, N. R. (1990). Autobiographical memory across the preschool years: Towards reconceptualizing childhood amnesia. In R. Fivush & J. A. Hudson (Eds.), *Knowing and remembering in young children* (pp. 223–248). Cambridge, UK: Cambridge University Press.

Fivush, R., Hazzard, A., Sales, J. M., Sarfati, D., & Brown, T. (2003). Creating order out of chaos?: Children's narratives of emotionally positive and negative events. *Applied Cognitive Psychology, 17,* 1–9.

Fivush, R., & Vasudeva, A. (2002). Remembering to relate: Socioemotional correlates of mother–child reminiscing. *Journal of Cognition and Development, 3,* 73–90.

Fonagy, P., & Target, M. (1997). Attachment and reflective function: Their role in self-organization. *Development and Psychopathology, 9,* 679–700.

Freud, S. (1960). *The ego and the id* (J. Riviere, Trans. & J. Strachey, Ed.). New York: Norton. (Original work published 1923)

Gallese, V. (in press). Embodied Simulation: From neurons to phenomenal Experience. *Phenomenology and the Cognitive Sciences.*

George, C., Kaplan, N., & Main, M. (1996). *The Berkeley Adult Attachment Interview Protocol.* Unpublished manuscript, University of California at Berkeley. (Original work done in 1984)

George, C., & Solomon, J. (1994/97). *The Experiences of Caregiving Interview.* Unpublished manuscript, Mills College, Oakland, CA.

Gloger-Tippelt, G., & König, L. (2000). *Kodier- und Auswertungsmanual für das Geschichtenergänzungsverfahren zur Erfassung der Bindungsrepräsentationen 5- bis 7-jähriger Kinder im Puppenspiel [Coding manual for the evaluation of doll play attachment representations of 5- to 7-year-old children].* Unpublished manual, Psychologisches Institut, Heinrich-Heine Universität, Dusseldorf, Germany.

Gloger-Tippelt, G., Gomille, B., Kšnig, L., & Vetter, J. (2002). Attachment representations in 6 year olds: Related longitudinally to quality of attachment in infancy and mothers' attachment representations. *Attachment and Human Development, 4,* 318–339.

Gloger-Tippelt, G., & König, L. (2003, August). Attachment representations in 6-year-old children from one- and two-parent families. In R. Miljkovitch (Chair), *The interface between real-life interactions and imaginary interactions during doll-play.* Symposium conducted at the 11th European Conference on Developmental Psychology, Catholic University, Milan, Italy.

Granot, D., & Mayseless, O. (2001). Attachment security and adjustment to school in middle childhood. *International Journal of Behavioral Development, 25,* 530–541.

Green, J., Stanley, C., Smith, V., & Goldwyn, R. (2000). A new method of evaluating attachment representations in young school-age children: The Manchester Attachment Story Task. *Attachment and Human Development, 2,* 48–70.

Grossmann, K. E. (1999). Old and new internal working models of attachment: The organization of feelings and language. *Attachment and Human Development, 1,* 253–269.

Grossmann, K. E., Grossmann, K., & Zimmermann, P. (1999). A wider view of attachment and exploration: Stability and change during the years of immaturity. In J. Cassidy & P. R. Shaver (Eds.), *Handbook of attachment: Theory, research, and clinical applications* (pp. 760–786). New York: Guilford Press.

Gullon-Rivera, A., & Bretherton, I. (2003). *Coding manual for self-representations in the Attachment Story Completion Task.* Unpublished manuscript, University of Wisconsin–Madison.

Hansburg, H. G. (1972). *Adolescent separation anxiety: Vol 1. A method for the study of adolescent separation problems.* Springfield, IL: Charles C. Thomas.

Heller, C. (2000). *Attachment and social competence in preschool children.* Unpublished masters thesis, Auburn University, Auburn, AL.

Herman, P., & Bretherton, I. (2001). "He was the best daddy": Postdivorce preschoolers' representations of loss and family life. In A. Gonçü & E. Klein (Ed.), *Children in play, story, and school* (pp. 177–203). New York: Guilford Press.

Hyman, I. E., & Billings, F. J. (1996). *Individual differences and the creation of false memories of childhood experiences.* Unpublished manuscript.

James, W. (1950). *Principles of psychology.* New York: Dover. (Original work published 1890)

Johnson-Laird, P. N. (1983). *Mental models.* Cambridge, MA: Harvard University Press.

Kaplan, N. (1987). *Individual differences in six-year-olds' thoughts about separation:*

Predicted from attachment to mother at one year. Unpublished doctoral dissertation, University of California at Berkeley.

Klagsbrun, M., & Bowlby, J. (1976). Responses to separation from parents: A clinical test for young children. *British Journal of Projective Psychology, 21,* 7–21.

Kuebli, J., Butler, S., & Fivush, R., (1995). Mother–child talk about past emotions: relations of maternal language and child gender over time. *Cognition and Emotion, 9,* 265–283.

Loftus, E. F., Coan, J. A., & Pickrell, J. R. (1996). Manufacturing false memories using bits of reality. In L. M. Reder (Ed.), *Implicit memory and metacognition* (pp. 195–220). Mahwah, NJ: Erlbaum.

Loftus, E. F., & Ketcham, K. (1994). *The myth of repressed memories.* New York: St. Martin's Press.

MacFie, J., Cicchetti, D., & Toth, S. (2001). The development of dissociation in maltreated preschool-age children. *Development and Psychopathology, 13,* 233–254.

Main, M. (1991). Metacognitive knowledge, metacognitive monitoring, and singular (coherent) vs. multiple (incoherent) model of attachment. In C. M. Parkes, J. Stevenson-Hinde, & P. Marris (Eds.), *Attachment across the life cycle* (pp. 127–159). London: Routledge.

Main, M. (1995). Recent studies in attachment. In S. Goldberg, R. Muir, & J. Kerr (Eds.), *Attachment theory: Social, developmental and clinical perspectives* (pp. 407–474). Hillsdale, NJ: Analytic Press.

Main, M., & Cassidy, J. (1988). Categories of response to reunion with the parent at age 6: Predictable from infant attachment classification and stable over a 1-month period. *Developmental Psychology, 24,* 1–12.

Main, M., & Goldwyn, R. (1984/1998). *Adult Attachment Interview scoring and classification system.* Unpublished manuscript, University of California at Berkeley.

Main, M., Kaplan, K., & Cassidy, J. (1985). Security in infancy, childhood and adulthood: A move to the level of representation. In I. Bretherton & E. Waters (Eds.), Growing points of attachment theory and research. *Monographs of the Society for Research in Child Development, 50*(1–2 Serial No. 209), 66–104.

Mandler, J. M., & Johnson, J. S. (1977). Remembrance of things parsed: Story structure and recall. *Cognitive Psychology, 9,* 111–151.

Metzinger, T. (2003). *Being no one: The self-model theory of subjectivity.* Cambridge, MA: MIT Press.

Miljkovitch, R., Pierrehumbert, P., Bretherton, I., & Halfon, O. (2004). Intergenerational transmission of attachment representations. *Attachment and Human Development, 6,* 305–325.

Mueller, E., & Tingley, E. (1990). The bears' picnic: Children's representations of themselves and their families. In I. Bretherton & M. Watson (Eds.), *Children's perspectives on the family* (pp. 47–65). San Francisco: Jossey-Bass.

Nelson, K. (1996). *Language in cognitive development: Emergence of the mediated mind.* New York: Cambridge University Press.

Nelson, K., & Gruendel, J. (1981). Generalized event representations: Basic building blocks of cognitive development. In M. E. Lamb & A. Brown (Eds.), *Advances in developmental psychology* (Vol. l, pp. 131–158). Hillsdale, NJ: Erlbaum.

Nelson, K., & Seidman, S. (1984). Playing with scripts. In I. Bretherton (Ed.), *Symbolic play: The development of social understanding* (pp. 45–71). Orlando, FL: Academic Press.

Newcombe, R., & Reese, E. (2004). Evaluations and orientations in mother–child narratives as a function of attachment security: A longitudinal investigation. *International Journal of Behavioral Development, 28,* 230–245.

Ongari, B., Tomasi, F., & Zoccatelli, B. (2003, August). Narrative representations of family relationships and socio-emotional adaptation to the educational context in pre-schoolers. In R. Miljkovitch (Chair), *The interface between real-life interactions and imaginary interactions during doll-play.* Symposium conducted at the 11th European Conference on Developmental Psychology, Catholic University, Milan, Italy.

Oppenheim, D. (1997). The Attachment Doll Play Interview for Preschoolers. *International Journal of Behavioral Development, 20,* 681–697.

Oppenheim, D., Nir, A., Warren, S., & Emde, R. N. (1997). Emotion regulation in mother-child narrative co-construction: Associations with children's narratives and adaptation. *Developmental Psychology, 35,* 284–294.

Oppenheim, D., & Waters, H. S. (1995). Narrative processes and attachment representations: Issues of development and assessment. In E. Waters, B. E. Vaughn, G. Posada, & K. Kondo-Ikemura (Eds.), Caregiving, cultural and cognitive perspectives on secure base behavior and working models. *Monographs of the Society for Research in Child Development, 60*(2–3, Serial No. 244), 197–233.

Page, T., & Bretherton, I. (2001). Mother– and father–child attachment themes in the story completions of preschoolers from postdivorce families: Do they predict relationships with peers and teachers? *Attachment and Human Development, 3,* 1–29.

Peterson, C. (1999). Children's memory for medical emergencies: 2 years later. *Developmental Psychology, 35,* 1493–1506.

Peterson, C., & Bell, M. (1996). Children's memory for traumatic injury. *Child Development, 67,* 3045–3070.

Piaget, J. (1951). *Play, dreams and imitation.* New York: Norton.

Piaget, J. (1952). *The origins of intelligence in children.* New York: Norton.

Piaget, J. (1954). *The child's construction of reality.* New York: Basic Books.

Pillemer, D. B. (1998). What is remembered about early childhood events? *Clinical Psychology Review, 18,* 895–913.

Pillemer, D. B., & White, S. H. (1989). Childhood events recalled by children and adults. In H. W. Reese (Ed.), *Advances in child development and behavior* (pp. 297–340). New York: Academic Press.

Poehlmann, J. (2004). *Narrative representations of attachment relationships in children of incarcerated mothers.* Manuscript submitted for publication.

Quas, J. A., Goodman, G. S., Bidrose, S., Pipe, M. E., Craw, S., & Ablin, D. S. (1999). Emotion and memory: Children's long-term remembering, forgetting and suggestibility. *Journal of Experimental Child Psychology, 72,* 235–270.

Reese, E., & Farrant, K. (2003). The social origins of reminiscing. In R. Fivush & C. A. Haden (Eds.), *Connecting culture and memory:The social construction of an autobiographical self* (pp. 29–48). Mahwah, NJ: Erlbaum.

Reese, E., Haden, C. A., & Fivush, R. (1993). Mother–child conversations about the past: Relationships of style and memory over time. *Cognitive Development, 8,* 403–430.

Robinson, J., Mantz-Simmons, L., MacFie, J., & the MacArthur Narrative Working Group. (1992). *The narrative coding manual.* Unpublished manuscript, University of Colorado, Boulder.

Schacter, D. L., & Tulving, E. (1994). What are the memory systems of 1994? In D. L. Schachter & E. Tulving (Eds.), *Memory systems* (pp. 1–38). Cambridge, MA: MIT Press.

Shouldice, A. E., & Stevenson-Hinde, J. (1992). Coping with security distress: The Separation Anxiety Test and attachment classification at 4.5 years. *Journal of Child Psychology and Psychiatry, 33,* 331–348.

Slough, N., & Greenberg, M. (1990). 5 year-olds' representations of separation from parents: Responses from the perspective of self and other. In I. Bretherton & M. Watson (Eds.), *Children's perspectives on the family* (pp. 67–84). San Francisco: Jossey-Bass.

Solomon, J., & George, C. (1999). The measurement of attachment security in infancy and childhood. In J. Cassidy & P. R. Shaver (Eds.), *Handbook of attachment: Theory, research, and clinical applications* (pp. 287–316). New York: Guilford Press.

Solomon, J., George, C., & DeJong, A. (1995). Children classified as controlling at age six: Evidence of disorganized representational strategies and aggression at home and school. *Development and Psychopathology, 7,* 447–464.

Spangler, G., & Zimmermann, P. (1999). Attachment representation and emotion regulation in adolescents: A psychobiological perspective on internal working models. *Attachment and Human Development, 1,* 270–290.

Steele, M., Steele, H., Woolgar, M., Yabsley, S., Fonagy, P., Johnson, D., & Croft, C. (2003). An attachment perspective on children's emotion narratives: Links across generations. In R. N. Emde, D. P. Wolf, & D. Oppenheim (Eds.), *Revealing the inner world of young children: The MacArthur Story Stem Battery and parent–child narratives* (pp. 163–181). New York: Oxford University Press.

Stein, N. L., & Glenn, C. G. (1979). An analysis of story comprehension in elementary school children. In R. O. Freedle (Ed.), *New directions in processing* (Vol. 2, pp. 53–120). Norwood, NJ: Ablex.

Steward, M. S. (1993). Medical procedures: A context for studying memory and emotion. In C. A. Nelson (Ed.), *Minnesota Symposia on Child Psychology: Vol. 26. Memory and affect* (pp. 171–225). Hillsdale, NJ: Erlbaum.

Suess, G. J., Grossmann, K. E., & Sroufe, L. A. (1992). Effects of infant attachment to mother and father on quality of adaptation in preschool: From dyadic to individual organization of self. *International Journal of Behavioral Development, 15,* 43–65.

Terr, L. (1983). Chowchilla revisited: The effects of psychic trauma four years after a school-bus kidnapping. *American Journal of Psychiatry, 140,* 1543–1550.

Terr, L. (1991). Childhood traumas: An outline and overview. *American Journal of Psychiatry, 148,* 10–20.

Toth, S. L., Cicchetti, D., MacFie, J., Maugan, A., & VanMeenen, K. (2000). Narrative representations of caregivers and self in maltreated pre-schoolers. *Attachment and Human Development, 2*, 271–305.

Toth, S. L., Cicchetti, D., MacFie, J., Rogosch, F. A., & Maughan, A. (2000). Narrative representations of moral-affiliative and conflictual themes and behavioral problems in maltreated preschoolers. *Journal of Clinical Child Psychology, 29*, 307–318.

Tulving, E. (1972). Episodic and semantic memory. In E. Tulving & W. Donaldson (Eds.), *Organization of memory* (pp. 381–403). New York: Academic Press.

van IJzendoorn, M. H., & Bakermans-Kranenburg, M. J. (1996). Attachment representations in mothers, fathers, adolescents, and clinical groups: A meta-analytic search for normative data. *Journal of Consulting and Clinical Psychology, 64*, 8–27.

Verschueren, K., Marcoen, A., & Schoefs, V. (1996). The internal working model of the self, attachment and competence in 5-year-olds. *Child Development, 67*, 2493–2511.

Waters, E. (1995). The Attachment Q-set (version 3.0). In E. Waters, B. E. Vaughn, G. Posada, & K. Kondo-Ikemura (Eds.), Caregiving, cultural and cognitive perspectives on secure base behavior and working models. *Monographs of the Society for Research in Child Development, 60(2–3*, Serial No. 244), 234–246.

Waters, E., & Deane, K. E. (1985). Defining and assessing individual differences in attachment relationships: Q-methodology and the organization of behavior in infancy and early childhood. In I. Bretherton & E. Waters (Eds.), Growing points of attachment theory and research. *Monographs of the Society for Research in Child Development, 50(1-2*, Serial No. 209), 41–65.

Waters, H. S., Rodrigues, L.M., & Ridgeway, D. (1998). Cognitive underpinnings of narrative attachment assessment. *Journal of Experimental Child Psychology, 71*, 211–234.

Wheeler, M., Stuss, D. T., & Tulving, E. (1997). Toward a theory of episodic memory: The frontal lobes and autonoetic consciousness *Psychological Bulletin, 121*, 331–354.

Wolf, D., Rygh, J. , & Altshuler, J. (1984). Agency and experience: Actions and states in play narratives. In I. Bretherton (Ed.), *Symbolic play: The development of social understanding* (pp. 195–217). Orlando, FL: Academic Press.

Young, J. Z. (1964). *A model of the brain*. London: Oxford University Press.

Zahn-Waxler, C., Cole, P. M., Richardson, D. T., Friedman, R. J., Michel, M. K., & Belouad, F. (1994). Social problem solving in disruptive preschool children: Reactions to hypothetical situations of conflict and distress. *Merrill-Palmer Quarterly, 40*, 98–119.

Zeahnah, C. H. (1989.). *The Working Model of the Child Interview*. Unpublished manuscript, Tulane University, New Orleans, LA.

Zimmermann, P. (1999). Structure and function of internal working models of attachment and their role in emotion regulation. *Attachment and Human Development, 1*, 291–306.

CHAPTER 3

Placing Early Attachment Experiences in Developmental Context

The Minnesota Longitudinal Study

L. ALAN SROUFE
BYRON EGELAND
ELIZABETH CARLSON
W. ANDREW COLLINS

The authors of this chapter developed their common interest in attachment theory and research via different pathways. We share in common a primary interest in the nature of development and the complex influences that govern it. In our view, development is nonlinear, hierarchical, and multifaceted. We have been, and continue to be, curious about the place of attachment within this broader view of development.

As attachment theory was emerging, Alan Sroufe was studying early emotional development, including its psychophysiological components, in the late 1960s and early 1970s. This work brought him into contact with two of the major advances in developmental psychology that launched attachment theory into prominence. The first was uncovering the inadequacy of learning models of the prior era to account for salient aspects of emotional life. In general, classical and operant conditioning played little role in the emergence and progressive changes in infant positive emotion. For example, infants' smiles to events waxed and waned due to internal cognitive and affective processes, not due to external reinforcement; particular events at a given age would evoke laughter over and over without extinction; and infants smiled more at full faces than at the profiles that would have been associated with nursing. Thus, when Ainsworth (1969) and Bowlby (1969) wrote that one was not attached to one's caregiver due to reinforcement or to association with feeding, but rather because evolution had prepared infants to do so merely given continued interactive presence, this struck a resonant cord with the emergent functionalist view of emotions (Campos, Mumme, Kermoian, & Campos, 1994; Sroufe, 1979; Sroufe & Waters, 1976; Sroufe & Wunsch, 1972).

The second theme that arose from the study of emotion was what is now called an "organizational perspective" on development. Infants may smile, look at, and interact with strangers as frequently as with mothers, but they combine looks, smiles, and vocalizations with caregivers in ways that are unique. In some circumstances, for example, when threatened or distressed, they preferentially seek contact with caregivers and even refuse contact with strangers. Moreover, the same external event (e.g., a brightly colored mask put on over the face) may elicit reactions ranging from squeals of laughter to frank fear (Sroufe, Waters, & Matas, 1974; Sroufe & Wunsch, 1972), depending on the agent, the setting, the order of events, and prior experiences. Thus, a mask will elicit more fear if put on by a stranger rather than the by mother, if the masking occurs in an unfamiliar situation, if the stranger puts on the mask prior to the mother wearing it, and if the baby was frightened moments before by another event. Clearly, it is the organization among behaviors and with regard to context that reveals the meaning of infant behavior, not mere occurrence or frequency. And attachment was the ultimate organizational construct, drawing upon all facets of development (cognitive, emotional, social) and being manifest in the balance between exploration and comfort seeking, with individual variations in patterns of behavior.

The second author, Byron Egeland, had an early interest in the origins and consequences of child maltreatment. Again, simple explanations and models had proven to be inadequate by the early 1970s. No linear cause, no single outcome, and no simple process had emerged from prior research (Egeland & Brunnquell, 1979). In terms of cause, it was clear that one could not simply attribute abuse to parental personality disorder. Many factors, including the stresses and supports available, proved to be important. Parental perceptions, expectations, and understandings regarding infants and their development seemed to be especially critical, and these often appeared to be carried forward from the parent's own developmental history (Brunnquell, Crichton, & Egeland, 1981). This converged perfectly with Bowlby's ideas concerning internal working models and his subsequent work on representation.

Likewise, not all children experiencing maltreatment were later aggressive, or anxious, or depressed, but rather they showed a variety of outcomes. The search for common core issues led Egeland to attachment. Many of these children had in common relationship difficulties and failures of self-integration (Egeland & Sroufe, 1981). In particular, emerging research on disorganized attachment meshed well with Egeland's interest in outcomes of abuse and neglect.

Finally, Egeland's interest in parental maltreatment as the outcome of a developmental process, the course of which could be altered by transforming experience, fit nicely with ideas of developmental pathways that were central to attachment theory. As it turned out, the major factors that enabled individuals to "break the cycle" of abuse were all relationship experiences: having an alternative responsive caregiver in childhood, a long-term therapy relationship in childhood, and a current supportive relationship with a partner (Egeland, Jacobvitz, & Sroufe, 1988). Each of these would follow from attachment theory.

By the mid-1970s Sroufe was conducting what would be the first longitudinal outcome study of attachment, in which children with known infant attachment quality were being seen in settings such as kindergarten, where the caregiver was not present. At the same time, Egeland launched a study of high-risk parents and their soon-to-be-born children. We then joined forces in 1977 to carry forward the Minnesota Longitudinal Study from birth to adulthood.

The third author, Elizabeth Carlson, became involved in attachment research while working on a short-term longitudinal project with teenage mothers in New York (Ward & Carlson, 1995). This was one of the first studies to utilize the Adult Attachment Interview (AAI) to predict infant attachment outcomes and was the first to do so with such a high-risk sample. Carlson came to Minnesota in 1990 with well-developed interests in disorganized attachment, representation processes, and their role in guiding behavior. She wrote a postdoctoral grant to study these issues within the Minnesota longitudinal project. By rescoring existing Strange Situation videotapes for disorganization, she ultimately produced the first empirical data on the longitudinal links between disorganization in infancy and dissociation in late adolescence (Carlson, 1998). Subsequently, she carried out the first analysis of the interplay of multiple measures of representation and behavior across the infancy, preschool, middle-childhood, and adolescent years (Carlson, Sroufe, & Egeland, 2004).

W. Andrew Collins, the fourth author, came to a specific interest in attachment research from a long history of research on parent–child interactions and relationships. The conceptual underpinnings of this work came from the then fledgling science of relationships (e.g., Kelley et al., 1983; Reis, Collins, & Berscheid, 2000). Given his long-standing interest in social relationships in middle childhood and adolescence and his emerging interest in romantic relationships and adult attachments, an infusion of the richer understanding of developmental process inherent in attachment theory was compatible with his long-term research goals. He joined the Minnesota longitudinal project in 1993 when we were studying adolescent development and contemplating the transition to adulthood. Developmental transitions had been a major focus of Collins's work, especially as they affected significant relationships (Collins, 1995). Moreover, he shared the view of the project that salient relationships are complex developmental constructions, drawing on the totality of one's history, as well as current supports and challenges. He has been especially intrigued with questions about links between early life and adult attachments and the contributory role of intervening peer relationships. These interests have contributed to our broadening view of attachment within a total developmental and relational context.

A VIEWPOINT ON ATTACHMENT

Attachment has proven to be perhaps the most important developmental construct ever investigated. At the same time, attachment researchers should be the first to acknowledge that early attachment experiences are not (and should not be) related to any and all outcomes. Likewise, it should be acknowledged that variations in attachment experiences are not the only vital influence on development, even in the domain of social relationships. Moreover, when they are related to outcomes, attachment variations are not properly viewed as linear, inevitable causes. From the outset, Bowlby (e.g., 1973) argued for a pathway/process model in which both early and later experiences of various kinds worked together to shape developmental outcomes and in which cause was viewed in probabilistic terms.

Attachment security is only one of many environmental influences on the developing child. Some important aspects of parenting, even in the early years, lie outside the purview of attachment. Attachment generally refers to provision of a haven of safety, a secure base for exploration, and a source of reassurance when the child is distressed. But parents do more than this. They also provide stimulation for the child that may or may not be appropriately modulated. They provide guidance, limits, and interactive support for problem solving. In addition, they support the child's competence in the broader world—for example, by making possible and supporting social contacts outside the home. While these functions are to some extent correlated with degree of attachment security, they are distinctive contributions of parents. A parent may be ineffective with regard to some of these, even when he or she has been a dependable secure base. For example, some parents who were sensitively responsive to their infants' signals of need may not be good at setting limits or structuring the child's encounters with the object world. These other aspects of early parenting at times predict to outcomes that attachment does not and vice versa.

The provision of a base of security for the child has been properly emphasized because this parenting issue arises early and remains in force throughout the child's development. It is always important. Still, new tasks for parents emerge age by age as the child's social world expands and as the child becomes increasingly autonomous. Many of these parenting issues, such as promoting the child's relationships with peers, are quite distinctive from providing a secure base. Again, while some links between provision for early attachment needs and later support for the child have been demonstrated, there is notable independence in these domains as well. For example, some parents who were very effective in helping their child establish a serviceable secure base in infancy are not effective in supporting the child's peer relationships or have great difficulty supporting autonomy at the transition to adolescence. They may, for example, lag behind in recognizing the child's readiness for more control at this age (Collins, 1995). (For a listing of just some of the many influences of parents, see Table 3.1.)

Beyond this range of direct parenting influences, many other family factors influence the development of the child. In our work we have found an impact from the quality of the parental relationship, the comings and goings of men in the home, the amount of general stress being experienced by primary parents, and experiences with siblings (Pianta, Egeland, & Sroufe, 1990; Pianta, Hyatt, & Egeland, 1986; Yates, Dodds, Sroufe, & Egeland, 1993). In addition, there also are important influences on development that lie outside of the family. Notable among these are relationships with peers. Again, as we discuss below, attachment experiences in early life are often related to various aspects of peer competence later. Nonetheless, peer experiences are by no means completely forecast by attachment history, and they exercise an influence on development that is at least somewhat independent of attachment history.

TABLE 3.1. The Tasks of Parenting

- Regulation of arousal
- Appropriately modulated stimulation
- Provision of secure base and safe haven
- Appropriate guidance, limits, and structure
- Maintenance of parent–child boundaries
- Socialization of emotional expression and containment
- Scaffolding for problem solving
- Supporting mastery and achievement
- Supporting the child's contacts with the broader social world
- Accepting the child's growing independence

In light of the complexity of development and the myriad of influences on it, it is to be expected that attachment history would not predict some important social outcomes at all well, nor would it *uniquely* predict more than a few outcomes of interest. Yet this in no way diminishes the importance of early attachment experiences. First, when early attachment does predict some outcome strongly and consistently, even in competition with other influences, such predictive power has great theoretical interest. For example, in our work we have found that early insecure attachment is strongly related to individual differences in dependency throughout the juvenile years (Sroufe, Fox, & Pancake, 1983; Urban, Carlson, Egeland, & Sroufe, 1991), just as specified by Bowlby (1973). In the psychopathology area, we found that anxious resistant attachment in infancy was the best predictor of anxiety problems in late adolescence, while avoidant attachment and disorganized attachment predicted conduct problems and dissociation, respectively (Carlson, 1998; Warren, Huston, Egeland, & Sroufe, 1997). Moreover, when we broaden our vision beyond simply cataloguing all of the outcomes related to attachment variation to the way attachment works in coordination with other aspects of experience or other developmental influences, it in fact has the potential for enhancing the value of attachment as a developmental construct.

The goal of this chapter is to illustrate this broadened view of attachment and its place in the developmental process by using primarily the examples of peer and romantic relationships. The capacity to effectively relate to peers is itself a developmental construct. Such a capacity is constructed age by age through a series of phases, beginning with a general orientation toward engagement and loosely coordinated interactions in the preschool period and culminating in highly sophisticated, reciprocal intimate relationships and integrated networks by early adulthood. This is a cumulative process in which success at each phase builds upon all preceding phases. As we discuss below, there is a place for early attachment relationships in this process but also for other experiences in the family and for peer experiences themselves. The picture that is emerging is multifaceted, dynamic rather than linear, and with considerable complexity in when, how, and in what particular aspect of social functioning attachment exerts its impact.

A BRIEF OVERVIEW OF THE MINNESOTA STUDY

Assessments made in the Minnesota study have been comprehensive. They have included cognitive, social, and behavioral development; measurement in homes, the laboratory, summer camps, and schools; and ongoing measures of the surrounding context. These have been described in a number of papers (Egeland & Brunnquell, 1979; Erickson, Egeland, & Sroufe, 1985; Roisman, Madsen, Hennighausen, Sroufe, & Collins, 2001; Sroufe, Egeland, & Carlson, 1999). They also will be detailed in a forthcoming book (Sroufe, Egeland, Carlson, & Collins, 2005). Here, only the most important assessments for the following discussion are summarized.

In the early childhood years, we carried out Strange Situation attachment assessments at ages 12 and 18 months. At age 2 years, we examined caregiver and child behavior in play, clean-up, and problem-solving situations, where ratings were made of caregiver support, assistance, and hostility and of child enthusiasm, positive and negative affect, and overall functioning. The focus was on how well the parent scaffolded the child's beginning movement toward autonomy and self-regulation. Similar ratings were made at age 3½ based on a series of laboratory teaching tasks. A subset of 40 children also was studied in detail in our own nursery school.

In the middle-childhood years, we collected comprehensive school assessments, including teacher rankings of peer competence at grades 1, 2, and 3. For a subset of 48 children, detailed observational measures and counselor ratings and rankings were made at a series of month-long summer day camps.

At age 13, we again carried out direct observation of parent and child. The variables were derived from videotaped parent–child interaction in the laboratory. Tasks involved planning an antismoking campaign together, the teen directing the parent to complete two puzzles while blindfolded, discussing together the possible results of imaginary events, and collaborating on a Q-sort description of "the ideal person" (Block, Block, & Gjerde, 1988; J. Sroufe, 1991). Research assistants coded these videotaped interactions using 11 scales developed by J. Sroufe (1991). The scales included affective components (positive affect, negative affect, anger, confrontive/ attacking), conflict and conflict resolution, parent–child boundary violations, and three "balance" scales that focused on the degree to which relationships (1) allowed spontaneous expression of positions and feelings by both partners, (2) served to scaffold the development of each individual, and (3) allowed the dyads to work together to meet the task demands. Some of these scales seem rather obviously related to attachment security; for example, Balance 1 is partly reflected in the capacity of the child to take a position and comfortably hold it, even in the face of parent disagreement. Others, such as the capacity to negotiate conflicts, are not so obvious. As a set we found that these observations were only modestly related to attachment history and therefore are justifiably viewed at least partly as an independent developmental influence.

In early adulthood we examined a variety of age-salient outcomes, including educational attainment, work competence, and parenting. We also administered the AAI at ages 19 and 26 years. A major focus to date has been adult romantic relationships. Between the ages of 20 and 26, participants who had been in relationships for at least 4 months ($n = 84$) were invited to complete a romantic relationship assessment with their partners either in their homes or at the laboratory. Tasks included completing the Current Relationship Interview (CRI; Crowell & Owens, 1996), filling out a battery of standard social psychological measures of participants' perceptions of their current romantic relationship, and participating in a sequence of two observational tasks with their partners. In these videotaped observations, dyads first discussed a couple-identified problem and subsequently collaborated on a Q-sort describing the ideal couple. Research assistants coded videotapes of the couple interactions using 10 dyadic rating scales of behavior and affect, developed to parallel the age-13 parent–child ratings described above (Aguilar et al., 1997; J. Sroufe, 1991) (ρ_I's ranged from .81 to .95, p's < .001). Coders were blind to the identity of the original participants within the couples or any aspect of the participants' history.

Romantic relationship quality has been previously operationalized in this research project using a composite measure of "romantic relationship process" derived from a principal components analysis of the rating scales mentioned above (Roisman et al., 2001). This quality measure is a standardized average of the Balance I, Balance II, Conflict Resolution, Overall Quality, Secure Base, and Shared Positive Affect rating scales (alpha = .95). Previously reported analyses have shown that participants coded as secure on the AAI (Main & Goldwyn, 1994) at age 19 were involved in higher quality romantic relationships at age 20–21 than those coded as insecure (Roisman et al., 2001).

Detailed demographic data for the full current follow-up longitudinal sample ($n = 170$) are available in several recent publications (Roisman et al., 2001; Roisman, Padrón, Sroufe, & Egeland, 2002). For the romantically involved subsample that is the focus of this report, 65.5% of the participants are Caucasian, 14.9% have mixed racial backgrounds (European American, African American, Latino, and/or Native American), 10.3% are African American, 1% are Native American or Latino, and 4.6% are unclassifiable due to missing data on their fathers' race. As described earlier, the mean duration of participants' romantic relationships was 2 years, 4 months (SD = 1 year, 10 months; range = 4 months–8.5 years). Only 24% of the couples had been romantically involved for less than a year, with over 50% dating 2 years or more.

ATTACHMENT AND PEER RELATIONSHIPS

In our organizational viewpoint (e.g., Sroufe et al., 1999), the capacity to relate to peers is a developmental construct. Attachment variations represent "initial conditions" in the unfolding of this system but they do not completely specify the outcome. Table 3.2 describes the changing issues in

TABLE 3.2. Changing Issues in Childhood Peer Relationships

Preschool: "Positive engagement of peers"

1. Selecting specific partners
2. Sustaining interactive bouts
   a. Negotiating conflicts in interaction
   b. Maintaining organization in the face of arousal
   c. Finding pleasure in the interactive process
3. Participation in groups

Middle childhood: "Investment in the peer world"

1. Forming loyal friendships
2. Sustaining relationships
   a. Negotiating relationship conflicts
   b. Tolerating a range of emotional experiences
   c. Enhancement of self in relationships
3. Functioning in stable, organized groups
   a. Adhering to group norms
   b. Maintaining gender boundaries
4. Coordinating friendships and group functioning

Adolescence: "Integrating self and peer relationships"

1. Forming intimate relationships
   a. Self-disclosing same-gender relationships
   b. Cross-gender relationships
   c. Sexual relationships
2. Commitment in relationships
   a. Negotiating self-relevant conflicts
   b. Emotional vulnerability
   c. Self-disclosure and self-identity
3. Functioning in a relationship network
   a. Mastering multiple rule systems
   b. Establishing flexible boundaries
4. Coordinating multiple relationships
   a. Same-gender and cross-gender
   b. Intimate relationships and group functioning

peer relationships from the preschool years through adolescence. An important lesson from this table concerns the way competencies at each phase draw upon competencies at each previous phase. For example, sustaining interactive bouts in the preschool period in the face of the inevitable conflicts that arise provides a foundation for sustaining relationships over time and negotiating conflicts in relationships in the middle-childhood period. Likewise, the intimate relationships of adolescence draw upon experiences with loyal friendships in middle childhood. Adult romantic relationships draw upon this entire history of interactive and emotional experiences with peers. In fact, it is reasonable to propose that prior peer experiences have indispensable and unique functions with regard to promoting adult relationships.

At the same time, effectiveness with peers is supported in part by experiences in the family, including early attachment experiences. Table 3.3 presents some of the rationale for why and how early attachment experiences support peer relationships. Attachment security provides five bases for later effectiveness with peers: (1) a motivational base, involving expectations of connectedness; (2) an attitudinal base, involving expectations of responsiveness; (3) an instrumental base centered on exploratory and play capacities; (4) an emotional base, including entrained capacities for arousal and emotional regulation; and (5) a relational base, involving empathy and expectations of mutuality (see Sroufe et al., 1999). By participating in a secure relationship during the infant period one begins to acquire the attitudes that support engagement with peers, the personal capacities to stay engaged and to be attractive to peer partners, and a fundamental inner understanding of what relationships require.

TABLE 3.3. How Attachment Security Promotes
the Development of Peer Relationships

The Motivational Base

- Positive expectations concerning relationships
- A basic sense of connectedness
- A belief that relationships will be rewarding

The Attitudinal Base

- The belief that one may elicit responses from others
- Expectations of mastery in the social world

The Instrumental Base

- Object mastery through support for exploration
- The capacity to enjoy play and discovery

The Emotional Base

- Modulated arousal
- Self-regulation of emotion

The Relational Base

- Expectations concerning reciprocity
- Empathic responsiveness deriving from empathic care

In our empirical studies we have made a number of important findings regarding the prediction of peer competence across time. First, important features of peer relationships are indeed predicted by attachment history from preschool to early adulthood. For example, attachment security in infancy accounts for 13% of the variance in middle-childhood friendship competence 9 years later, based on summer camp observations. These findings are consistent with those of the Grossmanns (K. E. Grossmann & K. Grossmann, 1991), who find that children with a history of secure attachment in infancy are less often ridiculed or excluded from group activities in middle childhood. In general, when peer measures have been based on direct observation, we have found clear links between infant attachment security and peer functioning at every age from preschool through adolescence (Sroufe et al., 1999). In fact, the predictions to adolescent functioning were as strong and in some cases stronger than predictions to peer variables at earlier ages. We have reasoned that this may be due to the special requirements for intimacy in adolescence.

Second, when we add other aspects of parenting to the predictive equation, there often is a substantial increase in the variance accounted for (Sroufe et al., 1999). Thus, when attachment assessments are combined with our assessments of appropriate stimulation and guidance between ages 2 and 3½, variance accounted for in the middle-childhood friendship score was doubled (with the multiple correlation now being .52). In a parallel manner, our assessments of support for emerging autonomy in early adolescence also supplement infant attachment in predicting later adolescent peer competence, and so forth.

Third, when prior peer competence measures at a given age are combined with attachment history, prediction of later peer competence generally is better than when using either predictor separately. In the example of predicting middle-childhood friendship competence that we have been using, adding preschool teacher peer competence ratings increases prediction beyond attachment history or even attachment and preschool parenting measures combined. The resulting multiple r is .62 ($R^2 = .40$).

Fourth, the strength and nature of the links between attachment or early peer measures and later assessments of peer competence depend on the particular aspect of peer functioning in question. For example, interactive competence with peers in middle childhood is predicted substantially better by earlier peer competence than by infant attachment security, though both are significant predictors. In contrast, attachment history is a better predictor of gender boundary maintenance among peers in middle childhood (a salient peer task in Western cultures), though it is also significantly predicted (but to a lesser degree) by earlier peer competence (Sroufe, Bennett, Englund, Urban, & Shulman, 1993). Often, emotional aspects of relationships have specific ties to attachment. In adolescence a feature of peer competence that we labeled the "capacity for emotional vulnerability" had clear links to attachment history, with a correlation of .41 over this 14-year interval. The camp counselors made ratings of this variable based on their observations of the young person's capacity to engage in the full range of camp experiences, including situations where feelings likely would arise and a chance of possible rejection was present. This finding is consistent with the idea that a core capacity for trust may be the legacy of early secure attachment.

The idea that strong prediction of outcomes comes when one uses attachment history in concert with other measures shows up in all areas of our work. Dramatic examples arise when we employ broadband competence constructs. One example is our measure of global competence at age 19 years. Following detailed coding of a lengthy interview covering all aspects of functioning, overall ratings were made of the degree to which the individual was functioning well with regard to the domains of (1) school/work; (2) family, peer, and romantic relationships; and (3) self-direction/personal responsibility. Attachment security in infancy was significantly related to this distal outcome, but it accounted for only 5% of the variance. But when we also used as predictors other aspects of early care and home environment quality, peer competence through the elementary school years, and parent–child support at the transition to adolescence, the variance accounted for approached 50%.

OUTCOME AND PROCESS

Increasingly, our interest is not simply in the question of whether early attachment predicts some outcome, or even how strongly it predicts it, but in the complex developmental processes in which attachment experiences work with and through other experiences in the course of development. We have now done a number of analyses in which we have examined early attachment experiences and other early care variables, later family variables, and peer experiences with regard to a range of adult outcomes (Collins & van Dulmen, in press; Roisman et al., 2001).

The picture that is emerging in each case is one of developmental complexity. For example, in previous research we found that both our early care variables, including infant attachment, and peer competence in elementary school predicted work competence in early adulthood (Collins & van Dulmen, in press). However, early care was no longer a significant predictor when peer competence was taken into account, and subsequent analyses supported the notion that the link between early care and work competence was partially mediated through the peer variable. Likewise, infant attachment significantly predicted an interview-based measure of relationship satisfaction at age 21 ($r = .32$), as did peer competence in elementary school (a composite of teacher rankings in grades 1, 2, and 3). Again, there was evidence for partial mediation, and with peer competence in the regression the link with attachment no longer was significant.

We now have been able to carry out direct behavioral assessments on 82 couples between the ages of 20 and 26 years. The results here are preliminary, and a number of interesting analyses await more of our participants forming partnerships. Still, the early findings provide additional support for the propositions put forward above. Attachment history is an important consideration, but the most interesting results come when we consider how attachment experiences work together with other aspects of experience. Infant attachment history does by itself predict numerous aspects of intimate relationship functioning, including the composite relationship process variable described earlier. Disorganized attachment (e.g., Main & Hesse, 1990) is an especially strong predictor, correlating with the composite process variable .35 and with hostility ratings .42. Insecurity composites from 12 and 18 months tend to yield significant correlations in the .20s and .30s with a range of relationship variables. Such relationships are impressive in that we are spanning two decades and numerous developmental phases.

The second point is that elementary peer competence measures (teacher rankings in grades 1–3) and parent–child interaction measures at age 13 also relate to the romantic relationship outcomes, and when either or both are added to the infant attachment measure prediction is often significantly increased (to the .30s or .40s). For example, when a composite of 13-year parent support measures (Balance I and II; see above) is added in predicting the capacity of the romantic couple to resolve conflict, the correlation rises from .27 to .36, with the change being significant. In this case there is also evidence for partial mediation. Some of the variance explained by infant attachment goes through the 13-year-old measure, and when it is included the link to infant attachment is no longer significant (see Figure 3.1). When conflict resolution between parent and child at age 13 is substituted, the result is very similar (with the multiple correlation slightly higher at .39). When teacher-rated peer competence was put into the regression following attachment, there was again a significant increment in predicting couple conflict resolution, but in this case there was no evidence for mediation.

In a similar manner, when couple observed hostility was the outcome, both 13-year parent–child interaction measures and elementary peer competence accounted for significant additional variance beyond that accounted for by infant attachment. In the case of the peer variable, the contributions seemed to be largely independent, even though the attachment and peer variables are related. There was no evidence for mediation in

Predicting Adult Conflict Resolution

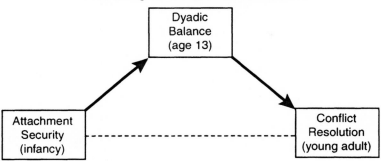

FIGURE 3.1. In some cases, as when examining both early attachment and parent support in early adolescence as predictors of couple conflict resolution, the impact of attachment is largely mediated through the later variable.

this case (see Figure 3.2). Various 13-year measures also accounted for variance beyond infant attachment in predicting couple hostility. With the composite 13-year parent support variable, there was again evidence for partial mediation. In this case, however, even with the evidence for an indirect effect for attachment, the direct effect also remained significant (see Figure 3.3). Thus, for this emotional aspect of young-adult romantic relationships, early attachment seemed to have *both* direct and indirect influences through its impact on later parenting.

To summarize, we have found great variety in the way attachment works, depending on the particular outcome and the other variables that

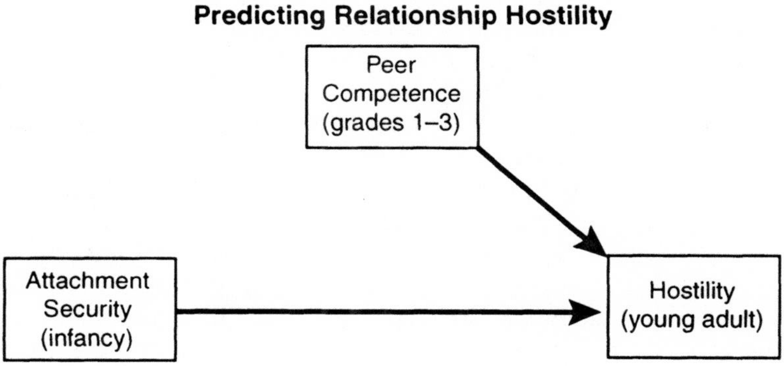

Predicting Relationship Hostility

FIGURE 3.2. In some cases, early attachment and other variables independently predict an outcome.

Predicting Relationship Hostility

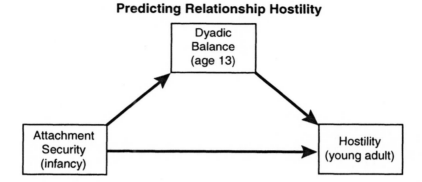

FIGURE 3.3. In some cases, early attachment appears to have both direct and indirect effects.

we also consider. At times, attachment does strongly predict outcomes, even in comparison with other more proximal variables. Almost always, however, when attachment history is combined with other variables, including peer experience at various ages and later experiences with parents, predictions of outcomes are enhanced. This is true even when the outcome variable in question is loaded with attachment relevance, such as hostility in couple relationships. With some combinations of variables attachment has primarily direct effects on outcomes, while with other combinations there are indirect effects. For at least some outcomes it seems to be the case that attachment promotes relationships with peers and that, subsequently, capacities are acquired in those encounters that in turn further promote later competence. Sometimes there are both direct and indirect effects. Infant attachment continues to contribute, especially with regard to capacities centering on emotional aspects of relating.

When we accumulate data on a larger number of couples, we expect that this emerging picture will become more coherent. Not only will an increase in sample size affect our power, it will enable us to do analyses based on our vastly more powerful observational measures of peer competence. Since the camp peer competence data are available only on a subsample, we need to have couple data on almost all of our participants to carry out the desired analyses. It remains our expectation that depending on the particular outcome and particular proposed mediator, all possible patterns will result. We expect some cases where early attachment has unique strength. One of these may be parenting in the next generation. Another may be specific measures of secure-base provision in adult relationships. There will likely be other cases where strength comes in combining attachment with other measures. Finally, there likely will be times when infant attachment drops out as a predictor after other measures are considered, even when our sample is complete.

Even when early attachment no longer predicts, its role in development is not trivialized once a process view is adopted. Beyond the indirect effects cited above, in previous papers we have documented many instances wherein early attachment variation predicts positive change following periods of troubled development in childhood (Sroufe, Carlson, Levy, & Egeland, 1999; Sroufe, Egeland, & Kreutzer, 1990). In addition, it should be pointed out that there are times when the process comes full circle and we show that attachment-related young adult variation (AAI and CRI measures) mediates earlier family or peer influences on later outcomes (Roisman et al., 2001).

TWO CASE EXAMPLES

While every case examined closely reveals the developmental complexity of influences over time, some underscore most clearly the major points we make in this chapter. Tony was a child who had been securely attached at both 12 and 18 months. In fact, throughout the preschool period his care was notably supportive. And this showed when he entered school. Teacher rankings of peer competence and emotional health, as well as ratings covering behavior problems and school performance, consistently indicated positive adaptation.

Unfortunately, things went very badly in subsequent years. His parents underwent a very acrimonious divorce, with a great deal of tension and conflict. His father, at least partly because of his anger toward Tony's mother, had visits with Tony's older brother and younger sister but not with Tony. In the next few years Tony's mother began relying on him a great deal—in our judgment putting him all too much in a spousal role and blurring the normal parent–child boundaries. In the face of this, as observed in our 13-year assessment, Tony began pushing away from his mother, even more so than is common among 13-year-olds. Normally, we would see this distancing as largely positive, a necessary effort to retain a degree of autonomy, when the form of connection being offered was compromising it. However, in this case the result was calamitous. Just at this point in development, Tony's mother died suddenly in an automobile accident, which would seem almost certain to have induced tremendous guilt in Tony. To be pushing away from a loved one when she or he died would be guilt-inducing, even for a mature adult. If this were not bad enough, Tony's father then decided to leave the state with the other two children, so that Tony quickly lost his mother, his father, and his siblings. He was taken in by an aunt and uncle, which was a good thing in that they cared about him; yet they were elderly and not prepared to properly supervise a teenage boy.

Considering these tragic and highly stressful events, it is not at all surprising that Tony's middle-adolescent and late-teenage years were very troubled. He had difficulties at school, was withdrawn from peers, and on a standard diagnostic interview at age 17½ clearly qualified for a diagnosis of conduct disorder. He was heavily involved in burglary, though largely in an "administrative" capacity, organizing the activities of other boys. When we had seen him at age 10, following the divorce, he already had a bit of an aggressive attitude (a "chip on his shoulder"); he was ready and even eager to be in conflict with other boys. But at that time he still was a very vibrant, lively child. When we saw him at age 15 he was literally unrecognizable as the child we had known. The light inside of him seemed to have gone out. He was visibly depressed and isolated.

Clearly, his history of secure attachment was not enough to protect him from the consequences of his middle-childhood and early-adolescent trauma. Knowing the history of early care alone was inadequate to predict this pattern of adaptation in adolescence. Does this mean, as some have at times suggested (Kagan, 1984; Lewis, 1997), that early attachment experiences are of trivial importance when later experience is divergent? Our past findings for the childhood and adolescent periods, wherein early positive care predicts resiliency following periods of difficulty (see above), make us think this is not so. While not enough data is yet available for adult outcomes to again test this hypothesis with group data, the case of Tony is instructive.

Recently, we had the opportunity to observe Tony with his 2-year-old daughter. Coders were, of course, totally blind to Tony's history. Their ratings revealed an extraordinarily supportive father. He was patient, involved, warm, and available, providing the structure, limits, and encouragement the child needed. Likewise, based on ratings made by another set of independent coders, his relationship with his wife was very positive, characterized by engagement, mutual understanding, and caring. His AAI at age 19 was classified as dismissing and included a clear statement that his mother's death did not have much import to him. By age 26, even though the transcript still was classed as dismissing, he was able to talk much more about his mother's death and surrounding feelings. His CRI, based on the relationship with his wife, was on the secure/dismissing boundary. There were clear statements of valuing his relationship (e.g., missing his partner when they are apart). With one case, it is not possible for us to conclude whether it was this spousal relationship that promoted Tony's fathering, or renewed relations with his father, or whether the history of secure attachment was the foundation for the marriage relationship, the fathering capacity, or both. But we do expect that when we have complete data it will again be demonstrable that the history of secure attachment is implicated for groups of participants who are able to make such dramatic recoveries of functioning.

There are parallel cases representing every other pattern of continuity and change. Our other example is the case of Anita who, in contrast to Tony, had an anxious/avoidant attachment with her mother at both our 12- and 18-month assessments. Moreover, her adaptation remained quite poor during the preschool years. She was extremely anxious, socially immature, and infantile. During one period, when teachers had made available baby carriages and large dolls, Anita herself spent 2 days in one of the carriages being treated as a baby by other girls. Teachers and staff wondered if she were prepsychotic. In further contrast to Tony, however, perhaps as a result of therapeutic help received by both mother and daughter, middle childhood was a dramatically more positive period. We were stunned to see this graceful, engaging child. A special strength was her social skill. She was clearly part of the popular girls group (the only child with an avoidant history where this was so in any of our three camps), and formal sociometrics showed her to be ranked near the top of the entire camp. Her transformation was so striking that following the camp, when camera operators and coders no longer had to be blind, many discussions ensued regarding whether this change was real and, if so, what happened to her former history. Is it still there? The answer, then and now, is that both are true. The change was real and the former history, of course, remains part of her. Children generally are not fooled. That they liked Anita followed from her engagement of them and sensitivity to them. She was a loyal friend. It is difficult to fake social competence as a 10-year-old. But even at this time of relatively positive functioning, shadows of the earlier adaptation were apparent. The most striking examples were her explicit statements of doubt that others would continue to like her, despite all the evidence to the contrary. She literally seemed to believe that when they got to know her better, they would no longer want to be her friend. She retained an extraordinary level of self-deprecation.

More compelling regarding the ongoing legacy of her early years were the negative changes witnessed during the adolescent years. She suffered from numerous behavioral and emotional problems. At age 17½ she qualified for diagnoses of conduct disorder, oppositional defiant disorder, obsessive–compulsive disorder, attention-deficit disorder, dysthymia, and social phobia. In other words, she was very angry, anxious, and depressed. (She also qualified for past major depression and various past substance abuse disorders.) Throughout the teenage years, her problems with drugs and authorities were serious, and she dropped out of school. She also engaged in self-abusive behavior. She had a female child at age 18, but the father of this child was not supportive and ultimately wound up in prison.

At age 19, her AAI was classified as U E3a, unresolved for abuse and preoccupied.

At the present time, she still has serious problems. She battles depression, has self-injurious inclinations, and shows some signs of thought disorder. Her global adjustment rating remains only 2 on a 5-point scale. But she completed a special program for dropouts and was awarded her degree. She lives with her daughter and is able to draw some emotional support from her grandparents. She is in regular contact with her mother, and their relationship seems to be improving. Here is what was said about her in the summary paragraph in the write-up of her interview at age 26:

> "It sounded to me like Anita is really trying to make her life better. She quit using drugs and alcohol a few years ago, and quit smoking as well. She is seeing a counselor and is hoping to get back to work. She volunteers at a local hospital. She is very concerned about and caring toward her daughter. She said that she works very hard at spending time with her, doing things they both enjoy, and in managing her anger toward her. She also seemed like she is insightful about her past, and seemed like a nice, though anxious, person. Although she is not doing great, I think that, given appropriate and caring professional help, she will get better over time."

The glimmers of hope we had seen in middle childhood seem to still be present in incipient form, but so too are the history of unresponsive care in the early years and repeated maltreatment in the years surrounding the transition to adolescence.

CONCLUSION

The attachment theory proposed by Bowlby was a thorough-going developmental theory. As attachment researchers, our goal is to understand not just correlated outcomes of early attachment but the process of development itself. Thus, our own interest has gone beyond direct linkages between infant attachment and ultimate functioning to the place of attachment in a broader developmental view.

In part, this has involved exploring early attachment as a foundation for later experience, both inside and outside of the family. Early on, reasoning like Ainsworth (Ainsworth, Bell, & Stayton, 1974), we found that where there had been anxious attachment in infancy, parents had more difficulty providing limits, boundaries, and support during the autonomy struggles of the toddler period (Matas, Arend, & Sroufe, 1978). We believe that those with secure histories are more accepting of parents' limits and guidelines at this time because a foundation of confidence in the parent's responsiveness already was laid out in infancy. But, of course, the struggles at age 2, if intractable, also now become part of the history for the next phase. This same thinking guided our choice of assessments and analyses at age 13.

Likewise, attachment experiences provide bases for entering into and negotiating the world of peers. As development continues, early attachment, later family experiences, and peer experiences together provide the foundation for the intimate relationships of maturity. These adult partner relationships, in turn, of course, are additional foundations for parenting and other tasks of later adulthood.

As intergenerational research comes to the fore, a prominent role for representational processes has been accepted. This was launched by the several studies showing that AAI classification predicted infant attachment pattern (Hesse, 1999; van IJzendoorn, 1995) and other studies showing that infant attachment variations were related to later differences in representation and, in some studies, later AAI classification. Our work leads us to adopt a dynamic view of this process also, as did Bowlby (1973). Early attachment experiences are apparently represented and carried forward, setting conditions for seeking, interpreting, and reacting to later experiences. But later experience also alters representations in an ongoing transactional manner (Carlson et al., 2004). Again, this in no way trivializes the importance of early attachment experiences; rather, it helps to situate attachment in a broader developmental viewpoint.

In many ways we are just at the beginning of this developmental understanding of attachment. But there is an outline of how to proceed, and we have the concepts, methods, and tools to take us forward.

REFERENCES

Aguilar, B., Christian, S., Collins, W. A., Cook, J., Hennighausen, K., Hyson, D., Levy, A., Meyer, S., Roisman, G., Ruh, J., Sesma, A., Vogeler-Knopp, T., & Wellman, N. (1997). *Romantic Relationship Assessment Observational Rating Scales.* Unpublished coding manual, Parent–Child Project, University of Minnesota.

Ainsworth, M. (1969). Object relations, dependency, and attachment: A theoretical review of infant–mother relationships. *Child Development, 40,* 969–1025.

Ainsworth, M., Bell, S., & Stayton, D. (1974). Infant–mother interaction and social development: Socialization as a product of reciprocal responsiveness to signals. In M. Richards (Ed.), *The integration of the child into the social world* (pp. 99–135). Cambridge, UK: Cambridge University Press.

Block, J., Block, J. H., & Gjerde, P. (1988). Parental functioning and the home environment in families of divorce: Prospective and concurrent analyses. *Journal of the American Academy of Child and Adolescent Psychiatry, 27,* 207–213.

Bowlby, J. (1969). *Attachment and loss.* New York: Basic Books.

Bowlby, J. (1973). *Separation.* New York: Basic Books.

Brunnquell, D., Crichton, L., & Egeland, B. (1981). Maternal personality and attitude in disturbances of child rearing. *American Journal of Orthopsychiatry, 51*(4), 680–691.

Campos, J., Mumme, D., Kermoian, R., & Campos, R. (1994). A functionalist perspective on the nature of emotion. In N. Fox (Ed.), *The development of emotional regulation: Biological and behavioral considerations. Monographs of the Society for Research in Child Development, 59* (2–3 Serial No. 240), 284–303.

Carlson, E. A. (1998). A prospective longitudinal study of attachment disorganization/disorientation. *Child Development, 69,* 1107–1128.

Carlson, E. A., Sroufe, L. A., & Egeland, B. (2004). The construction of experience: A longitudinal study of representation and behavior. *Child Development, 75,* 66–83.

Collins, W. A. (1995). Relationships and development: Family adaptation to individual change. In S. Shulman (Ed.), *Close relationships and socioemotional development* (pp. 128–154). New York: Ablex.

Collins, W. A., & van Dulmen, M. (in press). The significance of middle childhood peer competence for work and relationships in early adulthood. In A. Huston (Ed.), *Successful pathways from middle childhood to adulthood.* New York: Cambridge University Press.

Crowell, J., & Owens, G. (1996). *Current Relationships Interview.* Unpublished manuscript, State University of New York at Stony Brook.

Egeland, B., & Brunnquell, D. (1979). An at-risk approach to the study of child abuse: Some preliminary findings. *Journal of the American Academy of Child Psychiatry, 8,* 219–235.

Egeland, B., Jacobvitz, D., & Sroufe, L. A. (1988). Breaking the cycle of abuse: Relationship predictions. *Child Development, 59,* 1080–1088.

Egeland, B., & Sroufe, L. A. (1981). Developmental sequelae of maltreatment in infancy. In R. Rizley & D. Cicchetti (Eds.), *Developmental perspectives in child maltreatment* (pp. 77–92). San Francisco: Jossey-Bass.

Erickson, M., Egeland, B., & Sroufe, L. A. (1985). The relationship between quality of attachment and behavior problems in preschool in a high risk sample. In I. Bretherton & E. Waters (Eds.), Growing points in attachment theory and research. *Monographs of the Society for Research in Child Development, 50* (1–2, Serial No. 209), 147–186.

Grossmann, K. E., & Grossmann, K. (1991). Attachment quality as an organizer of emotional and behavioral responses in a longitudinal perspective. In C. Parkes, P. Marris, & J. Stevenson-Hinde (Eds.), *Attachment across the life cycle* (pp. 93–114). New York: Routledge.

Hesse, E. (1999). The Adult Attachment Interview: Historical and current perspectives. In J. Cassidy & P. R. Shaver (Eds.), *Handbook of attachment: Theory, research, and clinical applications* (pp. 395–433). New York: Guilford Press.

Kagan, J. (1984). *The nature of the child.* New York: Basic Books.

Kelley, H. H., Berscheid, E., Christensen, A., Harvey, J. H., Huston, T. L., Levinger, G., McClintock, E., Peplau, L. A., & Peterson, D. R. (1983). *Close relationships.* New York: Freeman.

Lewis, M. (1997). *Altering fate: Why the past does not predict the future*. New York: Guilford Press.

Main, M., & Goldwyn, R. (1994). *Adult attachment scoring and classification systems, Version 6*. Unpublished manuscript, University of California–Berkeley.

Main, M., & Hesse, E. (1990). Parents' unresolved traumatic experiences are related to infant disorganized attachment status: Is frightened and/or frightening parental behavior the linking mechanism? In M. Greenberg, D. Cicchetti, & M. Cummings (Eds.), *Attachment in the preschool years* (pp. 161–182). Chicago: University of Chicago Press.

Matas, L., Arend, R., & Sroufe, L. A. (1978). Continuity of adaptation in the second year: The relationship between quality of attachment and later competence. *Child Development, 49*, 547–556.

Pianta, R., Egeland, B., & Sroufe, L. A. (1990). Maternal stress and children's development: Prediction of school outcomes and identification of protective factors. In J. Rolf, A. Masten, D. Cicchetti, K. Neuchterlein, & S. Weintraub (Eds.), *Risk and protective factors in the development of psychopathology* (pp. 215–235). New York: Cambridge University Press.

Pianta, R., Hyatt, A., & Egeland, B. (1986). Maternal relationship history as an indicator of developmental risk. *Journal of Orthopsychiatry, 56*, 385–398.

Reis, H., Collins, W. A., & Berscheid, E. (2000). The relationship context of human behavior and development. *Psychological Bulletin, 126*, 844–872.

Roisman, G., Madsen, S., Hennighausen, K., Sroufe, L. A., & Collins, W. A. (2001). The coherence of dyadic behavior across parent–child and romantic relationships as mediated by the internalized representation of experience. *Attachment and Human Development, 2*, 156–172.

Roisman, G., Padron, E., Sroufe, L. A., & Egeland, B. (2002). Earned-secure attachment status in retrospect and prospect. *Child Development, 73*, 1204–1219.

Sroufe, J. (1991). Assessment of parent–adolescent relationships: Implications for adolescent development. *Journal of Family Psychology, 5*, 21–45.

Sroufe, L. A., Bennett, C., Englund, M., Urban, J., & Shulman, S. (1993). The significance of gender boundaries in preadolescence: Contemporary correlates and antecedents of boundary violation and maintenance. *Child Development, 64*, 455–466.

Sroufe, L. A., Carlson, E., Levy, A., & Egeland, B. (1999). Implications of attachment theory for developmental psychology. *Development and Psychopathology, 11*, 1–13.

Sroufe, L. A., Egeland, B., & Carlson, E. (1999). One social world: The integrated development of parent–child and peer relationships. In W. A. Collins & B. Laursen (Eds.), *Minnesota Symposia on Child Psychology: Vol. 30. Relationships as developmental contexts: Festschrift in honor of Willard W. Hartup* (pp. 241–261). Mahwah, NJ: Erlbaum.

Sroufe, L. A., Egeland, B., Carlson, E., & Collins, W. A. (2005). *The development of the person: The Minnesota Study of Risk and Adaptation from Birth to Adulthood*. New York: Guilford Press.

Sroufe, L. A., Egeland, B., & Kreutzer, T. (1990). The fate of early experience following developmental change: Longitudinal approaches to individual adaptation in childhood. *Child Development, 61*, 1363–1373.

Sroufe, L. A., Fox, N., & Pancake, V. (1983). Attachment and dependency in developmental perspective. *Child Development, 54,* 1615–1627.

Sroufe, L. A., & Waters, E. (1976). The ontogenesis of smiling and laughter: A perspective on the organization of development in infancy. *Psychological Review, 83,* 173–189.

Sroufe, L. A., Waters, E., & Matas, L. (1974). Contextual determinants of infant affective response. In M. Lewis & L. Rosenblum (Eds.), *Origins of fear* (pp. 49–72). New York: Wiley.

Sroufe, L. A., & Wunsch, J. P. (1972). The development of laughter in the first year of life. *Child Development, 43,* 1326–1344.

Urban, J., Carlson, E., Egeland, B., & Sroufe, L. A. (1991). Patterns of individual adaptation across childhood. *Development and Psychopathology, 3,* 445–460.

van IJzendoorn, M. (1995). The association between adult attachment representations and infant attachment, parental responsiveness and clinical status: A meta-analysis on the predictive validity of the Adult Attachment Interview. *Psychological Bulletin, 113,* 404–410.

Ward, M. J., & Carlson, E. A. (1995). Associations among adult attachment representations, maternal sensitivity, and infant–mother attachment in a sample of adolescent mothers. *Child Development, 66,* 69–79.

Warren, S., Huston, L., Egeland, B., & Sroufe, L. A. (1997). Child and adolescent anxiety disorders and early attachment. *Journal of the American Academy of Child and Adolescent Psychiatry, 36,* 637–644.

Yates, T., Dodds, M., Sroufe, L. A., & Egeland, B. (1993). Exposure to partner violence and child behavior problems: A prospective study controlling for child physical abuse and neglect, child cognitive ability, socioeconomic status, and life stress. *Development and Psychopathology, 15,* 199–218.

CHAPTER 4

Attachment Theory and Research in Ecological Perspective

Insights from the Pennsylvania Infant and Family Development Project and the NICHD Study of Early Child Care

JAY BELSKY

There is much about this chapter that would surely be different had I been able to pursue graduate studies at the Institute for Child Development at the University of Minnesota in the fall of 1974. But I was not, largely because my undergraduate mentor (who held me in the highest regard) reported (inaccurately), when writing on my behalf as part of the graduate school admission's process, that I was not particularly interested in research! So, instead of being at the institute just when Byron Egeland was launching his study of children at risk for child maltreatment and joining forces with Alan Sroufe and several graduate students to prospectively investigate the developmental antecedents and sequelae of infant–mother attachment security, I was at Cornell University's Department of Human Development and Family Studies learning all about the ecology of human development—but little about attachment theory and research. In fact, what I was learning about attachment theory was intended to turn me away from this perspective on early development that was eventually to shape so much significant research.

My first exposure as a graduate student to attachment theory came from reading Mary Ainsworth's (1973) outstanding essay delineating

Bowlby's theory, including her extensions of it with respect to the role of maternal sensitivity in promoting security, and summarizing the findings from her groundbreaking study. Some 2 years later I found myself working with Urie Bronfenbrenner, a major influence on my intellectual development at Cornell, on a review of research on the effects of daycare on children's social, emotional, and cognitive development, commissioned by the U.S. government. At this time Bronfenbrenner was just beginning to write about "the ecology of human development" and was highly critical of the Strange Situation procedure, describing all too much of developmental psychology as the study of the strange behavior of children in strange situations. In fact, when it came to publishing the report on the effects of child care, it reflected Bronfenbrenner's critique of the Strange Situation as "ecologically invalid" (Belsky & Steinberg, 1978; Bronfenbrenner, Belsky, & Steinberg, 1976). Because there was (as yet) no evidence validating the characterization of infants (or infant–mother relationships) as secure and insecure, it was fundamentally problematical to describe them in such value-laden terms on the basis of behavior manifest in a short laboratory procedure that required mothers to behave in a rather unmaternal manner—leaving their infant with a stranger in a strange place and episodically returning.

As it turned out, things were about to change, at least with respect to my thinking. In the very same issue of the journal *Child Development* in which our review of child care (Belsky & Steinberg, 1978) appeared, Sroufe and his associates (Matas, Arend, & Sroufe, 1978) published the first follow-up study of children seen in the Strange Situation, clearly demonstrating, in line with theoretical expectations, that children with secure attachment histories functioned more competently than those with insecure histories. When I read this groundbreaking report, I immediately appreciated the need to revise the Bronfenbrennarian critique of the Strange Situation that I had embraced. And I was not alone in my thinking. Within a few days of both the papers appearing in print, I received a letter from Alan Sroufe challenging the critique of the Strange Situation offered in our child care review. As I could not have agreed with him more (now that I had read his group's paper), I wrote back telling him so. In reply I received a lovely letter predicting that I would go far in my career because I showed every sign of being a rather unusual academic: one capable of changing his mind in response to data!

The Minnesota group's early research validating classifications of attachment security influenced me a great deal. Having received only minimal training in attachment theory at Cornell University, but a great deal on the role of family, community, cultural context, and historical situation in shaping human development (Bronfenbrenner, 1979), I found the prospect of integrating these two distinct research traditions pregnant with opportunity. In fact, because my doctoral research had focused upon parenting and infant development, with a special concern for fathering as well as mothering and husband–wife as well as parent–child relationships (Belsky, 1979a, 1979b), it proved rather easy to extend my research horizon to incorporate ideas from attachment theory into my ecologically oriented program of research on early human experience in the family. What was principally required was the inclusion of Strange Situation assessments into what developed into a series of four short-term longitudinal studies focused upon the opening years of life that I have come to refer to collectively as the "Pennsylvania Child and Family Development Project," which I directed over the first two decades of my career while I was at Penn State University (see Figure 4.1).

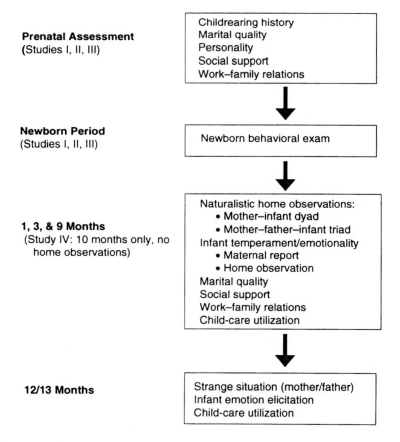

Prenatal Assessment
(Studies I, II, III)

> Childrearing history
> Marital quality
> Personality
> Social support
> Work–family relations

Newborn Period
(Studies I, II, III)

> Newborn behavioral exam

1, 3, & 9 Months
(Study IV: 10 months only, no home observations)

> Naturalistic home observations:
> • Mother–infant dyad
> • Mother–father–infant triad
> Infant temperament/emotionality
> • Maternal report
> • Home observation
> Marital quality
> Social support
> Work–family relations
> Child-care utilization

12/13 Months

> Strange situation (mother/father)
> Infant emotion elicitation
> Child-care utilization

FIGURE 4.1. Belsky's Pennsylvania Child and Family Development Project (four short-term longitudinal studies).

Inclusion of infant–mother and infant–father attachment assessments in these longitudinal studies enabled me to address a number of theoretically important questions. These concerned the determinants of individual differences in infant–parent attachment security, including infant temperament, quality of parenting, early child care, and the social context in which the parent–child dyad is embedded. At the same time that this work was going on in central Pennsylvania, my collaboration with colleagues in a 10-site study of infant daycare also enabled me to address issues of child care and attachment with greater precision than was possible in the Pennsylvania Child and Family Development Project and to extend my basic empirical research on attachment to examine the developmental sequelae of individual differences in infant–mother attachment security (see Figure 4.2).

In what follows, I summarize many of the results of these inquiries. First, I consider work pertaining to parenting and temperament influences on attachment security, before proceeding to address the broader ecological context in which attachment relationships are embedded. I next review my research on nonmaternal child care and infant–parent attachment security, as well as on the developmental sequelae of infant–mother attachment security. Finally, I draw some conclusions pertaining to a modern evolutionary perspective on attachment theory and research (Belsky, 1999b).

MOTHERING AND ATTACHMENT SECURITY

Even though Ainsworth (1973) had theorized and found that the sensitivity of maternal care during the first year of life predicted attachment security when the child was 1 year of age, there was need for additional research given her rather small sample of mother–infant dyads. Like others, I was fascinated by Ainsworth's sensitivity hypothesis and used my first longitudinal study of marital change across the transition to parenthood to examine the relation between mothering observed on three occasions during the first year of the infant's life and infant–mother attachment security assessed at 12 months. In this study, 56 Caucasian mothers and their infants from working- and middle-class families residing in and around the semirural central Pennsylvania community of State College where Penn State University is located were observed at home when infants were 1, 3, and 9 months of age. During each observation period, mothers were directed to go about their everyday household routine, trying as much as possible to disregard the presence of the observer. This naturalistic observational approach is one that I have used in all the work described here. In order to record maternal and infant behavior, we noted the presence or absence every 15 seconds of an extensive series of maternal and infant behaviors, and one particular kind of dyadic exchange in which the infant or mother emits a behavior, the

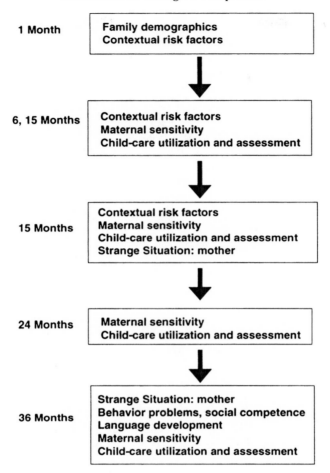

1 Month

Family demographics
Contextual risk factors

6, 15 Months

Contextual risk factors
Maternal sensitivity
Child-care utilization and assessment

15 Months

Contextual risk factors
Maternal sensitivity
Child-care utilization and assessment
Strange Situation: mother

24 Months

Maternal sensitivity
Child-care utilization and assessment

36 Months

Strange Situation: mother
Behavior problems, social competence
Language development
Maternal sensitivity
Child-care utilization and assessment

FIGURE 4.2. NICHD Study of Early Child Care.

other responds to it, and the first then contingently responds to the other (i.e., a three-step interchange).

Because we did not employ Ainsworth's (1973) rating system, we needed a way of conceptualizing and parameterizing the frequency scores of particular behaviors that we generated into indices of sensitivity. Toward this end, we theorized that more was not inherently better, and thus hypothesized that infants who established secure relationships with their mothers would experience neither the most frequent nor the least frequent levels of reciprocal mother–infant interaction. A composite measure of reciprocal interaction was derived from a factor analysis of individual parent and child behavior scores. Loading highly on this factor were measures of maternal attention and care (e.g., undivided attention, vocalize to infant, vocally respond to infant, express positive affection, stimulate/arouse infant), infant behavior (e.g., look at mother, vocalize to mother), and dyadic exchange (i.e., three-step interaction).

We theorized that insecure-avoidance might develop in response to intrusive, overstimulating maternal care (which would stimulate the child to turn away from the mother) and that insecure-resistance might be the consequence of insufficiently responsive, unstimulating care. Thus we predicted—and found—that mothers of secure infants would score intermediate on the composite index of reciprocal mother–infant interaction. Moreover, as anticipated, mothers of insecure-avoidant infants scored highest on this index, whereas mothers of insecure-resistant infants scored lowest (Belsky, Rovine, & Taylor, 1984). In fact, when the reciprocal interaction composite variable was decomposed into indices of maternal involvement and infant behavior, it was clear that it was the former rather than the latter that distinguished attachment groups.

On the basis of these results, Russ Isabella, a graduate student at the time, extended this work in our second and third longitudinal studies by focusing not solely upon the raw, composited frequencies of maternal and infant behavior on which our original index of reciprocal interaction was based, but rather on the close-in-time co-occurrence of mother and infant behaviors that were theorized to reflect synchronous and asynchronous exchanges in the dyad. Once again, mother–infant dyads ($n = 153$) were observed at home under naturalistic conditions for 45 minutes when infants were 6 and 9 months of age and the Strange Situation was administered in the university laboratory when children were 12 months of age. For his dissertation, Isabella pursued the hypothesis that dyads that fostered secure attachment would be characterized by interactions that appeared synchronous, whereas those that fostered insecurity would look asynchronous. And, based upon our earlier findings, it was predicted—and found—that insecure-avoidant dyads would be characterized by intrusive, overstimulating interactions and that insecure-resistant dyads would be characterized by unresponsive-detached caregiving (Isabella & Belsky, 1991; Isabella, Belsky, & von Eye, 1989). Thus, findings from the first inquiry were replicated and extended. In fact, not only had interaction processes reflective of overstimulation been related to insecure-avoidance and those reflective of unresponsive-detachment proven predictive of insecure-resistance in three separate samples that relied on similar approaches to recording mother–infant interaction (i.e., time-sampled behaviors), but dramatically different approaches to measuring interaction processes yielded similar results in related work carried out by others (e.g., Lewis & Feiring, 1989; Leyendecker, Lamb, Fracasso, Schoelmerich, & Larson, 1997;

Malatesta, Culver, Tesman, & Shephard, 1989; Smith & Pedersen, 1988). Significantly, all these findings were generally consistent with Ainsworth's (1973) original theorizing that linked sensitive and appropriately responsive care with the establishment of a secure attachment to mother by baby.

The same was true, it turned out, when the National Institute of Child Health and Infant Development (NICHD) Early Child Care Research Network (1997), of which I am a collaborating investigator, examined the developmental antecedents of infant–mother attachment security, measured when infants were 15 months of age, as part of its effort to examine the effects of early child care on child development (see below). As expected, it was found that higher levels of observed maternal sensitivity when infants were 6 and 15 months of age predicted increased likelihood of a child establishing a secure attachment to mother—in a sample of over 1,000 children. Clearly, just as Ainsworth (1973) had theorized and found herself in her original very small sample investigation, the nature of the child's interactional experiences with mother influenced whether an infant developed a secure or an insecure attachment.

THE ROLE OF TEMPERAMENT

An alternative explanation of individual differences in attachment to that proposed by Ainsworth (1973) emphasizing the quality of maternal care draws attention to the infant's temperament, especially the dimension of negative emotionality or difficulty (e.g., Goldsmith & Alansky, 1987). In particular, it was argued that insecurity reflects distress in the Strange Situation, which itself is a function of temperament (Chess & Thomas, 1982; Kagan, 1982). A fundamental problem with this interpretation, of course, was that infants classified as both secure and insecure manifest great variation in distress in the Strange Situation. Not only do some secure infants typically evince a great deal of distress in the Strange Situation (i.e., those classified B3, B4), whereas others do not (i.e., those classified B1, B2), but some insecure infants typically express a great deal of negativity in the Strange Situation (i.e., those classified C1, C2), whereas others do not (i.e., those classified A1, A2).

A possible way of bringing together competing perspectives on the role of temperament in the measurement of attachment security in the Strange Situation occurred to me upon considering results of findings generated by Thompson and Lamb (1984) and by Frodi and Thompson (1985). When it came to the expression and regulation of negative emotion in the Strange Situation, these investigators observed that secure infants receiving classifications of B1 and B2 looked more like insecure infants receiving classifications of A1 and A2 than like other secure infants (i.e., B3, B4); and that secure infants receiving classifications of B3 and B4 looked more like insecure infants classified C1 and C2 than like other secure infants (i.e., B1, B2). This observation raised the following question in my mind: Might temperament shape the way in which security or insecurity is manifested in the Strange Situation (A1, A2, B1, B2 vs. B3, B4, C1, C2), rather than directly determine whether or not a child was classified as secure? That is, might early temperament account for why some secure infants became highly distressed in the Strange Situation (i.e., those classified B3 or B4), whereas others did not (i.e., those classified B1 or B2), and why some insecure infants became highly distressed in the Strange Situation (C1, C2), whereas others did not (A1, A2). To address this question, we examined data available on 184 firstborn infants participating in our second and third longitudinal studies.

As theorized, we found that measures of temperament obtained during the newborn period, using the Brazelton Neonatal Behavior Exam, and when infants were 3 months of age, using maternal reports, discriminated infants classified as A1, A2, B1, and B2—that is, the ones who cried little in the Strange Situation—from those classified as B3, B4, C1, and C2 (i.e., those who tended to cry more). These measures did not, however, distinguish infants classified secure (B1, B2, B3, B4) from those classified as insecure (A1, A2, C1, C2) (Belsky & Rovine, 1987). More specifically, although secure and insecure infants did not differ on any of the temperament measures in either of the two longitudinal samples, those most likely to express negative emotion in the Strange Situation at 12 months of age scored lower as newborns on orientation (i.e., visual following, alertness, attention) and evinced less autonomic stability (i.e., regulation of state) and scored higher at age 3 months on a cumulative difficulty index. Thus, consistent with my theorizing and the Thompson, Lamb, and Frodi analyses of emotion expression within the Strange Situation, early temperament appeared to affect the degree to which infants became overtly distressed in the Strange Situation but not how they regulated—with or without the assistance of their mother—their negative affect. In sum, early temperament was systematically related to how much distress infants evinced in the Strange Situation, but not to whether they were secure or insecure.

In these first investigations, we, like all other investigators, focused solely upon temperament at a single point in time (i.e., during the newborn period or at 3 months of age). Such an approach was generally consistent with the then prevailing view of temperament as an inborn, stable, constitutional trait not particularly subject to change. Because we had obtained identical temperament reports from mothers when their infants were 3 and 9 months of age, we reconceptualized temperament as a characteristic of the infant that was subject to change. And when we examined change in temperament, as reported by mother, using data from our first longitudinal study, we discovered that infants who at 1 year of age were classified as secure became more predictable and adaptable from 3 to 6 months, whereas the exact opposite was true of infants who would develop insecure attachments to their mothers (Belsky & Isabella, 1988).

In subsequent work we extended this line of investigation. Theorizing that change in the manifestation of emotion over time might reflect emotion regulation processes, and thereby be related to attachment security, we examined, using 148 firstborn infants participating in our second and third longitudinal studies, stability and change in two separate dimensions of temperament, positive and negative emotionality, each based upon composited observational and maternal-report measures obtained when infants were 3 and 6 months of age (Belsky, Fish, & Isabella, 1991). Noteworthy is the fact that it was consideration of the emotional expressions in the Strange Situation of insecure-avoidant and some secure infants, especially those classified B1 and B2, that led us to think about positive emotions as well as negative emotions with respect to temperament change and attachment security. Central to such thinking was the observation that one thing that distinguished these two groups of children (i.e., A1/A2 vs. B1/B2) was that the secure children classified as B1 or B2 in the Strange Situation openly *greeted* their mothers upon reunion—with smiles, gestures and vocalizations—whereas insecure-avoidant infants classified A1 or A2 seemed to suppress such expressions of positive sentiment.

Relying upon our repeatedly measured (at 3 and 6 months) composites of infant positivity and negativity, we created four groups of infants with respect to each emotionality dimension: (1) those scoring high on the dimension in question at both points in time, (2) those scoring low at both points in time, (3) those who changed from high to low, and (4) those who changed from low to high. When we examined attachment security at 1 year of age as a function of these stability and change groups, several interesting findings emerged (Belsky, Fish, & Isabella, 1991). First, changes in negative emotionality were not as strongly related to later attachment as changes in positive emotionality. Consistent with the results of Malatesta, Culver, Tesman, and Shepard (1989), however, we discovered that it was infants who declined in the positivity they expressed between 3 and 9 months who were most likely to be classified as insecure in their attachment at 1 year of age. These data made intuitive sense in suggesting that children who ended up insecure at the end of the first year of life were the ones whose lives, at least while with their mothers, became less pleasurable over time. Further support for this line of thinking derived from the fact that we found that certain *combinations* of stability and change in negative *and* positive emotionality predicted attachment security. Specifically, insecurity was most likely to be observed (i.e., 53% of the time) when (1) infant negativity remained high over time (i.e., high-high group) *or* increased (i.e., low-to-high group) *and* when (2) infant positivity remained low over time (i.e., low-low group) *or* decreased (i.e., high-to-low group). In contrast, when none of these conditions obtained, insecurity was quite rare (i.e., 6%).

When considered in their entirety, all the findings summarized above regarding temperament and attachment dispel the notions that temperament determines attachment security in some simple, straightforward fashion or that there is no relation whatsoever between temperament and insecurity. Rather, they clearly and collectively suggest that the relation between these two constructs is complex. The fact, moreover, that stability and change in infant positive and negative emotionality between 3 and 9 months could be predicted using measures of the parent and family functioning obtained *before* the child was born and of parenting obtained when infants were 3 months of age strongly suggests that it is a mistake to presume that emotional features of temperament reflect, exclusively, some inborn characteristic of the infant (Belsky, Fish, & Isabella, 1991). Because they can change, and because such change appears tied to experiences in the family, understanding of such change may tell us as much about the development of attachment security as it does about presumed constitutional features of the child.

THE BROADER ECOLOGY OF ATTACHMENT SECURITY

Through this point I have considered what might be referred to as "classical" determinants of attachment security, namely, those considered in most developmental theorizing about the origins of secure and insecure attachment (Belsky, 1999a; Belsky, Rosenberger, & Crnic, 1995b). But an ecological perspective on human development, one that underscores the fact that the parent–child dyad is embedded in a family system (Belsky, 1981), which is itself embedded in a community, a cultural, and even a historical context (Bronfenbrenner, 1979), suggests that if one wants to account for why some infants develop secure and others insecure attachments to mother, father, or even child-care worker, then there is a need to look beyond the proximate determinants of mothering and temperament.

Toward this end, we undertook a series of inquires using data collected as part of our longitudinal studies based upon a contextual model of the determinants of parenting that highlights the role of parent, child, and social-contextual factors in shaping the parent–child relationship (Belsky, 1984). Central to the model was the presumption that parenting and thus the parent–child relationship is multiply determined and that the contextual factors of work, social support, and marriage can affect parenting both directly and indirectly (through personality). Also central to the conceptual model of the determinants of parenting is the notion that parenting, and thus the parent–child relationship, is a well-buffered system. Thus threats to its integrity stemming from any single source of influence (e.g., work) are likely to be compensated for by resources that derive from other sources of influence (e.g., marriage). Parenting and the parent–child relationship are most likely to be adversely affected when *multiple* vulnerabilities exist (e.g., difficult temperament plus conflicted marriage) that accumulate and undermine the effectiveness of other sources of influence in promoting parental functioning. It is just such thinking that led us to examine the cumulative impact of multiple determinants of parenting in affecting attachment security, not just the impact of one or another source of influence.

In the first work of this kind that we carried out using data collected as part of our first longitudinal investigation, linkages were examined between attachment security measured at 1 year and (1) mother's own childrearing history reported during the prenatal period; (2) mother's personality assessed using questionnaires at the same point in time; (3) change in mother-reported infant temperament between 3 and 9 months (already discussed above); (4) change in marital quality between the last trimester of pregnancy and 9 months postpartum (based upon self-reports obtained at both measurement occasions); and (5) prenatal reports by mothers of the friendliness and helpfulness of neighbors (i.e., social support). Results from univariate analyses revealed that mothers of secure infants scored higher than those of insecure infants on a personality measure of interpersonal affection, whereas mothers of avoidant infants scored lowest on a measure of ego strength; that, as indicated earlier, the (mother-reported) temperaments of secure infants became more predictable and adaptable over time, whereas the reverse was true of insecure infants; that insecure infants were living in families in which marriages were deteriorating in quality more precipitously than was so in the case of mothers of secure infants; and that the neighbors of secure infants were perceived as more friendly and helpful than those of insecure infants (Belsky & Isabella, 1988). More important than these univariate findings, however, was evidence that emerged when maternal, infant, and contextual stressors and supports were considered collectively: the more that the family ecology could be described as well resourced (i.e., positive maternal personality, positive change in infant temperament, less marital deterioration), the more likely the child was to develop a secure attachment to mother.

This work was then extended using data from the fourth longitudinal study, this one of a sample consisting exclusively of 125 firstborn sons whose families were enrolled when they were 10 months of age (rather than prenatally as in the first three investigations). Because of our interest in the multiple determinants of parent–child relations, extensive data were collected at enrollment on a variety of sources of influence (e.g., social support). At age 12 and 13 months, infants were seen in the laboratory to assess infant–mother and infant–father attachment, respectively, and to administer a series of emotion-evoking procedures following the Strange Situation. To create grand composite measures of overall family resources, three personality measurements were composited (extraversion + neuroticism – agreeableness), as were two measures of infant temperament/ emotionality (positivity – negativity), and four social-context measures ([social support satisfaction + number of people to provide support] + [work–family support – interference]). Results revealed that the greater the family resources across these domains of measurement, the more likely the infant–father relationship was classified as secure in the Strange Situation (Belsky, 1996), with rather similar results obtaining in the case of the infant–mother attachment relationship (Belsky, Rosenberger, & Crnic, 1995a). Thus, secure infant–parent relationships were more likely to develop when parents had personalities of the kind likely to foster sensitive parenting, when infants had temperamental dispositions that either made sensitive care easier to provide or had been fostered by such sensitive care, and when extrafamilial sources of support operated in a manner likely to enhance parental sensitivity.

NONMATERNAL CARE

Because of the role that lengthy child–parent separations played in Bowlby's original formulations of attachment theory, concern has been raised often about the consequences of more routine, short-term separations of the kind experienced on a daily basis by children cared for by someone other than a parent when mother is employed. The initial work addressing this issue focused almost exclusively upon children being cared for in very-high-quality, university-based centers and generally failed to reveal any consistent association between daycare and attachment insecurity (for reviews, see Belsky & Steinberg, 1978; Rutter, 1981). However, this first wave of attachment daycare research used as an index of security the extent to which the child became upset upon separation from parent, even though it was never clear conceptually whether greater or lesser distress should be considered a marker of security (or insecurity).

When we examined the issue of relations between nonmaternal care and security of infant–parent attachment in our second and third longitudinal studies, using the Ainsworth and colleagues (1978) reunion-based Strange Situation scoring system, two particularly interesting findings emerged. First, infants who experienced, on average, more than 20 hours per week of such care during their first year were more likely to develop insecure attachments than were children who experienced less nonmaternal care (Belsky & Rovine, 1988). In fact, when I compiled data from my own work and that from other studies of nonrisk samples that were published in the scientific literature (n = 491), the same pattern emerged (Belsky, 1988). Subsequently, Clarke-Stewart (1989) and Lamb and colleagues (Lamb, Sternberg, & Prodromdis, 1990) undertook similar analyses, drawing upon yet more published and unpublished data, and also chronicled a reliable, even if modest, association between more than 20 hours per week of nonmaternal care in the first year of life and attachment insecurity.

The second noteworthy finding to emerge from our own work concerned infant–father attachment security. Like Chase-Lansdale and Owen (1987) before us, we found that sons with more than 35 hours per week of nonmaternal care (in the United States) were more likely to develop insecure attachments to their fathers and thus have two insecure attachments (one to mother and one to father) than were other boys (Belsky & Rovine, 1988). These findings seemed particularly significant because earlier work in our lab (Belsky, Garduque, & Hrncir, 1984) and by others (Easterbrooks & Goldberg, 1987; Howes, Rodning, Galluzzo, & Myers, 1988; Main, Kaplan, & Cassidy, 1985; Main & Weston, 1981) indicated that children with two insecure attachment relationships functioned more poorly than did children with one or more secure attachments.

The evidence just summarized raised lots of questions as to whether nonmaternal care played a truly causal role in fostering attachment insecurity, and, if so, via what mechanisms, and about the contextual conditions under which nonmaternal care might contribute to the development of insecure attachment relationships (Fox & Fein, 1990). These and other unresolved issues pertaining to the effects of daycare on children's social, emotional, and cognitive development led to the establishment of the NICHD Study of Early Child Care (NICHD Early Child Care Research Network, 1994), a research project in which exactly the same research protocol is implemented at 10 different research sites across the United States. More than 1,300 children and their families were recruited into this work when infants were 1 month of age, after identifying children and families at their local hospitals shortly after their births. The sample is quite varied demographically and ethnically, but does not include any families in which mother does not speak English fluently or in which the mother is under 18 years of age. A rather extensive research protocol has been implemented to study infant and family development, as well as child care, in this extensive project which is following the children from age 1 month through middle childhood (with pending prospects for further extension). Most importantly, the quality of child care received is measured in detail using observational methods when the child is 6, 15, 24, 36, and 54 months of age. At these same ages, multiple features of the family are measured; most important for purposes of this chapter are assessments of the sensitivity of mothering based on mother–child interaction during semistructured free play and more naturalistic observations of maternal attentive responsiveness to the child while being interviewed. Strange Situations were administered when children were 15 months of age (and again when children were 36 months old).

Results from the NICHD Study of Early Child Care revealed that no feature of child care (e.g., quality, quantity, stability), when considered in isolation, predicted infant–mother attachment security (NICHD Early Child Care Research Network, 1997). Consistent with Bronfenbrenner's (1979, p. 38) dictum that "in the ecology of human development the principal main effects are likely to be interactions," we found, however, that child-care experience was related to attachment insecurity when certain ecological conditions co-occurred. That is, rates of insecurity were higher than would otherwise have been expected (on the basis of maternal sensitivity alone) when infants received poorer quality (i.e., insensitive) care from their mothers *and* (1) low-quality nonmaternal care, *or* (2) more than minimal amount of nonmaternal care (i.e., > 10 hours per week), *or* (3) more than one nonmaternal care arrangement in their first 15 months of life. In other words, it was under conditions of "dual risk" that early care was associated, for the most part, with attachment insecurity. Importantly, when infants were followed up at 3 years of age and seen again in the Strange Situation, only one of the dual-risk findings reemerged, that indicating that the combination of low levels of maternal sensitivity and lots of time in child care (irrespective of its quality) was related to elevated rates of insecure attachment (NICHD Early Child Care Research Network, 2001). When considered in their entirety, these child care findings are not only consistent with a controversial risk-factor conclusion drawn by me a decade earlier concerning the effects of infant daycare as currently experienced in the United States (Belsky, 1986, 1988), but with the results summarized above highlighting linkages between the accumulation of contextual risk and attachment insecurity.

THE DEVELOPMENTAL SEQUELAE OF INFANT–MOTHER ATTACHMENT SECURITY

In addition to affording an opportunity to evaluate the effects of early child care on infant–mother attachment security, data collected as part of the NICHD Study enabled me to explore individual differences in the future social and cognitive functioning of some 1,000 children studied in the course of investigating the long-term consequences of early child care experience. Drawing upon data gathered when children were age 3, I examined two separate issues with respect to the developmental sequelae of early attachment security. Each is discussed in turn.

Are the Consequences of Attachment Security Dependent upon Later Mothering?

Ever since the Minnesota investigators whose work was summarized earlier in this chapter started to chronicle the developmental consequences of attachment security and insecurity, demonstrating that early attachment predicted multiple aspects of later child development, there has been some confusion about the developmental process by which early security comes to be related to later child functioning. Although some have mistakenly attributed to students of attachment theory the view that attachment security/insecurity has some automatic or inevitable impact on the course of children's future development (Breur, 1999; Kagan, 1982; Lewis, 1997), attachment theorists have been clear that this represents a fundamental misreading of the theory (Belsky & Cassidy, 1994). Indeed, Sroufe (1983, 1988) has asserted for years that development is a function of early *and* continuing experiences, such that what happens after infancy (or any other developmental period) can mitigate the otherwise anticipated consequences of experiences earlier in life. In fact, early work by the Minnesota team of investigators showed that the effects of attachment security on later development were, to a large extent, dependent upon the quality of maternal care that children experienced after attachment security was assessed at the end of the first year of life (Erikson, Egeland, & Sroufe, 1985).

Drawing upon this earlier work and theorizing, Pasco Fearon and I set out to test the hypothesis that the developmental benefits of early security would be conditioned by the child's subsequent childrearing experiences, predicting that the most competent 3-year-olds participating in the NICHD Study of Early Child Care would be those who established secure attachments to their mothers by 15 months of age *and* whose mothers provided sensitive care to them when they were 24 months of age. Children who developed insecure attachments *and* experienced insensitive care subsequently were expected to function least competently, with all other children falling between these two extreme groups. And this is exactly what was found when data on socioemotional and cognitive-linguistic development gathered at 36 months of age was subjected to empirical assessment (Belsky & Fearon, 2002a). In other words, just as Sroufe (1983, 1988) had long argued, the developmental benefits of early security were dependent upon the continued experience of receiving emotionally supportive care and the developmental costs of insecurity were dependent upon the continued experience of receiving emotionally unsupportive care.

Do the Consequences of Attachment Security Vary by Contextual Risk?

In addition to addressing the question of whether the anticipated effects of early attachment security on later development were dependent upon the quality of maternal care experienced during toddlerhood, Fearon and I again drew upon the data collected as part of the NICHD Study of Early Child Care to see whether the effects of early attachment security varied as a function of the contextual conditions under which children grew up (Belsky & Fearon, 2002b). It seemed likely that the developmental benefits and costs of security/insecurity might vary as a function of whether children grew up under conditions expected to compromise their well-being (e.g., low income, maternal depression, single-parent home) rather than under more developmentally supportive circumstances. To address this possibility, we created measures of cumulative contextual risk, classifying children as experiencing low, moderate, high, and very high levels of risk depending upon the circumstances in which they grew up across the first 3 years of life and then examined the extent to which early security (at 15 months) predicted later development (at 36 months) across ecological conditions.

Although we found that secure attachment proved to be a developmental benefit with regard to understanding spoken language (but not more general cognitive development or the ability to express oneself) irrespective of whether a child grew up under conditions of high or low contextual risk, in the case of expressive language and socioemotional outcomes, the predictive power of early attachment security varied as a function of contextual risk. More specifically, children who had established secure attachment by 15 months of age scored higher in terms of language comprehension (i.e., receptive language) at 3 years of age than did children with insecure attachment histories.

In the case of expressive language development, the findings were consistent with what might be regarded as the simple risk-resilience model of attachment and later development in which security functions as a protective factor. That is, whereas the expressive language abilities of children with insecure attachment histories declined as contextual risk increased, this was not the case for children with secure attachment histories (see Figure 4.3). Security, therefore, appeared to play a clear protective function when it came to children's ability to use spoken language.

In the case of problem behavior and social competence, it was the insecure-avoidant group that appeared to be most affected by contextual risk, evincing adverse effects of cumulative contextual risk at a level of risk lower than that at which all other attachment groups "succumbed" to con-

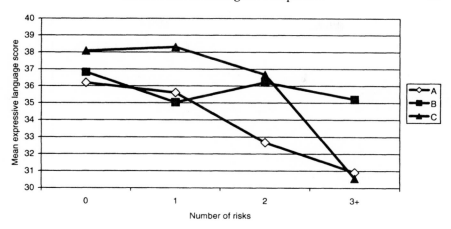

FIGURE 4.3. Mean expressive language scores as a function of attachment classification (A: Insecure-Avoidant, B: Secure, C: Insecure-Resistant) and degree of cumulative contextual risk (0: no risk, 1: low risk, 2: moderate risk, 3: high risk).

textual risk. In the case of behavior problems, whereas the attachment groups did not differ from each other at low levels of contextual risk (i.e., ≤1), and all groups were adversely affected by high levels of risk (i.e., ≥ 3), at moderate levels of risk (i.e., two risks) children with insecure-avoidant attachment histories showed the same level of poor functioning that the three other attachment groups evinced only at high levels of risk (see Figure 4.4). A similar pattern emerged for social competence, with the avoidant group showing a marked decrease in performance under conditions of two risks (see Figure 4.5). In a sense, then, the avoidant group proved more vulnerable to contextual risk—at least at a lower level of risk—than children in all other groups. When levels of risk became especially high, however, even a history of attachment security failed to protect children from the adverse effects of growing up in a developmentally adverse environment.

To summarize, then, it appears that security and insecurity afford children, respectively, developmental benefits and costs, but that in some cases these depend on (1) the type of insecurity the child manifests and (2) the ecological circumstances under which children grow up. Recall that when ecological circumstances were especially undermining of developmental well-being, even secure attachment did not always function to protect the child's well-being, and that it was a history of insecure-avoidant attachment that proved especially undermining of competent functioning, at least at 3 years of age.

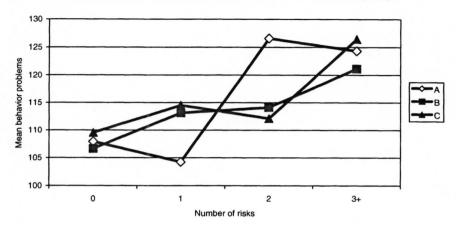

FIGURE 4.5. Mean social competence scores as a function of attachment classification (A: Insecure-Avoidant, B: Secure, C: Insecure-Resistant) and degree of cumulative contextual risk (0: no risk, 1: low risk, 2: moderate risk, 3: high risk).

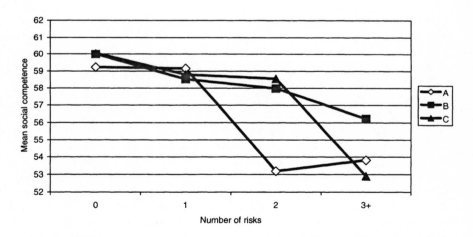

FIGURE 4.4. Mean problem behavior scores as a function of attachment classification (A: Insecure-Avoidant, B: Secure, C: Insecure-Resistant) and degree of cumulative contextual risk (0: no risk, 1: low risk, 2: moderate risk, 3: high risk).

CONCLUSION: A MODERN EVOLUTIONARY PERSPECTIVE ON EARLY ATTACHMENT

Almost two decades of research on infant–mother attachment security, coupled with an emerging interest in evolutionary biology that figured so importantly in Bowlby's original formulation of attachment theory, has led me to rethink the meaning of what I have found in my work, as well as what others have found in their related inquiries. Moreover, it leads me to question some of the implicit assumptions that guide the interpretation of much work on attachment. Central to this rethinking is the evidence I have summarized from my own work showing that (1) cumulative stresses and supports affect the probability that an infant will develop a secure attachment, (2) as does the sensitivity of the care provided by the child's principal caregiver, typically his mother; and that (3) changes in the infant's behavioral development, especially his emotional functioning, across the first year, also predict attachment security; and that (4) the predictive power of attachment theory often, though not always, varies as a function of the child's postinfancy childrearing circumstances (i.e., maternal sensitivity, contextual risk). When considered together, such findings raise the prospect of the following causal process: contextual stresses and supports affect the sensitivity of maternal care, which affects emotional and temperamental development, which affects whether or not the child develops a secure attachment and whether, and how, attachment security comes to forecast later development.

Although it is clearly the case that the causal linkages just detailed between contextual circumstances and attachment security and between attachment security and later development are probabilistic rather than deterministic, and thus that contextual effects and resulting developmental trajectories are not fixed, a question must be asked that is rarely raised by developmental psychologists: *Why* do developmental processes operate the way they do? What developmentalists usually ask are not such questions about ultimate causation, but ones about proximate causation: *How* does development operate? Such questions lead most developmentalists, myself included, to examine what predicts the quality of maternal care or attachment security, or what security of attachment is related to in terms of the child's future functioning. But when we find answers to these psychological and developmental questions, as we clearly have, we rarely stop to ponder why the developmental processes we have discerned should be present in the first place. In other words, we tend to take them for granted. But should we? And what might we be missing by doing so? Might we be too close to the phenomena we are studying to recognize, in some sense, what they are *all* about? I am beginning to believe that this might indeed be the case.

When Bowlby first discussed the evolutionary basis of attachment behavior, he stressed the survival (i.e., adaptive) value of the infant maintaining proximity to his or her caregiver. And when attachment researchers have written about the functioning of secure and insecure children, frequently they have spoken in terms of the adaptive functioning of the former and the maladaptive functioning of the latter. By using the same terminology to discuss evolutionary-biological and psychological-mental health phenomena, it is not surprising that some have come to equate the mental health benefits of a secure attachment with evolutionary benefits. Indeed, Ainsworth (1973, p. 45) herself seemed to imply as much when she argued "that 'securely attached' babies 'developed normally, i.e., along species-characteristic lines' " (Hinde, 1982, p. 69).

Yet, as Hinde (1982; Hinde & Stevenson-Hinde, 1991) has made abundantly clear, and as Ainsworth (1985) herself came to acknowledge, levels of analysis need to be distinguished when terms like "adaptation" are employed. Although it may be beneficial in the contemporary psychological or mental health sense to develop a secure attachment, it is certainly mistaken to presume that from an evolutionary or phylogenetic perspective that a secure attachment is better or more adaptive than an insecure attachment—however much we value contextual supports and maternal sensitivity, that is, determinants of attachment security—and positive interpersonal relations, a presumed sequelae of security. As Hinde (1982, pp. 71–72) noted,

> There is no best mothering (or attachment) style, for different styles are better in different circumstances, and natural selection would act to favor individuals with a range of potential styles from which they select appropriately. . . . Mothers and babies will be programmed (by evolution) not simply to form one sort of relationship but a range of possible relationships according to circumstances. . . . Optimal mothering (and attachment) behavior will differ according to . . . the mother's social status, caregiving contributions from other family members, the state of physical resources, and so on . . . a mother–child relationship which produces successful adults in one situation may not do so in another.

In other words, while it may be the case that securely attached children develop, in contemporary Western society (or perhaps just in middle-class U.S. society), more competently and are more likely to grow up into happy, mentally healthy adults in this ecology, it is completely inaccurate to infer from such evidence or to otherwise presume that, on the basis of natural selection theory, one attachment or mothering style is necessarily best. This is so even as we find that under supportive and less stressful contextual conditions, and when care is more sensitive, that infants and young children are more likely to develop secure attachments.

Such evolutionary thinking has led me to reconceptualize secure and insecure attachment in terms of reproductive and life history strategies that are flexibly responsive to contextual and caregiving conditions and which evolved in the service of evolutionary goals, not mental health ones pertaining to happiness or psychological well-being (Belsky, 1997, 1999b; Belsky, Steinberg, & Draper, 1991; see also Chisholm, 1996). From the perspective of evolutionary biology, the goal of all life is the replication of genes in future generations. Not only do species vary in terms of how they accomplish this task, but so do individuals within some species. Moreover, in certain species, humans included perhaps, such variation can be determined by concurrent or developmentally antecedent experiences. Depending upon the circumstances that organisms find themselves in, if they have the flexibility to adjust their behavior and development according to these life conditions, it may make sense to bear few offspring and care for them intensively, a tactic our value system tends to regard favorably, or to bear many and care for them less devotedly, an approach that contemporary norms tend to frown upon and discourage.

This suggests to me that the developing attachment system evolved to provide a means through which the developing child could turn information acquired from parents about prevailing contextual conditions—via the caregiving experience—into knowledge and "awareness" of the kinds of future he or she is likely to face. More specifically, the capacity to develop different patterns of attachment in response to the quality of care received evolved to provide a kind of "navigational" device to direct development in one direction or another depending upon what would have optimized reproductive success in adulthood in the environments of evolutionary adapatation. Might it be the case, then, that security represents an evolved psychological mechanism that "informs" the child, based upon the sensitive care he or she has experienced, that others can be trusted; that close, affectional bonds are enduring; and that the world is a more rather than a less caring place; and, as a result, that it makes reproductive sense to defer mating and reproduction; to be selective in pair bonding; and to bear fewer rather than more children, but care for them intensively, with a partner to whom one is committed? In contrast, might insecure attachment represent a similarly evolved psychological mechanism, also responsive to caregiving conditions, that conveys to the child the developing understanding that others cannot be trusted; that close, affectional bonds are unlikely to be enduring; and that it makes more sense to participate in opportunistic, self-serving relationships rather than mutually beneficial ones? In consequence, does a child who develops such a psychological orientation, in response to the caregiving he or she has received, which itself has been fostered by the less rather than the more supportive conditions that his or her parents have confronted, become inclined to mate earlier and more frequently, perhaps producing more offspring who are poorly cared for, because this approach to optimizing reproductive fitness makes more sense in the world as it is understood to be than by adopting the strategy more characteristic of those who have developed secure attachments? Or, even if this is no longer the case today, might these processes have operated in the environment of evolutionary adaptation, so that what we observe today are psychological mechanisms that have evolved and are still operative even if the reproductive "payoffs" that once were associated with them no longer obtain (Buss, 1995; Cosmides & Tooby, 1987)?

While I would not want to argue definitively on behalf of these speculative propositions, I do want to suggest that the reason that our work (and that of others) linking resourceful life circumstances and high maternal investment with attachment security generates the findings that it does may be because individual differences in attachment may be part of a complex developmental process that in human ancestral environments provided the means of directing development in particular ways that were reproductively strategic. To the extent that this was so, it suggests that findings linking contextual conditions and parenting processes to variation in attachment security, and variation in attachment security to variation in subsequent development, may be part of a developing system whose function was not originally understood or appreciated by Bowlby, Ainsworth, or many current students of attachment theory.

Like many others of his time, when Bowlby initially conceptualized the evolutionary basis of attachment, he wrote in terms of survival of the species. What he eventually came to understand, however, was that it is not survival alone that natural selection rewards but differential reproduction, defined in terms of the dispersion of genes in future generations. Moreover, what he also came to appreciate was that natural selection worked at the level of individuals as well as at the level of genes, not at the level of species; so the evolutionary payoffs accrued to those individuals who survived to reproduce and thus whose genes came to be disproportionately represented in future generations.

In conclusion, consideration of the centrality of differential reproduction among individuals in the Darwinian process of evolution by natural selection raises the prospect that the reason that individual differences in attachment may be related to rearing conditions, as my research and that of others has shown, as well as to future social and emotional development, is because patterns of attachment evolved as strategic alternatives for promoting reproductive fitness under varying circumstances in the environment of evolutionary adaptation. What this suggests is that it may be useful to move beyond a mental health orientation toward attachment to one that focuses upon reproductive functioning (i.e., mating and parenting).

What is particularly intriguing about such a reorientation is that it does not require the abandonment of much that has excited attachment researchers about the origins and especially the sequelae of individual differences in attachment. This is because a reoriented focus upon reproductive functioning involves many of the same processes that more mental health-oriented thinking about attachment directs attention to, namely, social and emotional development, particularly in the context of interpersonal relatedness and parenting. Thus, it is not so much that a modern evolutionary perspective on attachment suggests that attachment researchers—myself included—have been misguided in examining the antecedents and consequences of attachment that they have over the past several decades, but rather that they may have not fully appreciated how great the significance of the early attachment system may be. Thus, by moving beyond traditional psychological and developmental questions pertaining to *how* development operates, to ones that focus upon *why* it operates the way it appears to, increased insight into the developmental phenomena under investigation may be realized. This might provide new directions for research—in the case of attachment, most notably toward issues of mating and parental investment.

ACKNOWLEDGMENTS

Work on this chapter was supported by a cooperative agreement with the National Institute of Child Health and Human Development (U10-HD25420).

REFERENCES

Ainsworth, M. D. (1973). The development of infant–mother attachment. In B. M. Caldwell & H. N. Ricciuti (Eds.), *Review of child development research* (Vol. 3, pp. 1–94). Chicago: University of Chicago Press.

Ainsworth, M. D. (1985). Attachment across the lifespan. *Bulletin of the New York Academy of Sciences, 61,* 792–812.

Ainsworth, M. D., Blehar, M. C., Waters, E., & Wall, S. (1978). *Patterns of attachment: A psychological study of the Strange Situation.* Hillsdale, NJ: Erlbaum.

Belsky, J. (1979a). The interrelation of parental and spousal behavior during infancy in traditional nuclear families. *Journal of Marriage and the Family, 41,* 62–68.

Belsky, J. (1979b). Mother–father–infant interaction: A naturalistic observational study. *Developmental Psychology, 8,* 601–608.

Belsky, J. (1981). Early human experience: A family perspective. *Developmental Psychology, 17,* 3–23.

Belsky, J. (1984). The determinants of parenting: A process model. *Child Development, 55*, 83–96.

Belsky, J. (1986). Infant day care: A cause for concern? *Zero to Three, 6*, 1–7.

Belsky, J. (1988). The "effects" of infant day care reconsidered. *Early Childhood Research Quarterly, 3*, 235–272.

Belsky, J. (1996). Parent, infant, and social-contextual antecedents of father–son attachment security. *Developmental Psychology, 32*, 905–913.

Belsky, J. (1997). Patterns of attachment mating and parenting: An evolutionary interpretation. *Human Nature, 8*, 361–381.

Belsky, J. (1999a). Interactional and social–contextual determinants of attachment security. In J. Cassidy & P. R. Shaver (Eds.), *Handbook of attachment: Theory, research, and clinical applications* (pp. 249–264). New York: Guilford Press.

Belsky, J. (1999b). Modern evolutionary theory and patterns of attachment. In J. Cassidy & P. R. Shaver (Eds.), *Handbook of attachment: Theory, research, and clinical applications* (pp. 141–161). New York: Guilford Press.

Belsky, J., & Cassidy, J. (1994). Attachment: Theory and evidence. In M. Rutter & D. Hay (Eds.), *Developmental principles and clinical issues in psychology and psychiatry* (pp. 373–402). London: Blackwell.

Belsky, J., & Fearon, R. M. P. (2002a). Early attachment security, subsequent maternal sensitivity, and later child development: Does continuity in development depend upon continuity of caregiving? *Attachment and Human Development, 3*, 361–387.

Belsky, J. & Fearon, R. M. P (2002b). Infant–mother attachment security, contextual risk and early development: A moderational analysis. *Development and Psychopathology, 14*, 293–310.

Belsky, J., Fish, M., & Isabella, R. (1991). Continuity and discontinuity in infant negative and positive emotionality: Family antecedents and attachment consequences. *Developmental Psychology, 27*, 421–431.

Belsky, J., Garduque, L., & Hrncir, E. (1984). Assessing performance, competence, and executive capacity in infant play: Relations to home environment and security of attachment. *Developmental Psychology, 20*, 406–417.

Belsky, J., & Isabella, R. (1988). Maternal, infant, and social–contextual determinants of attachment security. In J. Belsky & T. Nezworski (Eds.), *Clinical implications of attachment* (pp. 41–94). Hillsdale, NJ: Erlbaum.

Belsky, J., Rosenberger, K., & Crnic, K. (1995a). Maternal personality, marital quality, social support and infant temperament: Their significance for infant–mother attachment in human families. In C. Pryce, R. Martin, & D. Skuse (Eds.), *Motherhood in human and nonhuman primates: Biosocial determinants* (pp. 115–124). Basel, Switzerland: Karger.

Belsky, J., Rosenberger, K., & Crnic, K. (1995b). The origins of attachment security: Classical and contextual determinants. In S. Goldberg, R. Muir, & J. Kerr (Eds.), *Attachment theory: Social, developmental and clinical perspectives* (pp. 153–184). Hillsdale, NJ: Analytic Press.

Belsky, J., & Rovine, M. J. (1987). Temperament and attachment security in the Strange Situation: An empirical rapprochement. *Child Development, 58*, 787–795.

Belsky, J., & Rovine, M. J. (1988). Nonmaternal care in the first year of life and the security of infant–parent attachment. *Child Development, 59,* 157–167.

Belsky, J., Rovine, M., & Taylor, D. G. (1984). The Pennsylvania Infant and Family Development Project, III: The origins of individual differences in infant–mother attachment: Maternal and infant contributions. *Child Development, 55,* 718–728.

Belsky, J., & Steinberg, L. (1978). The effects of day care: A critical review. *Child Development, 49,* 929–949.

Belsky, J., Steinberg, L., & Draper, P. (1991). Childhood experience, interpersonal development and reproductive strategy: An evolutionary theory of socialization. *Child Development, 62,* 647–670.

Breur, J. (1999). *The myth of the first three years.* New York: Free Press.

Bronfenbrenner, U. (1979). *The ecology of human development: Experiments by nature and design.* Cambridge, MA: Harvard University Press.

Bronfenbrenner, U., Belsky, J., & Steinberg, L. (1976). *Day care in context: An ecological perspective on research and public policy* (A report to the Department of Health, Education, and Welfare, Federal Interagency Day Care Requirements Policy Committee). Washington, DC: US Government Printing Office

Buss, D. (1995). Evolutionary psychology: A new paradigm for the psychological sciences. *Psychological Inquiry, 6,* 1–35.

Chase-Lansdale, P. L., & Owen, M. T. (1987). Maternal employment in a family context: Effects on infant–mother and infant–father attachments. *Child Development, 58,* 1505–1512.

Chess, S., & Thomas, A. (1982). Infant bonding: Mystique and reality. *American Journal of Orthopsychiatry, 52,* 213–222.

Chisholm, J. (1996). The evolutionary ecology of attachment organization. *Human Nature, 7,* 1–38.

Clarke-Stewart, K. (1989). Infant day care: Maligned or malignant? *American Psychologist, 44,* 266–273.

Cosmides, L., & Tooby, J. (1987). From evolution to behavior: Evolutionary psychology as the missing link. In J. Dupre (Ed.), *The latest and the best: Essays on evolution and optimality* (pp. 277–306). Cambridge, MA: MIT Press.

Easterbrooks, M. A., & Goldberg, W. (1987, April). *Consequences of early family attachment patterns for later social-personality development.* Paper presented at the biennial meeting of the Society for Research in Child Development, Baltimore.

Erickson, M., Egeland, B., & Sroufe, L.A. (1985). The relationship between quality of attachment and behavior problems in preschool in a high-risk sample. In I. Bretherton & E. Waters (Eds.), Growing points in attachment theory and research. *Monographs of the Society for Research in Child Development, 50* (1–2, Serial No. 209), 147–186.

Fox, N., & Fein, G. (1990). *Infant day-care: The debate.* Norwood, NJ: Ablex.

Frodi, A., & Thompson, R. (1985). Infants' affective response in the Strange Situation: Effects of prematurity and of quality of attachment. *Child Development, 56,* 1280–1291.

Goldsmith, H. H., & Alansky, J. A. (1987). Maternal and infant temperamental predictors of attachment: A meta-analytic review. *Journal of Consulting and Clinical Psychology, 55*, 805–816.

Hinde, R. A. (1982). Attachment: Some conceptual and biological issues. In C. Murray Parkes & J. Stevenson-Hinde (Eds.), *The place of attachment in human behavior* (pp. 187–214). New York: Basic Books.

Hinde, R., & Stevenson-Hinde, J. (1991). Perspectives on attachment. In C. M. Parkes, J. Stevenson-Hinde, & P. Morris (Eds.), *Attachment across the life cycle* (pp. 52–65). London: Routledge.

Howes, C., Rodning, C., Galluzzo, D. C., & Myers, L. (1988). Attachment and child care: Relationships with mother and caregiver. *Early Childhood Research Quarterly, 3*, 403–416.

Isabella, R. A., & Belsky, J. (1991). Interactional synchrony and the origins of infant–mother attachment: A replication study. *Child Development, 62*, 373–384.

Isabella, R. A., Belsky, J., & von Eye, A. (1989). Origins of infant–mother attachment: An examination of interactional synchrony during the infant's first year. *Developmental Psychology, 25*, 12–21.

Kagan, J. (1982). *Psychological research on the human infant: An evaluative summary*. New York: W. T. Grant Foundation.

Lamb, M. E., Sternberg, K., & Prodromdis, M. (1990). *Nonmaternal care and the security of infant–mother attachment: A reanalysis of the data*. Unpublished manuscript, National Institute of Child Health and Human Development, Bethesda, MD.

Lewis, M. (1997). *Altering fate: Why the past does not predict the future*. New York: Guilford Press.

Lewis, M., & Feiring, C. (1989). Infant, mother, and mother–infant interaction behavior and subsequent attachment. *Child Development, 60*, 831–837.

Leyendecker, B., Lamb, M., Fracasso, M., Schoelmerich, A., & Larson, C. (1997). Playful interaction and the antecedents of attachment. *Merrill-Palmer Quarterly, 43*, 24–47.

Main, M., Kaplan, N., & Cassidy, J. (1985). Security in infancy, childhood, and adulthood: A move to the level of representation. In I. Bretherton & E. Waters (Eds.), Growing points in attachment theory and research. *Monographs of the Society for Research in Child Development, 50* (1–2, Serial No. 209), 66–104.

Main, M., & Weston, D. (1981). The quality of the toddler's relationship to mother and father: Related to conflict behavior and readiness to establish new relationships. *Child Development, 52*, 932–940.

Malatesta, C. Z., Culver, C., Tesman, J., & Shepard, B. (1989). The development of emotion expression during the first two years of life. *Monographs of the Society for Research in Child Development, 54* (1–2, Serial No. 219), 1–104.

Matas, L., Arend, R., & Sroufe, L.A. (1978). Continuity of adaptation in the second year: The relationship between quality of attachment and later competent functioning. *Child Development, 49*, 547–556.

NICHD Early Child Care Research Network. (1994). Child care and child development: The NICHD Study of Early Child Care. In S. Friedman & H. Haywood (Eds.), *Developmental follow-up: Concepts, domains, and methods* (pp. 377–396). New York: Academic Press.

NICHD Early Child Care Research Network. (1997). The effects of infant child care on infant–mother attachment security: Results of the NICHD Study of Early Child Care. *Child Development, 68,* 860–879.

NICHD Early Child Care Research Network. (2001). Child care and family predictors of MacArthur preschool attachment and stability from infancy. *Developmental Psychology, 37,* 847–862.

Rutter, M. (1981). Socio-emotional consequences of day care for preschool children. *American Journal of Orthopsychiatry, 51,* 4–28.

Smith, P. B., & Pederson, D. R. (1988). Maternal sensitivity and patterns of infant–mother attachment. *Child Development, 59,* 1097–1101.

Sroufe, L. A. (1983). Infant–caregiver attachment and patterns of adaptation in preschool: The roots of maladaptation and competence. In M. Perlmutter (Ed.), *Minnesota Symposia on Child Psychology* (Vol. 16, pp. 16, 41–81). Minneapolis: University of Minnesota Press.

Sroufe, L. A. (1988). The role of infant–caregiver attachment in development. In J. Belsky & T Nezworski (Eds.), *Clinical implications of attachment* (pp. 18–40). Hillsdale, NJ: Erlbaum.

Sroufe, L. A., Fox, N. E., & Pancake, V. R. (1983). Attachment and dependency in developmental perspective. *Child Development, 54,* 1615–1627.

Thompson, R., & Lamb, M. (1984). Assessing qualitative dimensions of emotional responsiveness in infants: Separation reactions in the Strange Situation. *Infant Behavior and Development, 7,* 423–445.

CHAPTER 5

Early Care and the Roots of Attachment and Partnership Representations

The Bielefeld and Regensburg Longitudinal Studies

KARIN GROSSMANN
KLAUS E. GROSSMANN
HEINZ KINDLER

OUR DISCOVERY AND PURSUIT OF ATTACHMENT RESEARCH

Looking at the results of our longitudinal attachment research in Bielefeld and Regensburg, we feel that our dream has come true. When we started, we had not dared to hope for what we are now able to demonstrate: young adults' thoughts and feelings about close relationships are powerfully influenced by their early as well as their later relationships with mother and father.

Like many attachment researchers of our generation, we came to attachment study from other disciplines. Indeed, we discovered Bowlby's and Ainsworth's work only after we had completed our training. In the early 1960s, when behaviorism was still the dominant perspective in "respectable" U.S. psychology, Klaus accepted a Fulbright scholarship to study in the United States, married Karin, and went to New Mexico State University in Las Cruces. Within a year, Klaus became skilled at teaching rats to run through mazes and runways, a talent that gained him admission to the PhD program at the University of Arkansas in Fayetteville where Karin started to study mathematics.

At Hot Springs, Arkansas, we encountered seemingly obvious breaches in the behaviorist wall: Marian and Keller Breland were demonstrating that instinctual biases in animal's learning abilities and motivational systems imposed real boundaries on even the most rigorous stimulus control. From a mere conditioning perspective, their animals were misbehaving (Breland & Breland, 1961). And they weren't alone. The ethologists Konrad Lorenz and Niko Tinbergen were the first to challenge accepted canons of behaviorism, and they were joined by the comparative psychologists Frank Beach and Donald Hebb. Though we didn't know it at the time, this proved to be an excellent perspective from which to appreciate John Bowlby's insights into the nature and development of attachment relationships.

Together with the Brelands Klaus tested—for his dissertation work— behavioral differences between organisms in a combination Skinner box and runway. Rabbits (herbivores) and cats (carnivores) had to run down an alley 18 feet long and press a bar that released food pellets at the other end. The ratios of the running speed toward the bar as compared to the running speed back to the food reward box were the data. For the rabbits, the ratio was about 1:1, that is, the same speed in each direction; for the cats, however, the ratio was about 3:1. The cats displayed a strong reluctance to leave the food tray to get to the bar, meowing painfully and constantly checking back, and then ran back full speed to the tray. The rabbits, according to my naive interpretation, had no inborn fear that their vegetables would run away, but the cats were careful not to let their "prey"— food pellets, of course—out of eyesight, lest it escape (K. E. Grossmann, 1967). Klaus was cited, for the first time in his life, in a small book on animal behavior by Keller and Marian Breland (Breland & Breland, 1966), which was completed shortly before Keller's untimely death.

Upon our return to Germany in 1965 together with our 2-year-old U.S. citizen, Carol May, "from the Ozarks," Klaus accepted an assistantship at the department of zoology at the University of Freiburg to work with Bernhard Hassenstein. There he got a thorough training in ethology and conducted a series of operant conditioning experiments with honey bees (K. E. Grossmann, 1973). After our second child, Gerald, was born, Karin started to study psychology with a particular interest in adaptive behavioral processes.

Even before we met John Bowlby or Mary Ainsworth we had the good fortune to study animal behavior under the guidance of Konrad Lorenz. He took us along when he watched how greylag geese reestablish their rank order in a new location. We saw firsthand how a keen eye and patient observation could make sense of complex behavior in complex environments. Consequently, our first collaborative publication was a critique of the then prevailing early stimulation studies with rats from an ethological viewpoint (K. Grossmann & K. E. Grossmann, 1969). Funded by a grant, Karin collected and summarized papers on social development within the field of ethology. Her review included reports of early discussions between Jean Piaget, Konrad Lorenz, and John Bowlby in the 1950s (Tanner & Inhelder, 1963), Bowlby's report to the World Health Organization (WHO) (Bowlby, 1951), and Mary Ainsworth's (1967) observational studies of infants' attachment behavior in Uganda. Since this field seemed a fascinating new territory to explore, we accepted the challenge.

When Klaus received tenure in 1971 at the University of Bielefeld, he was free to choose his own field of investigation. In 1973 he traveled to Baltimore for a firsthand introduction by Mary Ainsworth to her observational methods and to the Strange Situation. This approach to the study of human infant behavior appeared natural to us because of its likeness to Lorenz's method of calling his geese away from their home territory to a new place to be able to observe the reestablishment of their rank order. Arguing likewise, Ainsworth put mothers and their infants in a "strange place" to observe the infant's organization of attachment behavior after separation.

It was apparent from long discussions with Mary Ainsworth and her students Mary Main, Inge Bretherton, Mary Blehar, and Russell Tracy that the success of attachment theory depended very much on the generality of her results across cultures. In addition, during that time, the concepts of maternal bonding and "early contact" were popular. Thus, we began our observations by attending the births of the infants we studied (K. Grossmann, Thane, & K. E. Grossmann, 1981). The initial goal of our study (which eventually became the Bielefeld Project) was simple: we wanted to replicate the link between maternal care and infant attachment security observed in Ainsworth's Baltimore study in a German middle-class sample. At first, our methods followed as closely as possible Ainsworth's own approach, which involved long hours of in-home observation, even though this degree of involvement limited our sample size, and still fell short of the many more hours of observation of each mother and child carried out in Baltimore.

Throughout our explorations of attachment theory and research, we had most generous intellectual support from many colleagues from Europe as well as from the United States. We received decisive and continuing help from Mary Main, who worked with us in 1976–1977 while attending a 9-month-long interdisciplinary workshop for biologists and psychologists at the Center for Interdisciplinary Research in Bielefeld (Immelmann, Barlow, Petrinovich, & Main, 1981). Mary Main coded our first infants in the Strange Situation procedure and taught us the method of analysis (K. E., Grossmann, K., Grossmann, Huber, & Wartner, 1981; see also Main, Hesse, & Kaplan, Chapter 10, this volume).

It may seem curious, but Mary Main's key results from her dissertation, which emphasized the relation between attachment, play, and exploration, were published first in German and only later in English (Main, 1977, 1983). In the early 1980s, Inge Bretherton spent a semester with us as a Humboldt fellow, supporting our efforts to "see" maternal sensitivity in written narratives of home observations. A few years later, Avi Sagi-Schwartz, also as a Humboldt fellow, and Nina Koren-Karie from Israel joined us for some time, encouraging our interest in cross-cultural studies that we followed up later in Japan and Papua New Guinea (K. Grossmann, Fremmer-Bombik, & K. E. Grossmann, 1990; K. E. Grossmann, K. Grossmann, & Keppler, in press).

As the children in our Bielefeld longitudinal study grew older, exchanges of ideas with Alan Sroufe and his research group in Minneapolis about preschool children became an additional source of inspirations for our own research (Suess, K. E. Grossmann, & Sroufe, 1992). The Minnesota study involved a high-risk group of young mothers and their infants. We were especially interested in determining whether in our samples of low-risk and much less stressed families early interactive and attachment experiences with the parents would have similar long-lasting effects on the children's social and emotional development during childhood and up to young adulthood. Our cooperation with Mary Main and Mary Ainsworth became particularly close when Ulrike Wartner, a former student of ours in Regensburg, assessed the Regensburg 6-year-olds for her dissertation at the University of Virginia, supervised by Mary Ainsworth (K. E. Grossmann & K. Grossmann, 1999; Wartner, 1987; Wartner, K. Grossmann, Fremmer-Bombik, & Süss, 1994).

As in so many studies reported in this volume, our project expanded far beyond these initial goals. Our measures included emotions during exploration, the father–child and sibling relationships, and interactions with friends. The Bielefeld Project led to the Regensburg Project and also to a few other short-term longitudinal studies. These were specifically designed to address new issues and questions that the advancing Bielefeld Project had left unanswered. During the early replication phases, observational methods were available but very soon it became quite obvious to us that German infants, children, and their parents had ways of expressing themselves that were captured insufficiently by the rating scales developed in the United States. We started to translate the concepts of attachment theory into our own empirical research strategy.

In addition, the core Bielefeld and Regensburg Projects were extended substantially by our doctoral students, each of whom added his or her special interests to the study of attachment (K. E. Grossmann, K. Grossman, & Zimmermann, 1999). They helped us to carry the projects to the threshold of adulthood. Despite the long term of the studies and the wide range of ages examined, we never gave up our commitment to anchoring our work in detailed observations in naturalistic settings. At times we felt we were placing an impossible burden on our students but their dedication produced rich returns.

Looking back, we are pleased with the intensity and frequency of our home observations. In this way we could follow the process of specific developments such as partnership orientation from infancy, through childhood and adolescence, to young adulthood. Documented interactions and recorded interviews also gave us continued opportunities to reanalyze attachment development from new perspectives as the knowledge base in attachment theory grew. Because of our ethological orientation, we had decided right from the start to limit use of questionnaires to the parents. Child data, we felt, should reflect observable experiences of the infants and children and the way the children talked about their experiences. The price we paid for this approach was that we and our students had to develop new and appropriate methods of analysis for almost each new assessment. These were developed from the attachment concept of adaptive functioning in situations that challenged the children's self and/or external organization of emotions. Our longitudinal studies contained material for creating and testing methods in more than 200 very labor-intensive *diplom*-theses. Such work proved to be a selection criterion providing us with many highly motivated and committed students. In addition, the scope of our studies was extended substantially by our more than 20 doctoral students who brought in their special interests and points of view. Their work has been extensively documented in a recent monograph, *Attachments* [note the plural!]: *The Composition of Psychological Security* (K. Grossmann, & K. E. Grossmann, 2004).

Initial generous funding for 5 years was provided by Stiftung Volkswagenwerk. Later support with funding by the German Research Council was less consistent. However, thanks to the personal help of Lotte Koehler and her Koehler Foundation, we were able to embark on our final assessments and complete the two major longitudinal projects as well as several supporting projects.

THE MAKING OF AFFECTIONAL BONDS

One of the central questions of attachment theory is, "How does the capacity to make affectional bonds develop?" Very early in our investigations this became the pivotal issue in our research. Attachment theory posits that the quality of the early parent/caregiver–child relationship has the most powerful influence on this development in the child. The mechanisms by which this extensive influence is exerted are thought to be the following:

1. Interactions and communications with the attachment figures during the early years become patterns of attachment and communication that organize the child's perceptions, thoughts, feelings, and behaviors, especially in times of distress. Experiencing understanding or rejecting responses of the attachment figures in distressing situations shapes the child's expectations, and thus his or her behavioral and mental strategies when dealing with adversity later in life. A healthy strategy is the ability to express thoughts and feelings to others and seek their comfort and help (Bowlby, 1991).

2. A person's mental models of close relationships also influence his or her capacity to make affectional bonds. Such inner working models of self and others in relationships are abstractions of attachment-related experiences with *both* parents. Although maternal behavior was the focus of many early attachment studies, attachment theory has since included the father as an important figure for the child's social and emotional development (see also K. Grossman et al., 2002a). In the second edition of *Attachment* Bowlby (1982) outlined the picture of personality development by stating: "A young child's experience of an encouraging, supportive and cooperative *mother*, and a little later *father*, gives him a sense of worth, a belief in the helpfulness of others, and a favourable model on which to build future relationships" (p. 378).

3. Parental respect for the child's attachment needs as well as his or her need to explore is a postulated third influence on the capacity to make affectional bonds. Bowlby (1987) formulated this as follows: "Complementary in importance to a parent's respect for a child's attachment desires is *respect for his desire to explore* and gradually to extend his relationships both with peers and with other adults" (p. 58). "By enabling him to explore his environment with confidence and to deal with it effectively, such experiences also promote his sense of competence" (Bowlby, 1982, p. 378).

Mary Ainsworth had continuously emphasized exploration and competence as complementary to attachment in social development (Ainsworth & Bell, 1974; Ainsworth, Bell, & Stayton, 1974). In her dissertation work, Mary Main was the first researcher to describe the influence of secure and insecure attachment on quality of exploration (Main, 1983). Following Main, we have stressed the theory that both a secure attachment and secure exploration are necessary when dealing with new challenges, when adapting to new circumstances, and when reconstructing working models from childhood that no longer fit one's current life (Bowlby, 1988b). In attachment research the inseparable connection and balance between the attachment system and the exploratory system for the development of inner working models has received too little attention. Without secure, non-defensive exploration, competencies and inner working models would fail to be continuously in contact with reality to the degree that the individual would be unable to deal constructively and enduringly with challenges that elicit negative emotions.

Furthermore, attachment theory considers all phases of development "during the years of immaturity—infancy, childhood and adolescence" (Bowlby, 1980, p. 41) as providing important influences along the pathway toward the adult personality. This belief requires attachment researchers to collect data as continuously as possible. In fact, Bowlby hesitated to accept the Strange Situation as a firm indicator of the child's future development. After inspecting data on stability of patterns, he wrote: "Thus too much prognostic significance must not be read into the statement that at the first birthday a couple is likely to have established a characteristic pattern of interaction. All that it means is that for most couples a pattern that is likely to persist is by that time present" (1982, p. 349). As it turned out, and as we show below, we were well advised to collect many interactional data during infancy beside patterns of attachment as assessed in the Strange Situation.

Our view of attachment has been a rather broad one and intentionally so (K. E. Grossmann & K. Grossmann, 1990). It includes parental support and emotions during exploration as well as the important role of fathers for the child's attachment development. This perspective provided us with a broader and more appropriate base for our studies of children in nonrisk families than would have a narrower focus solely on attachment and caregiving behaviors within the mother–child dyad (K. E. Grossmann et al., 1999; K. Grossmann & K. E. Grossmann, 2004). Our emphasis on collecting observations and interviews during toddlerhood, childhood, adolescence, and early adulthood also reflected the central role of two concepts that have guided our thinking about the development and quality of affectional bonds: (1) the child's response strategy when meeting emotional adversity and her response strategy when she meets challenging new situations that requires emotionally unrestricted exploration when searching for a solution, which parallels distressing situations that give rise to the attachment system; and (2) mothers' and fathers' caring, sensitive, supportive, and partnership-oriented interactions with their child that may serve as a positive model that the child can adopt toward others.

OVERVIEW OF OUR TWO LONGITUDINAL STUDIES

Mary Ainsworth inspired a number of young attachment researcher like Mary Main, Everett Waters, Alan Sroufe, Byron Egeland, and ourselves to start prospective studies in the early 1970s. We all were fortunate and per-sistent enough to follow our subjects into young adulthood. Naturally, each group chose a different approach depending on their background and resources. The following section gives an overview of the approach and research structures of our two major efforts, the Bielefeld and the Regensburg longitudinal studies.

The Bielefeld Project

The Bielefeld Project started in 1976 and 1977 (K. E. Grossmann & K. Grossmann, 1991; K. Grossmann, K. E. Grossmann, Spangler, Suess, & Unzner, 1985). The original sample consisted of 49 middle-class families from a middle-size town in northern Germany. Both parents were asked just prior to their child's birth to participate in a longitudinal study. Twenty-six families with infant sons and 23 families with infant daughters joined the study. All met the criteria of healthy pregnancy and birth and German as the mother's native tongue. The age of fathers at the time of birth ranged from 19 to 46 years and the age of mothers ranged from 18 to 42 years. All but two of the families were traditional in their division of labor. Mothers were primarily responsible for home and children, and fathers were the sole financial providers of the family. Thirty-eight (77.5%) young adults still participated at age 21–22.

With the exception of hospital observations at birth, of observations at the Strange Situation in infancy, observations in kindergarten, and the most recent assessments at age 22, all observations, interviews, and other data were collected in the families' homes. Lengthy home visits with interviews and observations of mother's and father's quality of interactions and communications with the infant, toddler, and child were the core elements of this study. Independent data were acquired by sending new research teams to the families at each subsequent visit.

The original design closely paralleled Ainsworth's Baltimore study. This allowed us to examine the cross-cultural generality of her results on maternal care and subsequent infant attachment patterns by using the Strange Situation (Ainsworth, 1973). We added observations of the births of the infants, newborn assessments, mother–newborn interactions, and observations of infant–father interactions to Ainsworth's basic design. Strange Situation assessments of attachment quality to both parents were done in the second year (K. Grossmann et al., 1985). In line with our broader view of attachment development (K. E. Grossmann & K. Grossmann, 1990), analyses of parental sensitivity and support of the child's exploratory behavior always paralleled measures of parental sensitivity to the child's attachment behaviors (K. E. Grossmann et al., 1999).

We kept our ethological commitment to observations throughout the childhood years, assessing both parents in interaction with their child and conducting interviews with both of them even though a few fathers missed some assessments. In our analyses of the videotaped materials, we focused on the probable subjective experience of the child during that particular interaction or individual exploration. In adolescence and young adulthood, open interviews about close relationships were designed to assess the subject's recollected experiences and evaluations of his or her relationships with parents and other supportive figures from a perspective of psychological adaptation. Figure 5.1 presents an overview of the major assessments of the Bielefeld longitudinal study.

The Regensburg Project

As the Bielefeld Project progressed into the preschool years, attachment research had produced new and challenging hypotheses. A few studies had explicitly included exploration as part of the quality of attachment (Main, 1983), and innovative methods of assessing attachment beyond infancy had been created (Main & Cassidy, 1988). These new developments prompted us to start a new study in our new home town of Regensburg, in southern Germany, again with infants from nonrisk middle-class families. The Regensburg longitudinal study started in 1980. Fifty-one 11-month-old infants from nonrisk families born between May and August 1979 were selected from the city's birth register, if the mother spoke German and if she had had a nonrisk pregnancy (Suess et al., 1992). It so happened that only girls—who outnumbered boys 2:1 because of the then-prevailing demographic gender distribution in the local birth register—experienced parental divorce in this sample. Thus, gender and parental divorce became confounded. That made replication of findings from the Bielefeld study less likely. At age 21–22, thirty-eight (74.5%) young adults still participated.

In contrast to the Bielefeld study, in which the majority of assessments from toddlerhood on were done in the families' homes, we asked the Regensburg families to our research rooms at the university. Figure 5.2 presents an overview of the major assessments of the Regensburg longitudinal study.

Although we began by employing assessment methods that were developed in the United States, we soon realized that we had to develop our own culturally appropriate criteria for judging nonverbal expressiveness; children's and parents' verbal responses indicating a secure state of mind, given the German manner of conversation, which tends to understate the intensity of emotions (Fremmer-Bombik, 1987); and culturally appropriate criteria for the Q-set evaluating security of partnership representation (see section below on assessing the outcome variables). The scoring used in U.S. research would have been less sensitive to individual differences in the levels of expressiveness and avoidance characteristic of our German sample.

Infancy Assessments

    Newborn period, first year, 24 and 36 months, predominantly home observations

    (1976–1980)

> Brazelton Neonatal Behavior Scales
> Ainsworth Maternal Sensitivity Scales
> Strange Situation with mother and father
> Mothers' and fathers' sensitive and challenging interactive play
> Other measures (e.g., Bayley Scales)

Childhood follow-up

    6- and 10-year assessments in Kindergarten and at home

    (1982–1987)

> Separation Anxiety Test
> Rutter Behavior Problem Scale
> Mothers' and fathers' sensitive and challenging interactive play
> Adult Attachment Interview (both parents)
> ACRI with child and each parent

Adolescent follow-up

    16-year assessments at home

    (1992–1993)

> Adult Attachment Interview
> Current Parent Relationship Interview
> Friendship Interview
> Emotion regulation vignettes
> Life events

Young adulthood follow-up

    22-year assessments at a lab

    (1998–2000)

> Adult Attachment Interview
> Current Relationship Interview
> Life events

FIGURE 5.1. Design of the Bielefeld longitudinal study.

Infancy Assessments

    11-, 12-, 17-, 18-month
lab observations

    (1980–1981)

> "Clown Situation" with each parent
>
> Play and obedience situations with each parent
>
> Strange Situation with each parent

Childhood follow-up

    4½-, 6-, and 8-year assessments

    in kindergarten and lab

    (1984–1987)

> Kindergarten observations
>
> California child Q-set
>
> Interview with mother about child
>
> Reunion situation with mother
>
> AAI with each parent

Adolescent follow-up

    16-year assessments with mother

    18-year assessments with father

    (1995–1999)

> AAI and computer game with a friend
>
> AAI with each parent
>
> Interactions with each parent
>
> Life events

Young adulthood follow-up

    20-year assessments

    (2000)

> Adult Attachment Projective
>
> Current Relationship Interview
>
> Life events

FIGURE 5.2. Design of the Regensburg longitudinal study.

APPROACH TO DATA ANALYSIS

Having looked forward into the lives of our participant families for so many years, we now adopt a retrospective view of the course we have traveled. Having assessed the young adults' state of mind with respect to attachment and their state of mind with respect to partnership as indications of their ability to make affectional bonds, what were the major influences on this capacity for these German children as young adults? Would we be able to find the mechanisms as postulated by attachment theory? We will focus on three key issues:

(1) child strategies when dealing with adverse experiences, (2) child experiences with both mother and father, and (3) parental respect and support for the child's attachment need as well as his or her desire to explore.

We begin by describing how we operationalized the young adult's ability to make affectional bonds. Our goals and the organization of our studies are most evident in the aggregated scores we used to combine related measures to better perceive patterns across infancy, childhood, and adolescence (see also Figures 5.1 and 5.2). These conceptual aggregations also helped us to track the influences of key mechanisms: child strategies when challenged emotionally, child interactive experiences with mother, and child interactive experiences with father. Figure 5.3 summarizes the variables in each of the key aggregate variables used in this report.

MEASURES

Assessing the Capacity to Make Affectional Bonds

We operationalized Bowlby's concept of young adults' "capacity to make affectional bonds" in terms of four dimensional variables scored from the Partnership Interview (PI) and the Adult Attachment Interview (AAI). For the Bielefeld sample, both interviews were conducted when the subjects were around 22 years of age. In the Regensburg sample, we administered the PI when the subjects were 20 years of age (Stöcker, 2003) and evaluated their state of mind with respect to attachment using the Adult Attachment Projective (George, West, & Pettem, 1999). The findings regarding this assessment are reported elsewhere (Keppler, 2004).

Aggregated variables	Infancy 0–3 years	Childhood 5–10 years	Adolescence 16–18 years
Child's strategy when meeting emotional adversity	Child Strange Situation 12–18 months	Child 5–10 years	Child 16–18 years
Mother's sensitivity and support	Mother during infancy	Mother during childhood*	Mother during adolescence*
Father's facilitation and support	Father during infancy	Father during childhood*	Father during adolescence*

*Available for only one of the two samples.

FIGURE 5.3. Structure of data aggregation for the current analysis: Three age levels and three pathways tested for each dependent variable.

The AAI was analyzed using Kobak's dimensional Q-sort approach (Strasser, in prep), as well as the traditional method of rating and classifying as taught by Mary Main. Classification agreement across these two methods was 87%. Correlations of the rated items with the criterion sorts provided by Kobak (1993) also yielded dimensional ratings for degree of security, degree of dismissiveness, degree of preoccupation, and degree of deactivation versus hyperactivation of the attachment system. In light of the very high correlations between security and dismissiveness ($r = -.97$) and between dismissiveness and deactivation ($r = .73$), we focus here on degree of security and preoccupation.

For the PI, our Regensburg research team had to create culturally adequate criterion Q-sorts. The PI is based on the Current Relationship Interview (Crowell & Owens, 1998) about "the recent best partnership" and was adapted for young German adults. The criterion sort was created by seven expert German attachment researchers who sorted the 100 items of the PI Q-set. Averaging the seven experts' Q-sorts yielded criterion sorts for degree of security, dismissiveness, and preoccupation of partnership representation (K. E. Grossmann, K. Grossmann, Winter, & Zimmermann, 2002). Again, degree of security and dismissiveness were highly negatively interrelated ($r = -.92$), allowing us to focus on degree of security and preoccupation for the current analysis only and treating dismissiveness as the opposite of security for the present purpose.

Security in Attachment and Partnership Representation

The five most important Q-sort items indicating security in the AAI and the PI were (1) the person values attachment or values an intimate relationship; (2) the person responds in a clear, well-organized fashion and provides realistic narrations of experiences; (3) the person is credible, easy to believe, and provides no contradictory information; (4) the person is confident that he or she could rely on parents or the partner and relates availability and commitment in the partnership as mutual; and (5) there is very little unwarranted idealization of parents, partner, or partnership.

Preoccupation in Attachment and Partnership Representation

The five most important Q-sort items indicating preoccupation in the AAI and the PI are (1) the person worries and ruminates about negative experiences with parents or in the partner relationship; (2) the person loses the topic during interview, fails to answer questions, and shows very little metacognitive monitoring of his or her own responses; (3) the person responds in excessive detail about attachment or partnership experiences;

(4) the reader must struggle to understand the person's statements; and (5) the person presents the self as passive, helpless, and very needy of support.

As expected, the dimensional scores for security in the AAI and the PI were significantly related ($r = .44$, $p < .01$), as were the dimensional scores for preoccupation in the two assessments ($r = .60$, $p < .01$). Still, the overlap was not complete, and apparently each interview was measuring different aspects of the young adult's state of mind with respect to close relationships.

Measures from Infancy, Childhood, and Adolescence in Bielefeld

During the children's infancy years, the families were seen at 0, 3, 6, 10, 12, 18, 24, and 36 months. During childhood, the families were seen at ages 5, 6, and 10 years. During adolescence, the families were seen at age 16 years (see Figure 5.1). For this analysis, the data sets were aggregated conceptually according to the three postulated mechanisms of influence: (1) strategies of the child when challenged emotionally; (2) interactive experiences with mother, or maternal sensitivity and support; and (3) interactive experiences with father, or father's facilitation and support. The descriptive word "facilitation" was chosen instead of father's "sensitivity" because in all of these families fathers were unlikely to alleviate distress signals of the infant with tender loving care themselves, but did respond by handing the distressed infant to the mother. Thus, they would facilitate a comforting response by the mother (see also K. Grossmann & K. E. Grossmann, 1991).

Data Aggregation for the Child's Strategy
When Challenged Emotionally

The upper section of Table 5.1 lists the composition of the aggregated variables for the Bielefeld Project according to the age periods. In infancy, the Strange Situation assessment of attachment quality to mother and father was conducted in both studies 6 months apart during the second year. This procedure emphasizes the infant's responses to mild stress induced by the novelty of the context and the departure of the mother (K. E. Grossmann et al., 1981). The infants' response patterns revealed secure, insecure-avoidant, and insecure-ambivalent qualities of attachment, as well as indications of disorientation and/or disorganization. For a composite index of an infant's strategy, the subpatterns of attachment were transformed into dimensional scores—with the subpattern B_3 receiving the highest score. The dimensional scores for each parent were added.

In childhood, the following five indicators of a child's strategy while meeting emotional adversity were collected for the Bielefeld children, when

TABLE 5.1. Composition of the Aggregated Variables of the Bielefeld Longitudinal Study

Aggregated variable	Age period at assessment	Specific measures
Child strategy when meeting emotional adversity	Infancy	1. Infant pattern of attachment to mother at 12 months and to father at 18 months in the Strange Situation: sum of the two dimensional security scores with B3 = 4, B2, B1, B4 = 3, etc.
	Childhood	1. Rating of behavior problems in preschool–age 5.5 years 2. Separation Anxiety Test security score—age 6 years 3. Scores for openness and person orientation when distressed—ages 6 years and 10 years 4. Score for active help seeking—age 10 years 5. Rating of behavior problems during home visit—age 10 years
	Adolescence (16 years)	1. Dimensional score for security on the AAI 2. Score for active help seeking 3. Rating for emotion regulation during responses to vignettes of peer rejection 4. Partnership orientation of friendship representation 5. Security of exploration (California Adult Q-Sort) 6. Anxiousness as rated by close others (CAQ)
Maternal sensitivity and support	Infancy	1. Maternal sensitivity (Ainsworth Scale), first year 2. Maternal cooperation (Ainsworth Scale), first year 3. Partnership orientation toward her 2-year-old 4. Score on the SCIP Scale at child's age of 24 months 5. Score on the SCIP Scale at child's age of 36 months
	Childhood	1. Score on the SCIP Scale at child's age of 6 years 2. Rating of guidance and scaffolding, 6 years 3. Child-reported maternal support, 10 years 4. Mother-reported support, 10 years 5. Mother-reported rejection, 10 years (negative)
Father's facilitation and support	Infancy	1. Caregiving index, first year 2. Score on the SCIP Scale at child's age of 24 months 3. Rating of guidance and scaffolding, 2 years
	Childhood	1. Score on the SCIP Scale at child's age of 6 years 2. Rating of guidance and scaffolding, 6 years 3. Child-reported support from father, 10 years 4. Father-reported support, 10 years 5. Father-reported rejection, 10 years (negative)

they were between 5 and 10 years of age (K. E. Grossmann & K. Grossmann, 1991): (1) the child's security score on the Separation Anxiety Test; (2) the 6- and 10-year-old's open expression of feelings and person orientation during distress as rated from interviews with them; (3) ratings of presenting the self as actively seeking help in interviews; (4) behavior problems in preschool as reported by the teacher; and (5) inappropriate behaviors during the home visit interview at age 10 years as reported by the interviewer (inverse of the standardized scores, respectively).

Strategy in adolescence was an aggregated score computed from six indicators: (1) score on the Security dimension in the AAI, (2) rating of strategy of turning to others for help, (3) appropriate emotion regulation when faced with (imagined) rejection from friends, (4) partnership-oriented friendship representation, (5) rating of Security of Exploration on the California Adult Q-Sort (K. Grossmann et al., 2002b), and (6) not anxious as judged by others (Zimmermann, 1999).

Data Aggregation for the Variables Indicating Maternal Sensitivity and Support

The second section of Table 5.1 lists the composition of the aggregated variables that indicated maternal sensitivity and support in attachment as well as in exploration-related situations. For the infancy period, the following indicators were aggregated: maternal sensitivity and cooperation during three home visits across the first year as rated with Ainsworth's scales (K. Grossmann et al., 1985), partnership orientation and understanding of her 2-year-old as rated from an interview (K. Grossmann, Fremmer-Bombik, Rudolph, & K. E. Grossmann, 1988), sensitive and challenging interactions during playful *explorations* (Sensitive and Challenging Interactive [SCIP] Scale) at 24 and at 36 months (K. Grossmann et al., 2002a). During childhood, maternal indicators of sensitivity and support were sensitive and challenging interactions during play with the 6-year-old, appropriate guidance and scaffolding during a mother–child task at age 6, child- and mother-reported maternal support as rated from separate interviews at age 10, and reported rejection by mother in an interview about the 10-year-old (inverse standardized scores).

Data Aggregation for the Variables Indicating Fathers' Facilitation and Support

The third section of Table 5.1 lists the respective variables for fathers. Fathers had been observed around the birth of the baby and at home during the first year, and mothers had provided information about their involvement. All these data were summarized in a paternal caregiving index for the first year (K. Grossmann et al., 2002). At the child's age of 24 months and 6 years, father's sensitive and challenging interactions during play were rated, as well as his appropriate guidance and scaffolding during a task that raised the child's curiosity and challenged his or her mastery. At 10 years, the child and the father were rated on paternal support from separate interviews and on fathers' reported rejection (inverse standardized scores).

FINDINGS

In the 22-year-long Bielefeld Project and the 20-year-long Regensburg Project we looked at children's experiences with both parents beginning in infancy and extending through adolescence for the roots of young adults' representation of close relationships. Sensitive, supportive, and appropriately challenging interactions with mother and father in situations that evoke the attachment system or the child's desire to explore were reflected in a secure, partnership-oriented strategy of the child and adolescent when meeting challenges. Early as well as continuing experiences with both parents and a history of emotionally secure strategies were strong roots of valuing close relationships as young adults.

Our key results will be presented in two parts. Part 1 focuses on the findings from the Bielefeld Project, part 2 adds some supporting and extending findings from the Regensburg Project.

The report of the findings from the Bielefeld Project has the following structure: pathways leading to security of attachment and partnership representation (and its inverse, dismissive partnership representation) are followed by parallel findings of pathways leading to preoccupation with attachment and partnership. First, zero-order correlations between the aggregated variables from the years of immaturity and the outcome variables will provide an overview for the interrelations between the variables. Second, results of regression and variance decomposition analyses are presented to show the relative contributions of later versus early child strategies, of mother's versus father's sensitive support, and of later versus early experiences with both parents to representations of close relationships in young adulthood.

Interrelations between the Earlier and Later Variables: Zero-Order Correlations

Figures 5.4a and 5.4b represent the network of zero-order correlations between the aggregated independent variables during infancy, childhood, and adolescence and (in Figure 5.4a) security of attachment and partner-

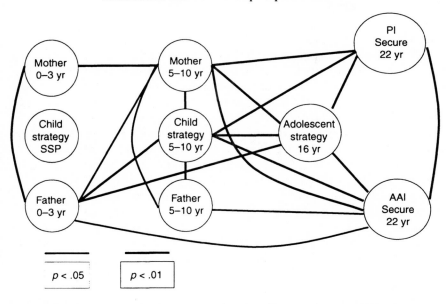

FIGURE 5.4a. Zero-order correlations between the aggregated variables and security of partnership and attachment representation.

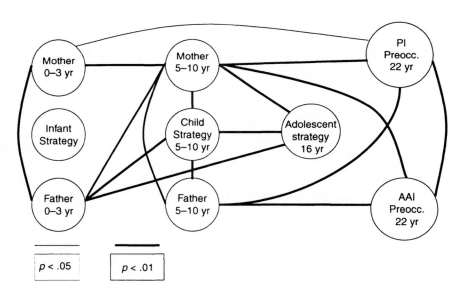

FIGURE 5.4b. Zero-order correlations between aggregated variables and preoccupation of partnership and attachment representation.

ship representation at age 22 years and (in Figure 5.4b) preoccupation with attachment and partnership representation.

The interrelations between the child's experiences with mother (upper path) and father (lower path) during infancy and childhood are highly significant, suggesting a similar parenting style of both parents. The infant's strategy (first circle of the middle path) as shown in his or her patterns of attachment to mother and father, however, did not relate significantly to the aggregated variables of maternal and paternal support. This finding has emerged because of the aggregation of both patterns, and because the aggregation of parental sensitivity across 3 years also contained ratings of support for the infant's and toddler's explorative play. Parental sensitive support of the toddler's play was unrelated to pattern of infant–parent attachment. In contrast, all aggregated variables for the childhood period were interrelated. The adolescent's strategy when meeting emotional challenges—as a composite of six indicators of his or her inner working models—was significantly influenced by maternal sensitivity and support during childhood, by fathers' behavior during infancy, and by the adolescent's strategy during childhood.

Security of attachment representation as well as partnership representation were significantly predicted by the adolescent's and child's strategy and by maternal sensitivity and support during childhood. Father's facilitation and support during childhood predicted security of attachment representation but not security of partnership representation at age 22 years. Correlational analysis even revealed a link between fathers' facilitation and support during the first 3 years of life ("infancy") and security of attachment representation at the age of 22 years (Figure 5.4a). This finding came as a surprise to us, given that all but two mothers were the infant's primary attachment figure and because father's facilitation and support was assessed only in play situations. It suggests that the pathway to a later secure/autonomous representation of attachment is influenced by father's behavior from the early years on.

Preoccupation with partnership and attachment was influenced differently (Figure 5.4b). Preoccupation with close relationships in young adulthood was not forecasted by the adolescent's or the child's strategy when meeting emotional challenges (middle path). Instead, maternal (upper path) and paternal support (lower path) during childhood, and even maternal sensitivity and support during the first 3 years of life, were important precursors. This provides suggestive evidence that low maternal sensitivity and support during infancy and toddlerhood increases the probability that the child may develop a preoccupied/enmeshed partnership representation as a young adult.

The Sensitive and Challenging Interactive Play (SCIP) Scale was developed to fill the need for a measure of parents' support of toddler explorations and their efforts to ensure that the child found appropriate challenges during play. It was applied to a 10-minute play session when the children were 23 months old. It proved to be an important variable in our longitudinal analyses. For example, regression analysis revealed that mother's SCIP score assessed at 24 months was related to lower degrees of preoccupation in partnership representation ($r = -.384$ [$p \leq 0.5$], $n = 38$). Furthermore, father's SCIP score assessed at 24 months was even related to *all four* outcome variables, the degree of security in partnership *and* adult attachment representation ($r = .36*$, $r = .35*$; $n = 38$), and to the degree of *non*preoccupation in their partnership *and* attachment representation ($r = -.40*$, $r = -.33*$; $n = 38$). Early paternal sensitive and challenging support of exploratory play seems to exert a powerful influence on later representations of close relationships (see also K. Grossmann et al., 2002a).

Figures 5.4a and 5.4b reveal also that in our study of middle-class families in which 75% of both parents remained in the family until the children became young adults, security of infant attachment to mother and father—using the Strange Situation procedure—did not predict security (or its opposite, dismissiveness), or preoccupation in young adulthood or any other of the aggregated variables at later ages. Separate analyses revealed that quality of early attachment to mother by itself predicted security of attachment up to the age of 10 years (see K. E. Grossmann & K. Grossmann, 1991, 2002b), but not if the aggregated variable of child strategy when meeting emotional adversity included attachment quality to father.

Predicting the Later Capacity to Make Affectional Bonds: Stepwise Multiple Regression Analyses and Variance Decomposition Analyses

A series of stepwise multiple regression analyses and variance decomposition analyses were applied to examine the pathways from early experiences and their relative contributions to later security or preoccupation in representations of partnership and attachment. Variance decomposition analysis is employed to partition the total explained variance of an outcome variable into three components: variance uniquely accounted for by one set of predictors, variance uniquely accounted for by the other set of predictors, and variance accounted for jointly by both sets of predictors. This procedure made it possible to investigate whether one of the predictors explained the same or different parts of the variance of the dependent variable as compared to the other predictor(s) (Amato, 1998).

The results of the first set of variance decomposition analyses appear in Figures 5.5a and 5.5b. Table 5.2 presents the exact percentages that are graphically indicated in Figures 5.5a and 5.5b. In these analyses, we com-

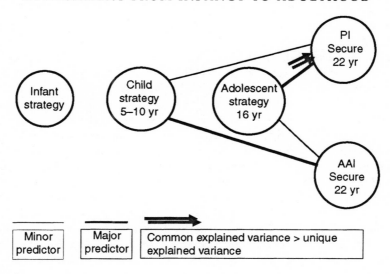

FIGURE 5.5a. Security of partnership and attachment representation as predicted from aggregated indicators of earlier child strategies when meeting emotional adversity.

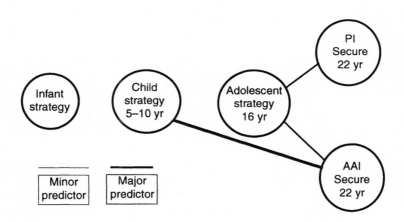

FIGURE 5.5b. Preoccupation of partnership and attachment representation as predicted from aggregated indicators of earlier child strategies when meeting emotional adversity.

TABLE 5.2. Percentage of Variance in Security and Preoccupation of Attachment and Partnership Representation of Young Adults Accounted for Uniquely and Jointly by Their Strategies When Meeting Adversity in Adolescence and Childhood (Aggregated Variables)

German criterion Q-sort scores at age 22 years	Secure attachment	Preoccupied attachment	Secure partnership	Preoccupied partnership
Total explained variance	39%	12%	20%	6%
Unique to child strategy at age 16	1%	0%	6%	4%
Unique to child strategy during childhood	21%	8%	2%	0%
Common explained variance	17%	4%	12%	2%

pared the early (childhood) versus the later (adolescence) strategy of the subject when challenged with emotional adversity as predictors of security and preoccupation of attachment and partnership representation.

Figures 5.5a and 5.5b and Table 5.2 show the roots of representations of close relationships in earlier strategies. The response strategies when meeting emotional adversity in adolescence and childhood predicted strongly whether the young adult would develop a secure attachment (39%) and/or partnership (20%) representation. A secure or preoccupied attachment representation in young adulthood was explained more strongly by the individual's strategy employed in childhood than by the strategy employed in adolescence. The child's strategy employed in childhood explained 21% of the variance of security of attachment representation and 8% of the variance of preoccupation with attachment (see Table 5.2). Although the corresponding figures for the adolescent's strategy alone are 1% and 0%, both strategies taken together added substantially to the explained variance (17% and 4%).

Ordinarily, measurements closer together in time are more closely associated. However, considering the nature of the assessments, and from a developmental point of view, these results are quite understandable. During childhood, the quality of parent–child relationship as evaluated by the child was central in all of our assessments, whereas in adolescence individual strategies when thinking about conflicts with parents as well as friends were more prominent.

In contrast, the joint contribution of child's strategies at both age periods, and to a degree the adolescent's strategy alone, accounted for more variance in the later secure partnership representation. The child's strategy when responding to emotional distress added very little to later partnership representation. The single variables that were aggregated suggest an interpretation. Among the assessments in adolescence, emotional response patterns within peer relationships occupied a much larger portion of the aggregated variable as compared to response patterns within the parent–adolescent relationship. The quality of relating to friends in adolescence seems to exert a stronger influence on later partnership representation than reported relationship with parents. Of course, adolescent and childhood strategies were, in turn, influenced by parental behavior, as Figures 5.4a and 5.4b indicate.

Figures 5.6a and 5.6b and the corresponding Tables 5.3 and 5.4 show the results of a second set of variance decomposition analyses, asking for the differential influence of mothers' and fathers' sensitive support during childhood (Table 5.3) and infancy (Table 5.4) on later representations of close relationships.

Sensitive and supportive experiences with both parents during childhood contributed very significantly to the child's later attachment representation, 34% to a secure attachment representation and 41% to a nonpreoccupied attachment representation (see Table 5.3). The unique contribution of each parent was far outweighed by their joint contribution, which was suggested by the strong intercorrelation of the aggregated indices (see Figures 5.4a or 5.4b). In contrast, the young adult's representation of partnership had much stronger roots in the sensitive support experienced from the mother than from the father. Preoccupation with partnership was also substantially rooted in both parents' behaviors.

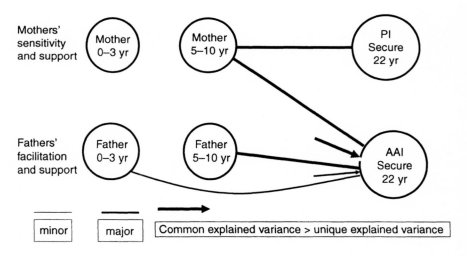

FIGURE 5.6a. Security of partnership and attachment representation as predicted from mothers' and fathers' sensitivity and support during infancy and childhood.

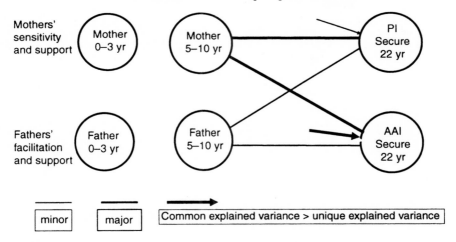

FIGURE 5.6b. Preoccupation of partnership and attachment representation as predicted from mothers' and fathers' sensitivity and support during infancy and childhood.

The findings presented in Table 5.3 provide strong support for the view that parental influence on evolving attachment and partnership representations is a continuing process throughout childhood.

Next, we tested whether the child's experiences with mother and father during the first 3 years were still influential 20 years later in his or her representation of close relationships. Table 5.4 shows the result of that specific variance decomposition analyses. It demonstrates that the roots go as far back as infancy. Early paternal facilitation and support, especially in combination with early maternal sensitivity and support, evidenced a signifi-

TABLE 5.3. Percentage of Variance in Security and Preoccupation of Attachment and Partnership Representation of Young Adults Accounted for Uniquely and Jointly by Mothers' and Fathers' Sensitivity and Support during Childhood (Aggregated Variables)

German criterion Q-sort scores at age 22 years	Secure attachment	Preoccupied attachment	Secure partnership	Preoccupied partnership
Total explained variance	34%	41%	26%	30%
Unique to mother's behavior during childhood	9%	9%	23%	15%
Unique to father's behavior during childhood	6%	9%	2%	1%
Common explained variance	19%	23%	1%	14%

TABLE 5.4. Percentage of Variance in Security and Preoccupation of Attachment and Partnership Representation of Young Adults Accounted for Uniquely and Jointly by Mothers' and Fathers' Sensitivity and Support during the First 3 Years (Aggregated Variables)

German criterion Q-sort scores at age 22 years	Secure attachment	Preoccupied attachment	Secure partnership	Preoccupied partnership
Total explained variance	12%	4%	4%	13%
Unique to mother's behavior during the first 3 years	1%	3%	0%	11%
Unique to father's behavior during the first 3 years	7%	0%	4%	0%
Common explained variance	4%	1%	0%	2%

cant influence on the young adult's security of attachment representation. In comparison, security of partnership representation was rooted only—albeit weakly—in early experiences with the father.

Preoccupation with partnership had significant roots in early experiences with mother but not with father, and preoccupation of attachment representation was hardly predictable from early experiences at all.

In separate analyses of all of those single variables that were aggregated in the above indices of mother's and father's behavior (see Table 5.1), the strongest single influences on the young adult's attachment representation regardless of age at assessment were tested (Strasser, in prep). In a stepwise multiple regression analysis, the dimensional score of secure attachment representation was best predicted by nonrejection of the mother rated from an interview when the child was 10 years old (24% explained variance) and father's play sensitivity (SCIP score) when the child was 6 years old (additional 11% explained variance). These two single variables predicted 35% of the variance of security of attachment representation at the age of 22 years (Strasser, in prep).

In contrast, only individual variables of father's facilitation and support predicted scores on the preoccupied attachment dimension. Father's rejection assessed with an interview when the child was 10 years old explained already 40% of the variance and father's play sensitivity (SCIP score) when the child was 2 years old added another 20%. As a result, a total of 60% of the variance of preoccupation in attachment was explained by these two aspects of fathering only. The discrepancy between these specific findings and the small relations between the aggregated indices of father's facilitation and support during infancy (see Table 5.4) and the dimensional score of preoccupation of attachment representation may be explained by the combination of three early father behaviors into the aggregated index.

We interpret the above findings as follows: High scores on the attachment preoccupation dimension reflect unclear, confused, and entangled responses in the AAIs. These include losing the topic easily, failing to answer questions, limited metacognitive monitoring, worrying and ruminating about negative experiences with parents, and presenting the self as passive, helpless, and requiring substantial support. It is notable that mainly two indicators of the child–*father* relationship, father's open rejection of his 10-year-old in the child interview and his low scores on the SCIP Scale, explained a very large proportion of the variance of this dimension of attachment representation. This finding clearly indicates that fathers' facilitation and support of their child's individuality and play exert an important influence on the clarity of mind with respect to the later attachment representation of their young adult sons and daughters.

SOME CONFIRMING AND EXTENDING FINDINGS FROM THE REGENSBURG LONGITUDINAL STUDY

We started our second major longitudinal study, the Regensburg Project, a couple of years after the Bielefeld Project. Common to both projects were the use of the Strange Situation procedure in infancy, the AAI in adolescence, and the PI with the young adults. Other assessments specific to this project are listed in Figure 5.2.

The Regensburg project does not quite match the Bielefeld Project in richness and detail, partly because data analysis is still in progress. Also, the Regensburg Project was started in order to, first, replicate selected important findings from the Bielefeld Project and second, to add newly developed relationship assessments to our attachment research such as the "Clown Situation" for 1-year-olds (Main & Weston, 1981), the Reunion procedure for 6-year-olds (Main & Cassidy, 1988), and mother–adolescent as well as father–adolescent interactions in a structured situation (Grotevant & Cooper, 1985). All assessments in the Regensburg Project were done in a university research room, which ensured a more standardized setting but had the disadvantage of lacking the richness of the "natural" home environment as a background. Still, the findings support the hypothesis that the inner working model of partnership in young adulthood has its roots in the interactive experiences of the subject with *both* parents throughout the years of immaturity.

Security and preoccupation of partnership representations were evaluated analogous to the Bielefeld Project, using the same criterion sorts of the German experts when the young adults were 20 years old (Stöcker, 2003). A few years earlier, subjects were observed in controlled interactions with their mothers and their fathers at 16 and 18 years of age, respectively. The parent–adolescent interaction tasks were patterned after Grotevant and Cooper's (1985) "Planning a Vacation Situation" and were videotaped and analyzed using the Autonomy and Relatedness Coding System created by Allen and Hauser (1996) (Becker-Stoll, 1997). This coding system groups adolescent and parent behaviors into four major categories: promoting or inhibiting autonomy and promoting or inhibiting relatedness.

Subjects who showed less relatedness to parents in the 16- and 18-year-old assessments were rated more dismissing and less secure in their partnership representations at age 20 years. Observed lack of relatedness in interactions with their parents seemed to have forcasted their model of partnership. Preoccupation with partnership had one of its roots in a preoc-cupied attachment representation in adolescence. Another root was found in their interactions with both parents. If granting autonomy to the adoles-cent in their joint "Planning a Vacation" task had been difficult for mothers and/or fathers and mostly inhibited by them 2 and 4 years earlier, the young adults were significantly more preoccupied with their partnerships and unclear in their discourse about it (Stöcker, 2003). Thus, augmenting the reported results from the Bielefeld Project about interactive experiences with parents in childhood, the Regensburg Project showed that experiences with both parents during adolescence still influenced the young adult's mental representations of partnership a few years later.

During the childhood years, both parents were interviewed separately when their child was 8 years old. They had to talk about their relationship to the child. If a father had talked convincingly about his positive involve-ment with his child—for example, his interest in, empathy with, and under-standing of his child—this child was very likely to receive a high rating in security of partnership representation as a young adult. It seemed as if the positive father–child relationship was now transferred to the adult partner. The parallel interview with the mother, however, did not predict the young adult's partnership representation.

Patterns of attachment shown by the 6-year-olds in the Reunion proce-dure (Main & Cassidy, 1988) had also been assessed. They had been scored and classified by the experts Mary Main, Jude Cassidy, and Mary Ainsworth in support of Ulrike Wartner in Charlottesville. Patterns of attachment at age 6 had been slightly predictable from patterns of attach-ment in infancy (Wartner et al., 1994). However, neither pattern of attach-ment at 1 year of age nor at 6 years of age forecasted later partnership rep-resentation. This finding seems to contradict the positive and significant relation found in the Bielefeld Project. However, in the Bielefeld Project, the indicator of child strategy when challenged emotionally was a composite score of five indices across 5 years, whereas in the Regensburg Project, the indicator was based only on the classification of the 6-year-olds' reunion behavior. The discontinuity found in the Regensburg Project suggests to us that patterns of separation/reunion behavior at early school age may have assessed only a small subset of the child's strategy when challenged emotionally and this subset was not able to predict later representations of close relationships.

Looking further back in our data, two sets of parent–infant interaction results were systematically related to later partnership representation. Both parents had been observed separately with their 1-year-olds during a play session and the "Clown Situation" that was stressful to all 1-year-olds (Main & Weston, 1981). As in the Bielefeld Project, father's play sensitivity with his infant forecasted later degree of security of partnership representation. Later preoccupation and unclear discourse about partnership in a young adult was significantly related to lower maternal and paternal sensitivity during play. In addition, higher degrees of preoccupation were also significantly predicted by higher scores of infant disorganization in the "Clown Situation" with mother though not with father. However, degree of disorganization in the Strange Situation with mother or with father was not related to later preoccupation at the age of 20 (Stöcker, 2003).

In sum, findings from the Regensburg Project also support the hypothesis of attachment theory that experiences with mother *and* father during infancy, childhood, and adolescence in attachment as well as exploration-related situations exert a strong influence on the child's later representation of a close relationship with a partner.

DISCUSSION

In both the Bielefeld and Regensburg Projects a child's attachment and exploratory experiences with mother *and* father in infancy, childhood, and adolescence structured the pathways toward representations of close relationships in young adulthood. Five sets of findings from both projects stand out. They provide empirical support for Bowlby's (1987) positions that there is "a strong causal relationship between an individual's experience with his parents and his later capacity to make affectional bonds" (p. 58).

1. A central finding of the Bielefeld Project was that security in attachment and partnership representation at the age of 22 years was significantly predicted from strategies in adolescence and childhood when faced with situations that challenged the attachment system. These strategies were characterized by a readiness (a) to communicate emotions and motives openly when in distress, (b) to turn actively to others for help, (c) to show appropriate emotional regulation during social challenges, (d) to value close relationships, and (e) to present a clear discourse when talking about attachment issues. This finding suggests that the ability to reflect on

close relationships from both partners' point of view is learned and practiced within the family starting at an age when partnership-corrected attachment behavior is cognitively possible. If, however, a relationship-oriented strategy of responding to distressing situations is not already developed during the childhood years, it does not emerge spontaneously in young adulthood when a love relationship could develop into a partnership in which each partner may serve as a secure base and haven of safety for the other when needed.

2. Mothers' as well as fathers' sensitive supportiveness, acceptance of the child, and appropriate challenging behaviors each in its own right *and* taken together were powerful predictors of internal working models of close relationships in young adulthood. These findings from both longitudinal projects reinforce Bowlby's (1982) position that "a young child's experience of an encouraging, supportive and cooperative *mother and father* gives her/him . . . a favorable model of close relationships" (p. 378).

3. Mothers' and fathers' sensitive and challenging cooperation *during joint play* with their child during the first 3 years contributed significantly to the child's later representation of close relationships. Parental sensitivity during play implies parental behavior that respects and supports the toddler's need to explore and to become competent. It also includes parental behaviors that promote cooperation, that facilitate the autonomous problem solving of the child, that pose appropriate challenges, and that give guidance and scaffolding. These findings support Bowlby's (1987) extended view of attachment development that includes the parent's respect for a child's desire to explore. This was assumed to be complementary in importance of responding in a caring way to the child's attachment desire (Bowlby, 1987, p. 58).

Two specific findings of both otherwise quite different longitudinal studies across 22 and 20 years provide additional support for the wider view that includes parental support of the child's need to explore. First, maternal and paternal sensitivity and support during play with the toddler (i.e. when the child's exploratory behavioral system was active), was directly related to less preoccupation and unclear discourse in partnership representation. This finding provides suggestive evidence that sensitive support, scaffolding, and age-appropriate challenges during the child's playful explorations, which are usually accompanied by fitting verbal comments, pave the way for a clear mental picture of close relationships. Second, interactions and experiences with father as well as father's acceptance of the child during childhood and/or adolescence influenced the inner working model of partnership and attachment in young adulthood were found to be as important as interactions with mother.

4. In contrast to the findings of some other studies reported in this volume, the patterns of attachment shown by the infants in the Strange Situa-

tion did not predict representation of attachment beyond childhood. Neither in the Bielefeld data nor in the Regensburg data did we find a statistical relationship between security of attachment in the Strange Situation procedure at 12 and 18 months with mother or father and adult measures of attachment or partnership representation.

Fortunately for the success of both studies, we did not rely solely on the Strange Situation as our only assessment in infancy and toddlerhood despite the dominating tendency in the 1970s and early 1980s in this direction. We had listened to Bowlby's warning against expecting too much prognostic significance from one measurement of attachment during the second year (Bowlby, 1982, p. 349). Mary Ainsworth had always stressed the validation nature of the Strange Situation for her previous home observations of maternal sensitivity and the infants' balanced behavioral strategy in response to the absence or presence of the attachment figure. With the Bielefeld Project, we could replicate her findings for the first year (K. Grossmann et al., 1985). However, the nature of attachment beyond infancy inferred from ethological observation in the child's "natural" environment and its developmental transformation(s) into standard assessment methods is a task still before us (Ainsworth, 1990; Solomon & George, 1999).

5. The Bielefeld longitudinal results illustrate the complexity of developmental pathways beyond infancy. At the end of the first year, 24 out of 49 (49%) infants had shown an avoidant pattern of attachment to their mother. This high proportion of avoidance in infancy had made this study a statistical "outlier" in cross-cultural comparison (van IJzendoorn & Kroonenberg, 1988). Thus, we had to ask, what will patterns of attachment forecast in the long run for this sample? We had noted back in 1985 that the pattern of avoidance in our infants was associated with higher maternal sensitivity and lower maternal rejection then reported by Ainsworth for her Baltimore sample. In fact, the average rating of maternal sensitivity of the "A-with-mother" group matched the average rating of maternal sensitivity of infants classified B1/B2 in the Baltimore group (see Figure 1 in K. Grossmann et al., 1985). This comparison allowed a more positive prognosis for the children. As it turned out, pattern of attachment at 12 months was indeed only a starting point for these infants. Subsequently, some of the avoidantly attached infants experienced supportive parenting in the domain of exploration whereas some of the securely attached infants experienced unsupportive parenting during the later years. Very important experiences that influenced the child's further socioemotional development were father's and mother's play sensitivity with their toddler, parental rejection during childhood, and parental divorce. Within the group of avoidantly mother-attached infants, one-half experienced a father who was above average in his play sensitivity a year later. In addi-

tion, half of the mothers who were relatively insensitive to their infant's signals (but by far not as insensitive as the mothers of "A-babies" in Ainworth's study; see K. Grossmann et al., 1985) became sensitively supportive and appropriately challenging toward their 2- and 3-year-old in play situations. Furthermore, only one-third of the "A-with-mother" infants experienced subsequent parental separation, compared to 50% of the "B-with-mother" infants. Parental separation had a great impact on adolescent representation of attachment (Zimmermann, Fremmer-Bombik, Spangler, & Grossmann, 1997). At the age of 22 years, however, many subjects had reflected on this experience such that parental divorce was no longer a major but only a mediating variable. In sum, infant pattern of attachment by itself did not forecast those parental and child behaviors that were predictive of later partnership and attachment representations.

Ainsworth (1990) asked attachment researchers to venture into creating methods that reflect the richness and the anthropological wisdom of attachment theory and its roots in evolution. We replicated her most influential finding that infants' balance of attachment and exploratory behaviors at home and in the Strange Situation is a developmental outcome of early experiences with mother. Beyond infancy and beyond assessing maternal ability to calm the infant's aroused attachment system by loving closeness, we explored a large variety of assessments and methods. What do attachment and exploration experiences with mother and father mean for the development of psychological security, that is, for the development of secure inner working models of self in relation to close others? If adults' inner working models have to be continuously aware of changes in the outside reality, and if a relative absence of negative psychological defenses that distort intolerable aspects of reality is required for healthy self-reliance and psychological security (Bowlby, 1980, 1988a), then we must explore influences from many sources during the long learning process as the child develops throughout the years of immaturity. Creating new methods of assessing psychological security was our attempt to understand the complexities of influences.

CONCLUSION AND REFLECTIONS FROM TODAY'S PERSPECTIVE: ADVOCATING THE CONCEPT OF PSYCHOLOGICAL SECURITY

We have defined psychological security in terms of a coherent, reflective, and balanced discourse about attachment and partnership relationships that is relatively free of psychological restrictions (K. E. Grossmann, 1999; Nelson, 1999). Our series of long-term longitudinal studies suggest that psychological security in early adulthood depends on a history of secure emotional organization *and* freedom to explore and evaluate past and present attachment relationships with parents and/or partners.

In both studies, psychological security was entrained by experiences with both parents throughout the years of immaturity. These experiences, in turn, shaped the child's and adolescent's strategy of thinking and behaving when meeting emotional challenges. Sensitive, supportive, and accepting mothers and fathers fostered their children's psychological security beginning in infancy and spanning across 20 years. In contrast, parental rejection and insensitivity were reflected in the young adult's disavowal of attachment and the value of close relationships; moreover, these youths lacked the freedom to explore, communicate openly, and rely on the help of others in times of distress.

In addition to our work's implications for attachment theory, 30 years' experience in longitudinal research has impressed us with the importance of appreciating (1) uncertainty, (2) attention to mechanisms, (3) philosophy of science, and (4) a lesson learned from ethology. We shall explain each issue in its own right.

Neither long-term longitudinal studies nor an individual child's development can be mapped in advance with much certainty. Much as every new phase of development offers the child a new perspective on his or her experience and on his or her possibilities, each new assessment in each of our studies was a challenge in exploring new methodologies and requiring interpretations from "a wider view" (K. E. Grossmann et al., 1999). For example, guided by the ethological perspective, we used a variety of methodological approaches in addition to standard assessments of quality of attachment to assess the quality of parental responsiveness to the infant's attachment and exploratory needs. Dealing with the uncertainty in this way, we increased the chances of making correct choices of measurements. When, indeed, we found no clear line of stable security or stable insecurity on the basis of the Strange Situation procedure, we still discovered an impressive series of relations between early parental behaviors and later representations of close relationships. In our studies, the Strange Situation remained a valuable tool validating the infants' previously experienced maternal sensitivity and it forecast attachment development during childhood. However, our measures of quality of parent–child interactions better predicted representations of close relationships in adolescence and young adulthood.

Searching for the mechanisms behind developmental processes in attachment, we did not only look at outcomes but kept asking and observing how different internalizations of experiences with attachment figures expressed themselves as different qualities of dealing constructively with challenges across a variety of situations. As part of our future work on mechanisms behind the processes of adjustment and maladjustment, psychological defenses as conceptualized by George Vaillant (2000) may play a central role as they are imbedded in the functioning of inner working models (Ainsworth, 1990; Bowlby, 1980). Our research group analyzed the AAI transcripts of the Regensburg adolescents for psychological defenses, in which we had asked how they viewed negative experiences with their attachment figures. Adolescents classified independently as secure gave significantly more indications of positive defenses such as "reflectivity," "altruism," "humor," and "sublimation" than were found for those classified avoidant or enmeshed in their state of mind with respect to attachment. High degrees of enmeshment revealed—unsurprisingly—an inclination to react impulsively and to use guilt-inducing techniques (Hetterich, 2004). The use of positive, instead of negative, restricting defenses may turn out to be one of the mechanisms that may enable insecure persons to overcome their constricted thinking and free them of the influence of old inner working models (Bowlby, 1988b, Chap. 8). We assume, however, that such a change outside psychotherapy can occur only with the help of a new supportive and caring partner.

In terms of philosophy of science, the ethological concept of behavioral adaptation of one individual to his close kin group, with its extension to mental adaptation as part of personality development, was already part of attachment theory (Ainsworth & Bowlby, 1991). We applied it to our empirical research. This kind of research is ideographic, inductive, and descriptive. It doesn't translate easily into experimental causation, which is the dominant paradigm in most of psychological research and which is appropriate for physiological analyses. However, the physiology of a person is functioning in the service of insecure as well as secure adaptations. Healthy psychological adaptation is related to a person's freedom to evaluate his or her psychological experiences on the basis of secure relationships. No single event is ever the cause for behaving in one way or another, but behaviors emerge from probable tendencies, depending on the person's social development, on the resulting organization of emotions, on current circumstances, and on the severity or inflexibility of psychological constraints. Such systems cannot be reduced to a few "independent" variables.

The lesson we learned from ethology is that intensive and detailed observations of adaptive/constructive or maladaptive/unconstructive behaviors to phylogenetically preprogrammed social systems, as we were taught by Konrad Lorenz, could be easily merged with Ainsworth's and Bowlby's visions of human adaptation. All three teachers gave us confidence to continue our emphasis on direct observation and to further explore the wider view of attachment development. Instead of relying on readily available methods of assessment constructed often for different samples, circumstances, or purposes and based on different theoretical backgrounds, we instead observed and analyzed how parents and children behaved in structured challenging situations more or less constructively, trustingly, or securely with each other.

Agreeing with Belsky (Chapter 4, this volume), we do not suppose that secure attachment is adaptive per se under every condition. Insecure attachment may at times serve an adaptive function when circumstances are difficult (Main, 1981), but only at the expense of less flexible adaptations to different circumstances and situations when they change. We see secure attachment as an optimal organization of emotions and behaviors around a—at least temporarily—stronger and wiser attachment figure (Ainsworth, 1985). This implies the greatest possible potential for (1) individual psychological strength and resilience by relying trustingly on others when in distress, and (2) for sympathetically communicating knowledge and insights with close others. Such communications enable each partner to act in a partnership-corrected manner that fosters close bonds. Ethological thinking as a principle helped us to identify limitations or ease of adaptation in a wide variety of circumstances related to inner working models of attachment due to different past experiences with attachment figures.

The influence of experiences primarily with both parents as attachment figures on individual differences in mental and behavioral development has now been firmly established. This knowledge has enriched psychology. We are happy to have had the stamina to carry through, with much support from our colleagues at home and all over the world, to overcome doubts, and to selectively ignore criticisms. Attachment theory indeed has profoundly changed developmental psychology, providing theoretical coherence within natural history that has never existed before. Attachment theory and research has successfully taken the individual out of his artificial isolated position within much of psychological experimental research. Attachment theory gave him back his social nature.

ACKNOWLEDGMENTS

In the longitudinal studies, our main coworkers and their foci were (1) young adulthood—Kerstin Stöcker, Karin Strasser, Monika Winter, and Anika Keppler; (2) adolescence—Peter Zimmermann and Fabienne Becker-Stoll; (3) middle childhood—Hermann Scheuerer-Englisch, Christine Stephan, and Petra August-Frenzel; (4) fathers—Heinz Kindler; (5) preschool age—Gerhard Suess; (6) parental attachment representation—Elisabeth Fremmer-Bombik; and many doctoral and masters students.

The Bielefeld Project was initially funded by a grant from the Volkswagen Foundation, followed by several grants from the German Research Council. The German Research Council also provided initial support for our second longitudinal study, the Regensburg Project. Extension and completion of our longitudinal work, as presented here, would not have been possible without the generous support by a private research foundation, the Dr. Lotte Koehler Foundation, Munich, which we acknowledge with deep gratitude.

We are grateful to Everett Waters, our coeditor, and Laura Specht Patchkofsky, Senior Production Editor at The Guilford Press, for their skill in transforming our German-English into an excellent English text.

REFERENCES

Ainsworth, M. D. S. (1967). *Infancy in Uganda: Infant care and the growth of love.* Baltimore: Johns Hopkins University Press.

Ainsworth, M. D. S. (1973). The development of infant–mother attachment. In B. M. Caldwell & H. N. Ricciuti (Eds.), *Review of child development research* (Vol. 3, pp. 1–94). Chicago: University of Chicago Press.

Ainsworth, M. D. S. (1985). Attachment across the life span. *Bulletin of the New York Academy of Medicine, 61* (9), 792–812.

Ainsworth, M. D. S. (1990). Some considerations regarding theory and assessment relevant to attachments beyond infancy. In M. T. Greenberg, D. Cicchetti, & E. M. Cummings (Eds.), *Attachment in the preschool years* (pp. 463–488). Chicago and London: University of Chicago Press.

Ainsworth, M. D. S. & Bell, S. M. (1974). Mother–infant interaction and the development of competence. In K. J. Connolly & J. Bruner (Eds.), *The growth of competence* (pp. 97–118). London and New York: Academic Press.

Ainsworth, M. D. S., Bell, S. M., & Stayton, D. J. (1974). Infant–mother attachment and social development: "Socialization" as a product of reciprocal responsiveness to signals. In P. M. Richards (Ed.), *The integration of a child into a social world* (pp. 99–135). Cambridge, UK: Cambridge University Press.

Ainsworth, M. D. S., & Bowlby, J. (1991). An ethological approach to personality development. *American Psychologist, 46* (4), 333–341.

Allen, J. P. & Hauser, T. H. (1996). Autonomy and relatedness in adolescent–family interactions as predictors of young adults' states of mind regarding attachment. *Development and Psychopathology, 8*, 793–809.

Amato P. R. (1998). More than money?: Men's contributions to their children's lives. In A. Booth & A. C. Crouter (Eds.), *Men in families: When do they get involved? What difference does it make?* (pp. 241–278). Mahwah, NJ: Erlbaum.

Becker-Stoll, F. (1997). *Interaktionsverhalten zwischen Jugendlichen und Müttern im Kontext längsschnittlicher Bindungsentwicklung* [Interactions between adolescents and their mothers in the context of longitudinal development of attachment]. Unpublished doctoral dissertation, Universität Regensburg, Regensburg, Germany.

Bowlby, J. (1951). *Maternal care and mental health.* Geneva: World Health Organization.

Bowlby, J. (1973). *Attachment and loss: Vol. 2. Separation, anxiety and anger.* New York: Basic Books.

Bowlby, J. (1980). *Attachment and loss: Vol. 3. Loss, sadness and depression.* New York: Basic Books.

Bowlby, J. (1982). *Attachment and loss: Vol. 1. Attachment* (2nd rev. ed.). New York: Basic Books.

Bowlby, J. (1987). Attachment. In R. L. Gregory (Ed.), *The Oxford companion to the mind* (pp. 57–58). Oxford, UK: Oxford University Press.

Bowlby, J. (1988a). Developmental psychiatry comes of age. *American Journal of Psychiatry, 145*, 1–10.

Bowlby, J. (1988b). *A secure base: Clinical applications of attachment theory.* London: Tavistock/Routledge.

Bowlby, J. (1991). Postscript. In C. M. Parkes, J. Stevenson-Hinde, & P. Marris (Eds.), *Attachment across the life cycle* (pp. 293–297). New York: Routledge.

Breland, K. & Breland, M. (1961). The misbehavior of organisms. *American Psychologist, 16*, 689–684.

Breland, K., & Breland, M. (1966). *Animal behavior.* London: Collier-Macmillan.

Crowell, J., & Owens, G. (1998). *Current Relationship Interview and scoring system.* Unpublished manuscript, State University of New York at Stony Brook.

Fremmer-Bombik, E. (1987). *Beobachtungen zur Beziehungsqualität im zweiten Lebensjahr und ihre Bedeutung im Lichte mütterlicher Kindheitserinnerungen* [Observations of attachment quality in the second year of life and its meaning with respect to maternal memories of childhood]. Unpublished doctoral dissertation, University of Regensburg.

George, C., West, M., & Pettem, O. (1999). *Adult attachment projective protocol and classification system.* Unpublished manuscript, Mills College, Oakland, CA.

Grossmann, K., Fremmer-Bombik, E., & Grossmann, K. E. (1990). Familiar and unfamiliar patterns of attachment of Japanese infants. In *Annual report, Research and Clinical Center for Child Development* (pp. 30–39). Sapporo, Japan: Hokkaido University.

Grossmann, K., Fremmer-Bombik, E., Rudolph, J., & Grossmann, K. E. (1988). Maternal attachment representations as related to patterns of infant–mother attachment and maternal care during the first year. In R. A. Hinde & J. Stevenson-Hinde (Eds.), *Relationships within families* (pp. 241–260). Oxford, UK: Oxford Science.

Grossmann, K., & Grossmann, K. E. (1969). Frühe Reizung und frühe Erfahrung: Forschung und Kritik [Early stimulation and early experience: Research and critique]. *Psychologische Rundschau, 20*(3), 163–175.

Grossmann, K., & Grossmann, K. E. (1991). Newborn behavior, early parenting quality and later toddler–parent relationships in a group of German infants. In J. K. Nugent, B. M. Lester & T. B. Brazelton (Eds.), *The cultural context of infancy* (Vol. 2, pp. 3–38). Norwood, NJ: Ablex.

Grossmann, K., & Grossmann, K.E. (2004). *Bindung. Das Gefüge psychischer Sicherheit* [Attachment: The composition of psychological security]. Stuttgart, Germany: Klett-Cotta.

Grossmann, K., Grossmann, K. E., Fremmer-Bombik, E., Kindler, H., Scheuerer-Englisch, H., & Zimmermann, P. (2002a). The uniqueness of the child–father attachment relationship: Fathers' sensitive and challenging play as the pivotal variable in a 16-year longitudinal study. *Social Development, 11*, 307–331.

Grossmann, K., Grossmann, K. E., Fremmer-Bombik, E., Kindler, H., Scheuerer-Englisch, H., Winter, M., & Zimmermann, P. (2002b). Väter und ihre Kinder—

Die "andere" Bindung und ihre längsschnittliche Bedeutung für die Bindungs-entwicklung, das Selbstvertrauen und die soziale Entwicklung des Kindes [Fathers and their children—a different attachment and its longitudinal signifi-cance for the child's attachment development, self-reliance, and social develop-ment]. In K. Steinhardt, W. Datler, & J. Gstach (Eds.), *Die Bedeutung des Vaters in der frühen Kindheit* [The significance of the father in early childhood] (pp. 43–72). Gießen: Psychosozial Verlag.

Grossmann, K., Grossmann, K.E., Spangler, G., Suess, G., & Unzner, L. (1985). Maternal sensitivity and newborns' orientation responses as related to quality of attachment in northern Germany. In I. Bretherton & E. Waters (Eds.), Growing points in attachment theory and research. *Monographs of the Society for Research in Child Development, 50*(1–2, Serial No. 209), 233–256.

Grossmann, K., Thane, K., & Grossmann, K. E. (1981). Maternal tactual contact of the newborn after various postpartum conditions of mother–infant contact. *Developmental Psychology, 17*(2), 158–169.

Grossmann, K. E. (1967). Behavioral differences between rabbits and cats. *Journal of Genetic Psychology, 111*, 171–182.

Grossmann, K. E. (1973). Continuous, fixed ratio and fixed interval reinforcement in honey bees. *Journal of the Experimental Analysis of Behavior, 20*, 105–109.

Grossmann, K. E. (1999). Old and new internal working models of attachment: The organization of feelings and language. *Attachment and Human Development, 1*, 253–269.

Grossmann, K. E., & Grossmann, K. (1990). The wider concept of attachment in cross-cultural research. *Human Development, 33*, 31–47.

Grossmann, K. E., & Grossmann, K. (1991). Attachment quality as an organizer of emotional and behavioral responses in a longitudinal perspective. In C. M. Parkes, J. Stevenson-Hinde, & P. Marris (Eds.), *Attachment across the life cycle* (pp. 93–114). London: Tavistock/Routledge.

Grossmann, K. E., & Grossmann, K. (1999). Mary Ainsworth: Our guide to attach-ment research. *Attachment and Human Development, 1*, 224–228.

Grossmann, K. E., Grossmann, K., Huber, F., & Wartner, U. (1981). German chil-dren's behavior towards their mothers at 12 months and their fathers at 18 months in Ainsworth's Strange Situation. *International Journal of Behavioral Development, 4*, 157–181.

Grossmann, K. E., Grossmann, K., & Keppler, A. (in press). Universal and culturally specific aspects of human behavior: The case of attachment. In W. Friedlmeier, P. Chakkarath, & B. Schwarz (Eds.), *Culture and human development: The impor-tance of cross-cultural research to the social sciences.* Amsterdam: Swetz & Zeitlinger.

Grossmann, K. E., Grossmann, K., Winter, M., & Zimmermann, P. (2002). Attach-ment relationships and appraisal of partnership: From early experience of sensi-tive support to later relationship representation. In L. Pulkkinen & A. Caspi (Eds.), *Paths to successful development* (pp. 73–105). Cambridge, UK: Cam-bridge University Press.

Grossmann, K. E., Grossmann, K., & Zimmermann, P. (1999). A wider view of attachment and exploration: Stability and change during the years of immaturity. In J. Cassidy & P. R. Shaver (Eds.), *Handbook of attachment: Theory, research, and clinical applications* (pp. 760–786). New York: Guilford Press.

Grotevant, H., & Cooper, C. R. (1985). Patterns of interaction in family relationships and the development of identity formation in adolescence. *Child Development, 56*, 415–428.

Hetterich, S. (2004). *Unterschiede in der Verwendung adaptiver und maladaptiver Abwehrmechanismen in narrativen Darstellungen früher Bindungserinnerungen* [Differences in applying adaptive and maladaptive defense mechanisms in narrations of early attachment memories]. Diplom Arbeit, Universität Regensburg, Regensburg, Germany.

Immelmann, K., Barlow, G., Petrinovich, L. & Main, M. (Eds.). (1981). *Behavioral development: The Bielefeld Interdisciplinary Project.* New York: Cambridge University Press.

Keppler, A. (2004). *Entwicklung sicherer und unsicherer internaler Arbeitsmodelle* [Development of secure and insecure inner working models]. Unpublished doctoral dissertation, Universität Regensburg, Regensburg, Germany.

Kobak, R. R. (1993). *The adult attachment Q-sort.* Unpublished manuscript, University of Delaware.

Main, M. (1977). Sicherheit und Wissen [Security and knowledge]. In K.E. Grossmann (Ed.), *Entwicklung der Lernfähigkeit in der sozialen Umwelt* [Development of the ability to learn in social context] (pp. 47–95.). Munich, Germany: Kindler.

Main, M. (1981). Avoidance in the service of attachment: A working paper. In K. Immelmann, G. Barlow, L. Petrinovich, & M. Main (Eds.), *Behavioral development: The Bielefeld Interdisciplinary Project* (pp. 651–693). New York: Cambridge University Press.

Main, M. (1983). Exploration, play, and cognitive functioning related to infant–mother attachment. *Infant Behavior and Development, 6*, 167–174.

Main, M., & Cassidy, J. (1988). Categories of response to reunion with the parent at age six: Predictable from infant attachment classification and stable over a one-month period. *Developmental Psychology, 24*(3), 415–426.

Main, M., & Weston, D. R. (1981). The quality of the toddler's relationship to mother and to father: Related to conflict behavior and the readiness to establish new relationships. *Child Development, 52, 932–940.*

Nelson, K. (1999). Event representations, narrative development, and internal working models. *Attachment and Human Development, 1*(3), 239–251.

Solomon, J., & George, C. (1999). The measurement of attachment security in infancy and childhood. In J. Cassidy & P. R. Shaver (Eds.), *Handbook of attachment: Theory, research and clinical applications* (pp. 287–316). New York: Guilford Press.

Stöcker, K. (2003). *Bindung und Partnerschaft* [Attachment and partnership]. Unpublished doctoral dissertation, Universität Regensburg, Regensburg, Germany.

Strasser, K. (in prep). *Einflüsse auf die Bindungsrepräsentation im frühen Erwachsenenalter über den Lebenslauf* [Influences on the attachment representation in early adulthood over the life course]. Unpublished doctoral dissertation, Universität Regensburg, Regensburg, Germany.

Suess, G., Grossmann, K. E., & Sroufe, L. A. (1992). Effects of infant attachment to mother and father on quality of adaptation in preschool: From dyadic to individual organization of self. *International Journal of Behavioral Development, 15,* 43–65.

Tanner, J. M., & Inhelder, B. (1963). Discussions on child development. A consideration of the biological and cultural approaches to the understanding of human development and behavior. In *Proceedings of the Meetings of the World Health Organization Study Group on the Psychobiological Development of the Child* (vols. 1–4). London: Tavistock.

Vaillant, G. E. (2000). Adaptive mental mechanisms: Their role in a positive psychology. *American Psychologist, 55,* 89–98.

van IJzendoorn, M. H., & Kroonenberg, P. M. (1988). Cross-cultural patterns of attachment: A meta-analysis of the Strange Situation. *Child Development, 59,* 147–156.

van IJzendoorn, M. H., & Sagi, A. (1999). Cross-cultural patterns of attachment: Universal and contextual dimensions. In J. Cassidy & P. R. Shaver (Eds.), *Handbook of attachment: Theory, research and clinical applications* (pp. 713–734). New York: Guilford Press.

Wartner, U. G. (1987). *Attachment in infancy and at age six, and children's self-concept: A follow-up of a German longitudinal study.* Unpublished doctoral dissertation, University of Virginia, Charlottesville.

Wartner, U. G., Grossmann, K., Fremmer-Bombik, E., & Suess, G. (1994). Attachment patterns at age six in south Germany: Predictability from infancy and implications for preschool behavior. *Child Development, 65,* 1014–1027.

Zimmermann, P. (1999). Structure and functions of internal working models of attachment and their role for emotion regulation. *Attachment and Human Development, 1,* 291–306.

Zimmermann, P., & Becker-Stoll, F. (2002). Stability of attachment representations in adolescence—the influence of ego-identity status. *Journal of Adolescence, 25,* 107–124.

Zimmermann, P., Fremmer-Bombik, E., Spangler, G., & Grossmann, K. E. (1997). Attachment in adolescence: A longitudinal perspective. In W. Koops, J. B. Hoeksma, & D. C. van den Boom (Eds.), *Development of interaction and attachment: Traditional and non-traditional approaches* (pp. 281–292). Amsterdam: North-Holland.

CHAPTER 6

Understanding and Resolving
Emotional Conflict

The London Parent-Child Project

HOWARD STEELE
MIRIAM STEELE

In this chapter we review what strikes us the common thread in our findings from 12 years of longitudinal attachment research, that is, the enormous value for parents, and in turn children, to understand and resolve emotional conflict within and between people. Individual differences in this essential psychological capacity may be reliably identified with the research methods we use, including the Adult Attachment Interview (AAI), the Strange Situation, and emotion narrative tasks we have relied on with older children. As we see it, these methods capture individual differences in the ways parents and children approach, understand, and try to resolve the inevitable emotional conflicts that lie at the heart of family life. Thus, the chapter takes this theme as its title, and we revisit it throughout as we work our way through summarizing what we observed earliest in our research through to what we have found most recently, in the context of our 11–12 year follow-up. We begin with personal reflections on how our careers as longitudinal attachment researchers began, along with some notes on where, and from whom, we gained our inspiration.

CONTEXT

We came to attachment theory and research through our interest in psychoanalysis, firmly rooted in the context of our experience as graduate students at Hebrew University in Jerusalem in 1983–1984. Freud attended the opening of the Hebrew University in 1925, when he had expressed the hope that psychoanalysis would become a core topic of study at the institution. However, when the psychology department was set up, it's members understandably sought to establish their scientific *not* psychoanalytic credibility. Thus, when we arrived in Jerusalem in 1983, Miriam with her undergraduate degree in psychology, and Howard with his undergraduate degree in history and M.A. in religious studies from University of British Columbia (UBC) in Vancouver, Canada—we were surprised and delighted to find the recently established Sigmund Freud Centre for Research and Study in Psychoanalysis at the Mount Scopus campus of Hebrew U. The first incumbent of the Chair in the Freud Centre was from London, England—Professor Joseph Sandler—who, together with his wife Anne-Marie Sandler, made Freud's dream (and ours to study psychoanalysis!) a reality. From the Sandlers we soaked up a range of psychoanalytic thinking, including their object relational assumption that every wish arising in the mind involves a mental model of the self and the other, and a wished-for interaction (Sandler & Sandler, 1978). We also learned about the powerful role assigned to early experiences as an organizer of later development via psychological structures, including defensive processes, that are resistant to change.

We left Jerusalem in 1984 nourished by the invitation Anne-Marie Sandler had extended when Miriam professed her interest to train as a child psychotherapist—very plainly, Anne-Marie said, "Come to Hampstead." We would do so, but not before spending a year working as research assistants on developmental and clinical research projects in the UBC Psychology Dept (Miriam with Tannis Macbeth and Howard with Peter Suedfeld), and a subsequent year (1985–1986) in New York at Teachers College where each of us completed an MA degree in developmental psychology. Larry Aber, then at Barnard College, made us familiar with how certain core psychoanalytic ideas about the significance of early experience were supremely well articulated in John Bowlby's attachment theory and well validated by Mary Ainsworth's observational research. We were not, at first, it should be said, deeply enthused by the approach that placed all children in one of three attachment categories. Didn't this approach deny the individuality of the child better appreciated by more traditional psychoanalytic authors like Anna Freud or Donald Winnicott? Persuaded that a fuller set of psychoanalytic training opportunities were available in London, we began PhD studies in 1986 at University College London where Howard was to work with Joe Sandler on psychoanalytic theories of conflict and defense, and Miriam was to work with Peter Fonagy, who agreed to supervise her intended work on the transition to parenthood.

We returned to the Society for Research in Child Development monograph (Main, Kaplan, & Cassidy, 1985) we had brought from New York on "growing points of attachment theory and research" concentrating on Main, Kaplan, and Cassidy's "move to the level of representation" and their seminal report on intergenerational links between infant–parent attachment and attachment interviews collected 5 years later. This work provided the rubric under which we would work together on a study of the transition to parenthood, taking a systematic account of both expectant mothers' and fathers' psychological conflicts, anxieties, and defensive strategies stemming from their own childhood experiences. We were thus launched on the longitudinal attachment study we referred to as the London Parent–Child Project, which we have pursued from our institutional "secure" bases in London, namely, the Psychology Department at University College London and the Anna Freud Centre. Presently, in the summer of 2004, we are bidding farewell to London and returning to New York, in order to accept academic posts in the Graduate Faculty of the New School for Social Research, where our theoretical orientation—exploring the psychoanalytic roots and applications of attachment theory—has been warmly welcomed.

Our luck in beginning our longitudinal attachment work in London was greatly augmented by the experience of receiving advice on a regular basis, during the early stages (1986–1990), from John Bowlby. In the late 1980s, he still maintained his office at the Tavistock Clinic where he had been based for more than 40 years. His office served as a central clearinghouse for all matters to do with attachment manuscripts in preparation, in press, and published. Bowlby facilitated our attendance at the 1987 Adult Attachment Interview Institute, convened by John Byng-Hall, and taught by Mary Main and Erik Hesse, in London at the Tavistock Clinic. This valuable training enabled us to reliably rate and classify the 200 AAIs we collected from 100 expectant mothers and their partners, the expectant fathers.

When we asked John Bowlby where we should go to learn about the Strange Situation, he said, "Go to Regensburg"—and so we did! In the summer of 1988, we observed the intricately organized hierarchy of "working models," including coteaching, coworking, cosupervising, and remarkable cooperation, within the diverse research team of undergraduates, graduates, and postdoctoral researchers directed by Karin and Klaus Grossmann. We shared stories about how best to cultivate the interest and commitment of participants in longitudinal attachment research. Such simple things as sending birthday cards can consolidate participant–researcher relationships, and help researchers track addresses of participating families. With respect to how to administer the Strange Situation, the Grossmanns helpfully pointed out: "Go by the child, not by the clock." A 12-month-old does not need to be left distressed in a separation for 3 minutes—15–30 seconds of distress is ample evidence that the attachment system is activated. We went on to collect 96 Strange Situation observations of 12-month-old infants with their mothers, and 90 observations of 18-month-old infants with their fathers. Following formal training from the expert teacher of Mary Jo Ward (in 1989) concerning the rating of Strange Situation tapes, we arrived at reliable classifications and ratings, first of the infant–mother, and later of the infant–father, attachment relationship.

Ours was the first report of a prospective link between pregnant women's responses to the AAI and their infants' attachment to them at 1 year, findings that we rushed to publish (Fonagy, Steele, & Steele, 1991). Similarly, we provided the first report of an independent link between the AAI responses of expectant fathers and their infants' attachments to them at 18 months of age (H. Steele, M. Steele, & Fonagy, 1996). While there had been previous reports of such intergenerational links, these prior studies had been based on interviews collected from parents 6 years after the transition to parenthood (K. Grossmann & K. E. Grossmann, 1988; Main, Kaplan, & Cassidy, 1985). Hence, with respect to this pioneering work with the AAI, it could be claimed that the levels of coherence and valuing of relationships observed in the attachment interviews from these parents may have resulted, in part, from *becoming and being a parent* (i.e., an influence of the child upon the parent). Our early work sought to show that intergenerational patterns of attachment could be demonstrated even when the AAI was administered *before* there was any child on the scene. Indeed, we found that the cross-generational link was similarly, and distinctively, evident for both mothers and fathers (H. Steele et al., 1996).

IMPLICATIONS OF INTERGENERATIONAL PATTERNS OF ATTACHMENT: SOCIAL OR GENETIC TRANSMISSION PROCESSES?

Our powerful cross-generational evidence bolstered the understanding of the nature and determinants of attachment security during infancy. While the pioneering studies including assessments of infant–mother and infant–father attachment had demonstrated statistical independence of these relationships (K. E. Grossmann & K. Grossmann, 1981; Main & Weston, 1981), controversy has endured over the extent to which attachments to parents are learned or somehow given at birth by our genetically based emotional predispositions as some have argued (e.g., see Fox, Kimmerly, & Schafer, 1991). We have sought to understand this link across generations between attachment narratives of the parents and their infants' attachments in terms of psychoanalytic ideas about emotion regulation and the social influences of parents upon their children. Bowlby (1973) had drawn attention to this intergenerational phenomenon, highlighting how social influences may be as important, if not more so, than genetic influences. However, it was a long time before this assumption was systematically explored (O'Connor, Croft, & H. Steele, 2000). Recent twin studies have addressed this question for the first time. These studies underline probable social origins for infant–mother patterns of attachment, namely, that shared environmental effects, not heritability, account for the vast majority of variance in concordance of child–mother attachments among a large number of monozygotic and dizygotic twins studied in independent laboratories (Bokhorst et al., 2003; O'Connor & Croft, 2001). This work gives considerable additional weight to claims that attachment during early childhood is a relationship-specific construct. But what in the parent is being transmitted to what in the child? To fill in the canvas, we have found it useful to draw widely from psychoanalytic object relations theories (e.g., Bowlby, 1979; Sandler & Sandler, 1998; Winnicott, 1971) and convergent theories of emotional development (Gottmann, Katz, & Hooven, 1997; Tomkins, 1963).

OBJECT RELATIONS THEORIES
AND EMOTION REGULATION

Object relations theories share the assumption that the principal emotional motivation in human life is the wish to form and maintain relationships to others, for the survival value and satisfaction provided by significant enduring relationships. In the first place, it is typically mothers who are this "other" but, in time, fathers, grandparents, and indeed anyone able and willing to play an ongoing caregiving role toward the child is likely to be the intense focus of the child's relationship needs. Bowlby documented how early child–caregiver relationships reflect the environment in which we evolved. He saw newborns' gestures and heard the newborns' cries as component instincts of the attachment behavioral system. Bowlby jettisoned Freudian instinct theory in favor of his more contemporary ethological, cognitive, yet also psychoanalytic theory of child development. We have discussed in detail the sense in which, for his psychoanalytic colleagues in the early 1960s, this was a step too far, such that Bowlby was widely shunned by other psychoanalysts including other object relations theorists, especially the group who followed the thinking of Melanie Klein (for a full discussion, see H. Steele & M. Steele, 1998, 1999). Nonetheless, Bowlby remained a psychoanalyst all his long professional life and continued to regard attachment theory as an object relations theory (see Bretherton, 1998). He desisted from talking about the child's "internal world," abandoning this term to the Kleinians whom he perceived as giving far too little attention to external "lived" reality. In the service of his evolutionary perspective, Bowlby (1969/2000) incorporated from cognitive psychology the term "internal working model" to refer to the process by which children arrive at (in the best of circumstances) "tolerably accurate" internal representations of their relationship experiences. The internal working model concept, and its meaning-making capacities, has been most thoroughly excavated and extended (see Bretherton, 1999) to show that "lived" experiences are represented at various levels of specificity within the mind, serving as guides to perception of the self and others, including strategies for how to interpret negative emotions and engage in behavioral strategies for managing these.

The relationship specificity of this process during infancy is nothing less than remarkable. Decades of research by ourselves and others confirms the probable nature of this amazing social process, the behavior displayed by young children in the Ainsworth Strange Situation, particularly upon reunion, reflects internalized strategies they have learned *from the specific caregiver they are being observed with* for displaying and sharing negative affect or psychic conflict. Infants with an avoidant attachment to mother have learned to reveal as little as possible about their inner experiences of negative affect, which makes sense against the background of their mothers who have been observed to be singularly nonresponsive to negative affect (K. E. Grossmann, K. Grossmann, & Schwan, 1986). Infants with avoidant attachments have learned that it doesn't pay to acknowledge conflict, that it is better to pretend that all is well even when deep down (at identifiable psychophysiological levels) pronounced and enduring distress can be discerned (Spangler & K. E. Grossmann, 1993). The infant with a resistant attachment has learned to overtly display what are often intense negative emotions, doing so in a petulant/fighting or passive/withdrawn manner without any clear expectation of his or her needs being met, which in fact go unmet over the 20-minute observation (see Cassidy & Berlin, 1994). For these infants, they cannot help showing themselves to be in an acute emotional conflict, conveying a sense of confusion as to from where, and from whom, a strategy out of their painful circumstances may come. This is consistent with the observational work of Haft and Slade (1989), who posit that such resistant babies are likely to have been cared for by parents who ignore or misconstrue their emotional signals. In contrast to these insecure (avoidant or resistant) patterns, the infant with a secure attachment is often joyful in the presence of the parent, openly displays negative emotion, and shows confidence in his or her needs being met by the caregiver. Securely attached infants have been repeatedly shown to have parents who have helped them to achieve an emerging sense of balance and control with respect to the management of negative and positive emotions. In other words, securely attached infants appear to have learned that unmanageable feelings of distress can be resolved with the help of the caregiver. Finally, infants who show disorganization at 1 year of age with the parent are shot through with either hopelessness or helplessness (Lyons-Ruth & Jacobvitz, 1999), even as they also give evidence of a more organized avoidant, resistant, or secure strategy. We know from the Spangler and K. E. Grossmann (1993) report that this disorganized group is also likely to be distressed long after the 20-minute observation period is over. In our longitudinal work, we predicted these infant patterns of attachment to mother (at 12 months) and to father (at 18 months) from AAIs obtained from their parents prior to the children's birth. Notably, no infant we observed, of 96 infants seen with their mothers, and 90 seen with their fathers, was disorganized in their attachments to *both* parents. Hence, all four infant patterns of attachment are arguably social in origin, relationship-specific, and stemming from experiences internalized by the child concerning how to regulate emotional conflict.

Before Bowlby had fully launched himself toward attachment theory, with its own distinctive model of human motivation, including aggression as essentially a reaction to frustrated unmet attachment needs, he wrote vividly about the inevitable daily presence in children's lives of intense "libidinal" and "aggressive" feelings, love and hate (Bowlby, 1956/1979). While he would later drop all reference to libido, he did retain it in this lecture, delivered on the anniversary of Freud's birth, in his 1979 collection of lectures, titled *The Making and Breaking of Affectional Bonds*. He placed the 1956 lecture, titled "Psychoanalysis and Child Care" at the front of this slim accessible volume, which merits much reading and rereading. In this lead chapter, he credits Freud (as expected for the occasion) with drawing our attention to the inevitability of ambivalence in human life: "There is nothing unhealthy about conflict. Quite the contrary: conflict is the normal state of affairs in all of us. Every day of our lives we discover afresh that if we follow one course of action we have to forgo others which are also desired" (Bowlby, 1979, p. 6). He also cites Konrad Lorenz, noting that in this respect humans are not unique, since "all animals are constantly beset by impulses which are incompatible with one another, such as attack, flight and sexual approach" (Bowlby, 1979, p. 7). What distinguishes healthy from unhealthy individuals is the extent to which the inevitable conflict between feelings of love and hate, often directed toward the same person, are controlled, regulated, and so resolved. For children, Bowlby tells us this will develop naturally if young children have the loving company of their parents who put up with outbursts of hostility by showing that they are not afraid of hatred and conveying a belief that it can be contained and controlled. Such is "the tolerant atmosphere in which self-control can grow"

(Bowlby, 1979, p. 12). Bowlby maintained then, and throughout his later writings, that a child's need for love and care is paramount and that "provided these needs are met, frustrations of other kinds will be met with well" (Bowlby, 1979, p. 13). Fellow psychoanalysts Dorothy Burlingham and Anna Freud (1944) made a related observation when they remarked on how the positive appraisals made by new mothers about their babies was out of all proportion to reality, adding that this is well and good because soon after, in the toddler years, these mothers will have to be relentlessly nagging their young children in order to instil a moral sensibility. Against the bedrock of early experiences of having one's needs for care and love met, later limit-setting responses from one's parents are frustrations that can be easily accommodated, and are indeed sought after so that the natural wish to explore may be pursued within an environment felt to be safe. Recent attachment research, including our own longitudinal study, strongly suggests that parents capable of mentally and emotionally exploring—*with balance and coherence*—the meaning of their attachment histories are best able to meet their children's social and emotional needs.

THE POWER OF THE ADULT ATTACHMENT INTERVIEW

Meeting the child's needs for love and care in the first year requires a leap of faith on the caregiver's part as babies are inevitably experienced, at least at times, as taking more than they are giving (Hrdy, 1999). We investigated this evolutionary-based social and psychic conflict at 1 year by asking mothers and fathers to describe what they liked best and what they liked least about becoming parents and about their baby. We posed these questions in the context of a 20-minute audiorecorded interview. We transcribed the maternal responses verbatim before training a group of graduate students to rate the transcriptions on a series of scales pertaining to the mothers' thoughts and feelings regarding their babies, and the experience of becoming parents. The students were kept blind to the Strange Situation data and the parents' AAI data. They independently and reliably arrived at ratings of how loving, rejecting, ambivalent, and coherent the mother was when speaking about her baby. Interestingly, when these ratings were correlated with our observations of infant–mother attachment security, there were modestly significant correlations in predicted directions, with mothers of securely attached infants being more loving and coherent, and less rejecting and ambivalent. *But* these interviews, collected concurrently with the Strange Situation, did not enhance the more robust prediction of infant–mother attachment security we could make from the AAIs collected *before* the babies were born (M. Steele, H. Steele, & Fonagy, 1992).

Time and again in our research we have been sent back to consider the significance of parents' responses to the AAI, as it frequently correlates better with later child outcomes than any other parent measure of interest we have obtained from a wide list (see Figure 6.1), including the AAI, and questionnaire measures of marital satisfaction, parents' self-esteem, or parents' neuroticism or extroversion. In addition, the AAI has also often proved to be a much better predictor of longer term child emotion variables than the infant–mother or infant–father Strange Situation data we have collected (e.g., M. Steele, H. Steele, & Johansson, 2002).

Phase 1: Infancy Assessments

   3rd trimester of first pregnancy and 12–18 months later

   (1987–1989)

Expectant parents: AAI, with mood assessmed before and after interview
Strange Situation: Each infant with mother at 12 months and father at 18 months

Phase 2: Early Childhood

   5- and 6-year laboratory assessments

   (1992–1994)

MacArthur Story Stem Battery (5 years)
Theory of Mind (5 years)
Affect Task (6 years)
Other measures: Verbal IQ, life events, repeat parent AAIs

Phase 3: Middle/Late Childhood

   11- to 12-year home visits

   (1999–2001)

Friends and Family Interview (FFI), developed, administered, validated
Modified/extended Affect Task, treated as a clue to social cognition
Verbal IQ, Strengths and Difficulties Questionnaire

Phase 4: Long-term follow-up

   16-year assessments

   (2004–2006) *in progress*

AAIs to 16-year-olds
FFIs to next-born siblings
Questionnaires assessing quality of sibling relationships and mental health

FIGURE 6.1. Overview of London Parent–Child Project: Selected assessments over 4 phases and 17 years.

WHAT DOES
THE ADULT ATTACHMENT INTERVIEW MEASURE?

At the earliest stages of our research, we systematically investigated the psychometric properties of the AAI, which have been the subject of a number of empirical reports (Bakersman-Kranenburg & van IJzendoorn, 1993; Sagi et al., 1994; H. Steele & M. Steele, 1994; Waters & Crowell, 1995). Our own efforts in this direction corroborate the conclusion that the AAI is a uniquely valid measure of competence in the parenting role—that is, it points to the adult who will or will not be likely to meet the child's needs for care and love in the first year, and to manage effectively most if not all later parenting tasks appropriate to each developmental stage in the child's life. Moreover, the parent who does well on the AAI—that is, the adult who is highly coherent regarding his or her attachment experiences (whether favorable or adverse), and credibly valuing of attachment—is not necessarily more verbally intelligent, nor less neurotic, nor more likely to be in a good mood before being interviewed (H. Steele, 1991). The latter finding is worthy of brief elaboration, because it gives further clues as to the emotional profile linked with providing an autonomous-secure as opposed to an insecure (dismissing, preoccupied, or unresolved) response to the AAI. We began our work at a time when effects of mood on memory were popular (Bower, 1984), such that it may have been the case, we posited, that adults who are judged to tell a "good" or a "coherent" attachment story were perhaps in a better mood *before* the interview. We investigated this possibility by asking the pregnant women and their male partners to complete a single-item mood grid with 64 squares illustrating various shadings of mood arrived at by cross-tabulating arousal level and hedonic tone (Russell, Weiss, & Mendelsohn, 1989). Prior to being interviewed with the AAI, the expectant parents we were about to interview had a wide range of mood states, from moderately miserable (low on arousal and low on pleasure) through to moderately positive (high on arousal and high on pleasure). We observed no relation between mood prior to being interviewed and whether or not the AAI that would follow was judged autonomous-secure or insecure. The significant effect we did observe concerned the greater than chance probability that someone who provided a coherent autonomous-secure interview was more likely to be in a good mood *after* the interview. Hence, it seems, *being able to reflect in a coherent manner* upon childhood experiences of being upset, ill, separated from caregivers, rejected, and possibly having suffered loss or abuse—all *contributes to a positive emotional state.*

In other words, it feels good to have discussed openly and in an organized manner how one has managed and resolved emotional conflicts in one's attachment history. This may be the single defining feature of AAIs judged high on coherence and classified autonomous-secure. These interviews show a spontaneous capacity to acknowledge distress in one's past attachment experiences, and to show a range of strategies, both interpersonal and intrapersonal, for managing and resolving negative emotions. By contrast, the speaker who provides an interview classified insecure-dismissing may give a positive picture of his or her attachment history but this lacks credibility (Ds1), or is perhaps peppered with a highly derogating response with respect to one or both parents (Ds2), or is perhaps a cognitive retelling of difficulties that lacks emotional engagement (Ds3). These are the three main subtypes of insecure-dismissing responses, and all tend to leave the speaker feeling exhausted and in a correspondingly negative mood. In ego psychological terms, when there is an overreliance on defensive strategies of denial, isolation of affect, projection, and intellectualization (A. Freud, 1936), the person concerned is likely to be aware of the emotional strain via symptoms of anxiety or impoverished mood, without being able to make the connections to the underlying emotional conflicts causing the symptoms. In the contemporary language of interpersonal strategies for emotion regulation, these dismissing speakers show their tendency to rely on avoidance, contempt, or turning away (e.g., Gottman, 1993), and feel the worse for it. The insecure-preoccupied pattern of response to the AAI suggests a different yet also restricted and burdensome strategy of dealing with negative emotion, namely, one of escalation (the E2 angry stance) or of quiet despair (the E3 passive stance). These speakers too were in a much less positive mood after the interview, according to their own report, and presumably this was also manifestly clear to the interviewer.

IMPLICATIONS OF PARENTS'
ADULT ATTACHMENT INTERVIEW RESPONSES
FOR THEIR CHILDREN'S DEVELOPMENT

Mothers

Though an interview with an expectant parent, or an actual parent, comes to an end after about 45–75 minutes, the responsibility of the parent to the child, and the child's need for the parent, is ongoing. In our follow-up research beyond the assessments of attachment to mother and father in infancy, we have concentrated on obtaining as far as possible the child's view of family life and matters to do with the resolution of inevitable emotional conflicts inherent to family life. At 5 years of age, we found that a most fruitful strategy for accessing the inner world of the child was via presentation of story stems, depicting a domestic emotional conflict via the use of dolls and story beginnings where the child was asked to "show me and tell me what happens next." These emotion narrative stems came from the battery of stories known as the MacArthur Story Stem Battery (Emde, Wolf, & Oppenheim, 2003). We administered 11 different stems to 86 children, taperecorded and videotaped their 956 story completions, and successfully reduced their responses through data-reduction techniques to three internally consistent emotional themes: (1) limit setting (2) prosocial, and (3) antisocial (M. Steele et al., 2003). The most powerful finding to emerge from the statistical analyses was the significantly elevated levels of limit-setting responses (e.g., most commonly evident when children depicted a parent who exercised authority with verbal discipline) among children whose mothers had provided autonomous-secure AAIs more than 5 years previously, before the birth of the children.

This was the first report demonstrating that maternal attachment interviews identified as coherent and secure predict a central organizing feature of 5-year-olds' child narratives, that is, the extent to which they resolve social and emotional dilemmas by referencing an authoritative parent (after Baumrind, 1967). Where maternal interviews were observed to be insecure, either dismissing or preoccupied regarding attachment, their children were much less likely to depict their mothers (in story-stem doll-play responses) as possessing this authoritative characteristic long recognized as an attribute of effective parenting.

Interestingly, it appears that the concept of parental authority was systematically reviewed from an attachment perspective for the first time only in the 1990s (see Bretherton, Golby, & Cho, 1997; Richters & Waters, 1992), despite much previous attention given to parental authority and warmth in the broader literature on childrearing and socialization (e.g., Baumrind, 1967). As Bretherton and colleagues (1997) point out, Bowlby (1973) himself noted that aspects of the parenting style described as *authoritative* in the socialization literature (Baumrind, 1967, 1971) are compatible with the sensitive, accepting, and cooperative parenting behaviors held up as optimal by attachment theory and research. Authoritative parents resembled responsive attachment figures in paying attention to their children's needs and point of view, and tended to use negotiation and reasoning to engage their children's cooperation. In addition, authoritative parents were firm, self-confident, and did not allow themselves to be coerced or manipulated by their children. As Bretherton and colleagues put it, authoritative parents are leaders not dictators. Our results confirm and extend this line of thinking in showing that children's narratives depicting mothers with authoritative characteristics were most likely to come from children whose mothers provided (some 5-plus years previously) an attachment interview likely to be called autonomous-secure, organized, balanced, and coherent.

There is, of course, a deep psychological meaning to *limit setting* in a context of social and emotional arousal and uncertainty, such as is created by the presentation to children of the MacArthur Story Stem Battery. The wider psychoanalytic literature from which attachment theory arose provides some clues. For example, limit setting has much to do with normal development conceived in terms of ego skills including frustration tolerance, delay of gratification, and impulse control (A. Freud, 1965). Further, the normative development of these affect-regulatory and cognitive skills may be seen to depend upon the bedrock provided by a consistent and caring adult (normally the mother) who provides the growing child with a background sense of safety (Sandler, 1958). Interestingly, the title of Joseph Sandler's (1987) collection of his published papers dating from this early paper through the mid-1980s bears the title *From Safety to Superego*, suggesting that moral development depends on a sufficient amount of early attachment experiences that provide an enduring sense of safety. The child whose aggression is not safely limited will be vulnerable to unlimited aggressive impulses.

Understanding Mixed Emotions

One of our most consistent findings over the years of our longitudinal research is related to the influence of the early mother-child relationship, indexed by the AAI from—or the Strange Situation with—mother, upon the child's later ability to imaginatively and resourcefully describe and explain the emotional reactions of others. In our research, these "others" have typically been doll figures, puppets, or characters presented in cartoons. For example, when the children in our study were age 6, we presented them with a series of cartoons depicting social interactions that involved an emotional dilemma or conflict. In the final panel of each cartoon set (there were 12 in total) the characters were drawn without any facial expression. We would then ask the children to assign a face to the characters. Figure 6.2 is an example of one of the cartoon sets and the emotion faces we supplied to the children in transparency form so that they could place them on top of the cartoon drawings. We would probe for a narrative about why the characters(s) were feeling in the manner suggested by the child, inviting consideration of whether more than one feeling might be relevant for any character, and we would also probe for information about whether anyone's feelings might soon change. One child presented with the school block-building drama (see Figure 6.2) described how the successful builder felt "happy" but also "sad" for the friend who was not doing so well. Furthermore, this child suggested that the unsuccessful builder felt "sad" and the teacher felt "happy" for the child who was doing well but "worried" for the other child. Accordingly, the teacher was depicted as praising the child who was doing well and as offering

Teacher: "See what you two
can do with these blocks"

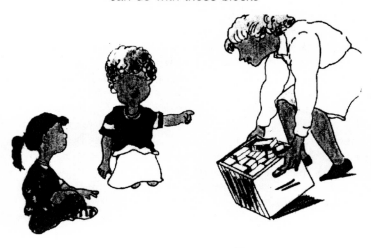

One girl is having an easier time
than the other

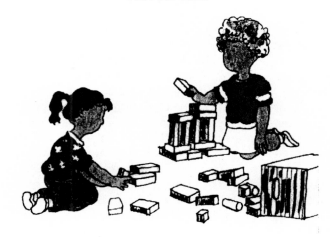

(continued)

FIGURE 6.2. Illustration from the Affect Task.

Whoever drew these pictures forgot to put faces on.
What do you think they are feeling?

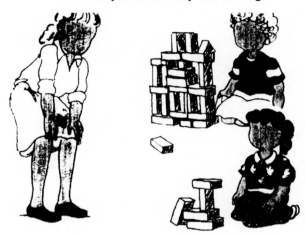

Emotions children were asked
to attribute to cartoon drawings in the Afffect Task

- Fear
- Anger
- Sadness
- Disgust (protruding tongue)
- Angry eyes and sad mouth = mischief
- Surprised eyes and sad mouth = disappointment
- Neutral
- Happy
- Surprised

FIGURE 6.2. *(continued)*

help to the child having trouble. When asked if anyone's feelings might change soon, it was suggested that the "sad" unsuccessful builder would become "happy" because she would soon "get the hang of it." This sensitive and hopeful response would score well on our scale indexing "understanding of mixed emotions," which we consider to be closely linked to interpersonal and intrapersonal conflict-resolution skills. Notably the extant literature at the time of undertaking this work suggested that an understanding of mixed emotions was normally obtained at around 11 years of age (Harter & Buddin, 1987). Yet among the group of 63 6-year-old children who were administered our cartoon-based Affect Task, 40% achieved moderate to high scores for mixed emotion understanding, providing at least one response that resembled the emotionally complex one given above (H. Steele et al., 1999). This group was significantly more likely to have been securely attached to mother at 1 year, and significantly more likely to have a mother whose AAI had been classified autonomous-secure prior to the child's birth. Taken together with convergent evidence from Judy Dunn and her colleagues, these longitudinal findings suggest that the pregnancy AAIs we administered to the mothers, and our subsequent observations of infant–mother attachment at 1 year, were each markers of the kinds of mother–child relationships that would be typified by open and flexible conversations about emotion in the self and others over the early childhood years.

The AAIs we had collected from the fathers, and the infant–father attachments observed at 18 months, did not enhance our prediction of mixed emotion understanding at 6 years. Hence we were led to conclude that children's understanding of emotion may be specifically linked to the history and current status of the mother–child relationship. This was a perspective underscored by our 11-year follow-up when we readministered a version of the Affect Task (M. Steele et al., 2002) in the home setting, and also collected interviews probing for negative and positive feelings about self and relationships to parents, siblings, and best friend (H. Steele & M. Steele, 2004a). When the Affect Task responses at 11 years were coded for evidence of an ability to acknowledge the distress of the central character, and to propose a resourceful coping strategy, it was the early mother–child relationship (indexed by autonomous-secure responses to the pregnancy AAIs) which alone (from our early attachment measures) predicted this emotion understanding outcome that we deemed to be a core feature of social cognition. Concurrent maternal warmth, indexed by a self-report questionnaire completed by the mothers, also correlated with this 11-year child outcome. Notably, however, in the regression analysis (see M. Steele et al., 2002), the pregnancy AAI made a significant and independent contribution to the model even after taking into account the current level of warmth mothers expressed. Thus, the power of longitudinal attachment

research, and in particular of responses to the AAI obtained during pregnancy, was plainly evident in the domain of children's coping with emotional conflict at the cusp of adolescence.

Fathers

Having included fathers, as much as mothers, in the early stages of our
research, we have watched carefully for any distinctive results linking
fathers' AAI responses to their children's social and emotional development. With the single very important exception of individual differences in
fathers' AAI responses being significantly and uniquely associated with
individual differences in their 18-month-old children's attachments to
them, we had a long wait of 10 years before we observed further distinctive
father-related results.

It was in the context of our 11-year follow-up research that we came
across powerful and unique results concerning the early and probably
ongoing father–child relationship upon their children's mental health (H.
Steele & M. Steele, 2001) and social conflict-resolution strategies involving
siblings and peers. In the context of home visits, we interviewed 11-year-
olds about their most favorite and least favorite aspects of themselves, and
their relationships to mother, father, sibling(s), and best friends. We called
this 30-minute audio- and film-recorded task "The Friends and Family
Interview" (H. Steele & M. Steele, 2004b).

The preamble to the interview declared to the young people that
"something we have learned from studying children and families over time
is that some of the strongest feelings we have, good and bad ones, arise in
the context of our family relationships." We further added that "there are
ways in which we like things the way they are, and ways in which we
would like things to change," suggesting "we will be asking you about
these things as we talk about yourself, your family and your best friend." In
the usual way, we assured the young people of confidentiality and advised
them of their ethical right not to answer any questions or indeed to with-
draw at any time if they wished. In fact, each of the more than 50 young
people we interviewed answered all the questions. Their responses were
coded in terms of five global categories:

1. coherence
2. understanding of self and others
3. secure-base availability of parents
4. peer relations and social skills
5. pride in school achievement
6. anxiety and defense

These scoring categories were chosen because of their relevance to normative social and emotional development at the transition between middle childhood and early adolescence. While we looked for evidence of the young person's ability to provide a coherent narrative, and also evidence of each parent's emotional availability, we did not score "attachment security." This is significant because we have routinely believed that the point of longitudinal attachment research should be to study attachment during infancy, when this is the most important developmental task, and in later childhood to focus on the most relevant developmental tasks, whether this be the understanding of emotion, mental health, peer relationships, self-esteem, and indeed any other considerations concerning optimal adaptation.

With respect to the construct of coherence, we were particularly interested in the extent to which these young peoples' narratives would show evidence of being linked to the early mother–child as well as to the father–child attachment relationships. Interestingly, the correlations that appeared significant over the 12-year interval pertained to links between the parents' AAIs and the children's own attachment narratives, with the earlier Strange Situation assessments not figuring prominently in these results. The aspect of the 11-year-olds' coherence that was most strongly related to their parents' AAIs was truthfulness or credibility. Truthfulness has recently been highlighted as a core aspect of attachment security across the lifespan (Cassidy, 2001). Those young people who told the most convincing or "truthful" accounts of the positive and negative aspects of their views of self and others were likely to have had mothers whose pregnancy AAIs had been judged autonomous-secure. Additionally, for boys only, they were also likely to have had fathers whose AAIs were judged autonomous-secure. Hierarchical regression results suggested that both parents' early AAIs were relevant to the levels of truthfulness in the sons' interviews at age 11, but this was not evident for the interviews from the daughters, where the significant correlation with their mothers' AAIs appeared unique. We interpreted this (H. Steele & M. Steele, 2004b) in terms of the sociological and psychoanalytic account of development provided by Chodorow (1978). It is Chodorow's claim that the developmental task for boys requires immediate involvement of father as well as mother (who they must separate from) in order to achieve a coherent self-identity. For girls and daughters, by contrast, fathers may be less relevant to their self-understanding because identity involves defining themselves in relation to their gender-mate and mother, from whom they never separate in the early and deep sense that is required of sons.

We did observe long-term connections between the AAIs collected from expectant fathers and their daughters' and sons' interviews at age 11, but, interestingly, these were in the domains of relations to siblings and friends. In other words, when it came to discussion of social concerns and conflicts with age-mates (within and beyond the family), links to the early (and ongoing?) father–child relationship became evident. The most coherent and resourceful accounts of how social disagreements are negotiated and resolved came from those young people whose fathers had provided autonomous-secure AAIs many years before. We inferred that these fathers had helped their children across the early childhood years to think and feel resourcefully about how to manage the emotions that arise in close relations with siblings and peers, the world beyond the intimate mother–child sphere.

Our speculations about the distinctive influence of fathers upon children's development, from our interviews with the 11-year-olds, were further supported by our findings when we asked the 11-year-olds to complete a standard mental health screening tool (Goodman, 1997). Some of our young participants were experiencing strain in the domains of peer relations, conduct problems, and hyperactivity. Notably, higher scores on these indices of behavioral perturbance (if not disturbance) were reported by those young people whose fathers had provided AAIs many years before judged insecure (either dismissing or preoccupied). This influence of fathers' AAIs held even after we statistically controlled for the influence of recent life events (young person's response) and the influence of reported behavioral problems (by mother) at age 5 (H. Steele & M. Steele, 2001). Interestingly, when we recently reexamined this data, we found that included in the archive of longitudinal information we hold is a brief self-report measure of marital satisfaction administered to the parents during the initial pregnancy phase. We have noticed that the link between fathers' AAI security and children's self-reported mental health is mediated by mothers' (pregnancy) report of "current" marital satisfaction. The power and dynamics of longitudinal attachment research appear to be an open-ended process of discovery!

Time and again we have observed and reported how our longitudinal research underlines distinctive long-term contributions made by mother and father to their firstborn child's social and emotional adaptation. It may be that the inner world of emotion understanding, and the capacity to speak freely and openly about negative and positive feelings, is uniquely related to the mother–child relationship. By contrast, the father–child relationship may be more relevant to the negotiation of social interactions with siblings and peers and to the maintenance of emotionally and socially appropriate behavior. Children need to learn (from mothers perhaps) to appreciate the intentions of others and negotiate inner emotional conflicts while also learning (from fathers perhaps) how to achieve and maintain conventionally appropriate behavior that enables one to feel successful in negotiating interactions with siblings, peers, and others.

THE THERAPEUTIC POWER
OF ATTACHMENT THEORY AND RESEARCH

The power of longitudinal attachment research ultimately lies in the positive consequences it may have for our understanding of well-being within individuals and relationships. Not surprisingly, many developmental attachment researchers (ourselves included) are either clinicians or consult with, mentor, or facilitate the work of therapists working with individuals, couples, and families (Dozier, Stovall, Albus, & Bates, 2001; Slade, 1999; H. Steele & M. Steele, 2003; M. Steele & Baradon, 2004). This work is intrinsic to attachment theory, formulated by a clinician aiming to improve his understanding of, and potential to help, individuals and families with severe emotional disturbances (Bowlby, 1979). Attachment research, certainly in the fashion we have pursued it, has aimed to understand patterns and individual differences in how children and parents regulate emotional conflict as each of us negotiates the essential human needs to both explore the world (i.e., be autonomous) and remain in intimate contact with significant others (i.e., be related). Maintaining a sense of cohesion, within ourselves and between people, as we pursue these potentially competing tasks is a lifelong challenge.

One of the conundrums in clinical work has been, and will remain, the question of how best to turn things around for a child, adolescent, or adult who has suffered loss or trauma? We have branched out to study these questions in our work with mentally disturbed adolescent inpatients (Wallis & H. Steele, 2001), as well as with "hard-to-place" late-adopted children (M. Steele et al., 2003). But, interestingly, there was robust evidence of how people turn things around for the better, following loss or trauma, within the nonclinical sample on which our longitudinal findings are based. Resolutions of a traumatic past, it appears, is achieved via new relationships that move one toward a renewed belief in the usefulness of depending on others and a lively interest in social exploration. How does this happen? We stumbled on this conclusion from reviewing carefully the AAIs we collected from the pregnant women and their partners, and then comparing these afresh to our observations of the infant–parent relationship.

In many cases the baby appeared securely attached to the parent and the parent appeared to have been well loved during his or her own childhood. But in other cases—a significant minority—the baby was securely attached but the parent's early attachment experiences included significant adversities, such as loss or trauma. The Main, Goldwyn, and Hesse (2003) scoring system permits one to give high scores for coherence to such interviews and call them autonomous-secure, putting them in the much admired "earned" secure group. We sought to understand this group further by perusing how they used language in the AAI. We noticed that a defining feature of their narratives was the *way* they relied on language as a tool for giving meaning to experience, including the attribution of mental states (beliefs and desires) to attachment figures whose behavior they did not fully understand, and were threatened by, as children, but have come to understand (if not forgive) as adults. Initially, we called this the "internal observer," as we thought this term captured the sense in which adult speakers could observe how family life was when they were children, and distinguish this from the understanding they gained through later relationships across development. Evidence of the "internal observer" in maternal AAIs was indeed a powerful correlate of infant–mother attachment security (see Fonagy, M. Steele, H. Steele, Moran, & Higgitt, 1991). We had arrived at the term "internal observer" by way of extending, and elaborating upon, the scale termed "metacognition" in the classic Main and colleagues (2003) rating and classification system introduced to us in 1987. This became in our writings "self-reflection" and then modified to "reflective functioning" because we were describing a capacity to monitor thought processes and motivations *in others* as well as the self. Reflective functioning, we showed, was especially important for parents to achieve if there was significant adversity in their past. Without it, there appeared to be little or no chance of having a securely attached infant; by contrast, where reflective functioning was present, the toxic cross-generational effect of emotional conflicts, past trauma, or loss was almost completely eliminated (Fonagy, M. Steele, H. Steele, Higgitt, & Target, 1994).

For those people who have had the luxury or good fortune of having a stable childhood, relatively free of negative life events or difficulties, the demand for developing a reflective capacity is lessened. This pattern of functioning works well so long as experience confirms the good expectations of the individual. However, when a major life event occurs, the fragility implicit in this "secure" mode of functioning may be suddenly revealed. We found this perspective helpful in explaining the apparent mismatch in our early findings between some "autonomous-secure" mothers who surprisingly had insecurely attached infants (see Fonagy et al., 1991). This group of 14 mother–child pairs shared an AAI profile of elevated levels of idealization (usually more indicative of dismissal) and apparently *more* positive childhood experiences, compared to the autonomous-secure group who successfully passed on security to their infants. Correspondingly, this group of mothers who appeared especially vulnerable to the challenges of becoming a mother led us to think of them as the "fragile-secure" group. This finding urges caution toward those who present convincingly rosy descriptions of childhood experiences, as they imply a lack of character-building experiences, such as knocks and disappointments, which temper optimism with realism.

By contrast, in response to an environment consistently placing enormous stress and challenges on the attachment system, the individual may urgently need to reflect upon the minds of sometimes—or frequently—malevolent caregivers, and challenging sibling relationships. Being able to predict forthcoming hostility directed at the self, that is, to have a theory of the malevolent other's mind, may prove essential to survival.

ATTACHMENT AND THEORY OF MIND

In addition to the importance of predicting potential attacks upon the self, our longitudinal research has shown advanced theory-of-mind skills in 5-year-old children with a previously observed highly anxious/fearful, disorganized attachment to mother, as well as among those children with a history of a secure attachment (Fonagy, H. Steele, M. Steele, & Holder, 1997; H. Steele, in press). Notably, these successful predictions from infant–mother attachment security at 1 year to theory of mind performance at age 5 were in respect of belief–desire reasoning skills, that is, where the child was required to guess correctly the *feeling state* of a deceived puppet. Attachment security did not predict belief–belief reasoning, that is, where the child was required to guess correctly the *behavior* of a doll acting on information that is no longer valid. Thus the relations between infants' social experiences and the evolution of their theory of mind skills are likely to depend on the extent to which the context loads more on the social-emotional register as opposed to the cognitive-behavioral one. Also, given the similar performance we have observed for children with organized-secure and disorganized early attachments, we must not assume that similar phenotypic outcomes share the same social determinants. In one case, a child may be advanced in theorizing about emotion because one or both parents have provided much helpful talk about emotion and mind (after Dunn, Brown, & Beardsall, 1991). In another case, the child may be advanced because the parent was liable to unpredictable and frightening behavior such that the child needed to know when to run or hide. The value of quickly detecting (on the caregiver's face) the imminent rise of anger *before* it reaches its full-blown potential (when this has previously led to abusive behavior from the caregiver) cannot be underestimated (see Pollak & Sinha, 2002).

CONCLUSION

Our own longitudinal work on firstborn children living in traditional mother–father–child homes points to possibly distinctive contributions to be made by mothers, as opposed to fathers, in respect of their children's social and emotional development. Our data suggests that children's understanding and resolution of emotional conflict *within themselves* is perhaps uniquely influenced by the mother–child relationship, while understanding and resolving emotional conflict in the *outer world* of human interaction— for example, with siblings and peers—is perhaps uniquely influenced by the father–child relationship. Yet there can be no simple division between inner and outer conflicts. There is a dynamic interplay between these domains that longitudinal research can at times successfully map. Provocative in this respect is our recent finding (to be reported at SRCD 2005) that mother's reports of marital satisfaction during pregnancy mediate the longitudinal link between fathers' attachment security and their children's self-reported mental health at 11 years of age.

Inevitably threats to our own health and safety, or to our loved ones, give rise to acute and possibly ongoing concern. To cope with our worries, we may need help in the struggle to organize thoughts, feelings, and behaviors in personally satisfying and socially constructive ways. The source of assistance may come from diverse sources, including mother, father, or observations of how mother and father negotiate their conflicts. Longitudinal attachment research is well equipped to specify the nature of the support young children need, and that all of us require in differing amounts, across the lifespan. Interviews of parents about their own attachment histories and observations of parent–child interactions amply demonstrate that a parent wishing to promote a secure attachment, and in the longer term a coherent, stable, and healthy sense of self, must reflect upon the probable emotional states of his or her infant, "hold" the infant with sensitivity and respect, so as to guide the child toward ownership of his or her feelings, and the related capacity of more autonomous affect regulation. Bowlby, Anna Freud, Winnicott, and other object relations theorists have said and written as much, many times, over the last half-century or more. The power of longitudinal attachment research, as we regard it, has been demonstrated in the empirical support attachment research findings have provided for so many vital psychodynamic ideas concerning the social and psychological processes underpinning affect regulation, the facilitating "good enough" environment on which human development depends, and the natural emergence, or (re) acquisition following trauma, of a balanced sense of self.

Currently, with the help of a talented team of doctoral research students (Emma Goldman, Alejandra Peres, and Francesca Segal), we are conducting a 16-year follow-up to retrieve more data from the sample. When it came to deciding what methods to include, foremost among those we are employing is, not suprisingly, the AAI. The AAI responses from these first-born children should give us fresh and vital information about the range of individual differences in understanding and resolving emotional conflicts during the midadolescent years, the ways in which representations of mother and father are distinct yet integrated, and how these aspects of psychological development may be related to mental health, as well as to earlier attachment experiences in the family, both in the current and in the previous generation.

ACKNOWLEDGMENTS

The research on which this chapter was based was supported in part by generous grants from the Köhler Stiftung, Germany. A generous project grant was also received from the Economic and Social Research Centre of the United Kingdom (No. R000233684). The work reported here has also benefited from a grant from the MacArthur Network node studying the Transition from Infancy to Early Childhood. And, very usefully, postgraduate fellowships to research students working on the study have been received from the Economic and Social Research Council, the Medical Research Council of the United Kingdom, the British Council, the Social Sciences and Humanities Research Council of Canada, and the Overseas Studentship Awards in the United Kingdom. Our greatest debt of gratitude is owed to the families participating in the research, who freely share their time and interest.

REFERENCES

Ainsworth, M. D. S., Blehar, M. C., Waters, E., & Wall, S. (1978). *Patterns of attachment: A psychological study of the Strange Situation*. Hillsdale, NJ: Erlbaum.

Bakermans-Kranenburg, M. J., & van IJzendoorn, M. H. (1993). A psychometric study of the Adult Attachment Interview: Reliability and discriminant validity. *Developmental Psychology, 29*, 870–879.

Bakermans-Kranenburg, M. J., & van IJzendoorn, M. H. (in press). No association of the dopamine D_4 receptor (DRD$_4$) and -521 C/T promoter polymorphisms with infant attachment disorganization. *Attachment and Human Development, 6*, 211–218.

Baumrind, D. (1967). Child care practices anteceding three patterns of preschool behaviour. *Genetic Psychology Monographs, 75*, 43–88.

Baumrind, D. (1971). Current patterns of parental authority. *Developmental Psychology Monographs, 4*, 1–103.

Bokhorst, C. L., Barkermans-Kranenburg, M. J., Fearon, R. M. P., van IJzendoorn, M. H., Fonagy, P., & Schuengel, C. (2003). The importance of shared environment in mother–infant attachment security: A behavioral genetic study. *Child Development, 74*, 1769–1782.

Bowlby, J. (1956/1979). *Psychoanalysis and child care* in The Making and Breaking of Affectional Bonds. London: Routledge.

Bowlby, J. (1969/2000). *Attachment and loss: Vol. 1. Attachment*. New York: Basic Books.

Bowlby, J. (1973). *Attachment and loss: Vol. 2. Separation*. New York: Basic Books.

Bowlby, J. (1988). *A secure base: Clinical applications of attachment theory*. London: Routledge.

Bretherton, I. (1998). Attachment and psychoanalysis: A reunion in progress. *Social Development, 7*, 132–136.

Bretherton, I., Golby, B., & Cho, E. (1997). Attachment and the transmission of values. In J. Grusec & L. Kucszynski (Eds.), *Handbook series: Parenting and children's internalization of values.* New York: Wiley.

Bretherton, I., & Munholland, K. A. (1999). Internal working models in attachment relationships: A construct revisited. In J. Cassidy & P. R. Shaver (Eds.), *Handbook of attachment: Theory, research, and clinical applications* (pp. 89–111). New York: Guilford Press.

Burlingham, D., & Freud, A. (1944). *Infants without families.* New York: International Universities Press.

Cassidy, J. (2001). Truth, lies, and intimacy: An attachment perspective. *Attachment and Human Development, 3,* 121–155.

Cassidy, J., & Berlin, L. J. (1994). The insecure/ambivalent pattern of attachment: Theory and research. *Child Development, 65,* 971–991.

Dozier, M., Stovall, K. C., & Albus, K. E. (1999). Attachment and psychopathology in adulthood. In J. Cassidy & P. R. Shaver (Eds.), *Handbook of attachment: Theory, research, and clinical applications* (pp. 497–515). New York: Guilford Press.

Dozier, M., Stovall, K. C., Albus, K. E., & Bates, B. (2001). Attachment for infants in foster care: The role of caregiver state of mind. *Child Development, 28,* 101–104.

Dunn, J., Brown, J., & Beardsall, L. (1991). Family talk about feeling states and children's later understanding of others' emotions. *Developmental Psychology, 27* 448–455.

Emde, R. N., Wolf, D. P., & Oppenheim, D. (Eds.). (2003). *Revealing the inner worlds of young children.* Oxford, UK: Oxford University Press.

Fonagy, P., Steele, H., & Steele, M. (1991). Maternal representations of attachment during pregnancy predict the organization of infant–mother attachment at one year of age. *Child Development, 62,* 891–905.

Fonagy, P., Steele, H., Steele, M., & Holder, J. (1997). Attachment and theory of mind: Overlapping constructs? *Association for Child Psychology and Psychiatry Occasional Papers, 14,* 31–40.

Fonagy, P., Steele, M., Steele, H., Moran, G., & Higgitt, A. (1991). The capacity for understanding mental states: The reflective self in parent and child and its significance for security of attachment. *Infant Mental Health Journal, 12,* 201–218.

Fonagy, P., Steele, M., Steele, H., Higgitt, A., & Target, M. (1994). The Emmanuel Miller Memorial Lecture 1992: The theory and practice of resilience. *Journal of Child Psychology and Psychiatry, 35,* 231–257.

Fox, N. A., Kimmerly, N. L., & Schafer, W. D. (1991). Attachment to mother/attachment to father: A meta-analysis. *Child Development, 62,* 210–225.

Freud, A. (1936). The ego and the mechanism of defense.

Freud, A. (1965). *Normality and pathology in childhood.* Harmondsworth, UK: Penguin Books.

Gervai, J., & Lakatos, K. (2004). Comment on "No association of dopamine D_4 receptor (DRD$_4$) and −521 C/T promoter polymorphisms with infant attachment disorganization" by M. J. Bakermans-Kranenburg and M. H. van IJzendoorn. *Attachment and Human Development, 6,* 219–222.

Goodman, R. (1997). The Strengths and Difficulties Questionnaire: A research note. *Journal of Child Psychology and Psychiatry, 38,* 581–586.

Gottman, J. M., Katz, L. F., & Hooven, C. (1997). *Meta-emotion: How families communicate emotionally.* Mahwah, NJ: Erlbaum.

Grossman, K., Fremmer-Bombik, E., Rudolph, J., & Grossmann, K. E. (1988). Maternal attachment representations as related to patterns of infant–mother attachment and maternal care during the first year. In R. A. Hinde & J. Steveson-Hinde (Eds.), *Relationships within families* (pp. 241–260). Oxford, UK: Oxford University Press.

Grossman, K. E., Grossman, K., Huber, F., & Wartner, U. (1981). German children's behavior toward their mothers at 12 months and their fathers at 18 months in Ainsworth's Strange Situation. *International Journal of Behavioral Development, 4,* 157–181.

Grossman, K. E., Grossman, K., & Schwan, A. (1986). Capturing the wider view of attachment: A reanalysis of Ainsworth's Strange Situation. In C. E. Izard & P. B. Read (Eds.), *Measuring emotion in infants and children* (Vol. 2, pp. 124–171). New York: Cambridge University Press.

Haft, W., & Slade, A. (1989). Affect attunement and maternal attachment: A pilot study. *Infant Mental Health Journal, 10,* 157–172.

Harter, S., & Buddin, B. (1987). Children's understanding of the simultaneity of two emotions: A five-stage developmental acquisition sequence. *Developmental Psychology, 23,* 388–399.

Hrdy, S. B. (1999). *Mother nature: A history of mothers, infants, and natural selection.* New York: Pantheon Books.

Lakatos, K. Toth, I., Nemoda, Z., Ney, K., Sasvari-Szekely, M., & Gervai, J. (2000). Dopamine D$_4$ receptor (DRD$_4$) gene polymorphism is associated with attachment disorganization in infants. *Molecular Psychiatry, 5,* 633–637.

Lyons-Ruth, K., & Jacobvitz, D. (1999). Attachment disorganization: Unresolved loss, relational violence, and lapses in behavioral and attentional strategies. In J. Cassidy & P. R. Shaver (Eds.), *Handbook of attachment: Theory, research, and clinical applications* (pp. 520–554). New York: Guilford Press.

Main, M., Goldwyn, R., & Hesse, E. (2003). *Adult attachment interview scoring and classification system (Version 7.2).* Unpublished manuscript, Department of Psychology, University of California, Berkeley.

Main, M., Kaplan, N., & Cassidy, J. (1985). Security in infancy, childhood, and adulthood: A move to the level of representation. In I. Bretherton & E. Waters (Eds.), Growing points of attachment theory and research. *Monographs of the Society for Research in Child Development, 50,* (1–2, Serial No. 209), 66–104.

Main, M., & Weston, D. R. (1981). The quality of the toddler's relationship to mother and father: Related to conflict behavior and the readiness to establish new relationships. *Child Development, 52,* 932–940.

Natale, M., & Hantas, M. (1982). Effect of temporary mood states on selective memory about the self. *Journal of Personality and Social Psychology, 42,* 927–934.

O'Connor, T. G., & Croft, C. M. (2001). A twin study of attachment in preschool children. *Child Development, 72,* 1501–1511.

O'Connor, T. G., Croft, C. M., & Steele, H. (2000). The contributions of behavioral genetic studies to attachment theory. *Attachment and Human Development, 2,* 107–122.

Pollak, S. D., & Sinha, P. (2002). Effects of early experience on children's recognition of facial displays of emotion. *Developmental Psychology, 38,* 784–791.

Richters, J. E., & Waters, E. (1992). Attachment and socialization: The positive side of social influence. In M. Lewis & S. Feinman (Eds.), *Social influences and behavior.* New York: Plenum Press.

Russell, J.A., Weiss, A., & Mendelsohn, G.A. (1989). Affect grid: A single-item scale of pleasure and arousal. *Journal of Personality and Social Psychology, 57,* 493–502.

Sagi, A., van IJzendoorn, M. H., Scharf, M. H., Koren-Karie, N., Joels, T., & Mayseles, O. (1994). Stability and discriminant validity of the Adult Attachment Interview: A psychometric study in young Israeli adults. *Developmental Psychology, 30,* 771–777.

Sandler, J. (1960). The background of safety. *International Journal of Pscyhoanalysis, 41,* 352–356.

Sandler, J. (1987). *From safety to superego.* London: Karnac Books.

Sandler, J., & Sandler, A. M. (1998). *Internal objects revisited.* London: Karnac Books.

Slade, A. (1999). Attachment theory and research: Implications for the theory and practice of individual psychotherapy with adults. In J. Cassidy & P. R. Shaver (Eds.), *Handbook of attachment* (pp. 575–594). New York: Guilford Press.

Spangler, G., & Grossmann, K. E. (1993). Biobehavioral organization in securely and insecurely attached infants. *Child Development, 59,* 1097–1101.

Steele, H. (1991). *Adult personality characteristics and family relationship patterns: The development and validation of an interview-based assessment.* Unpublished PhD dissertation, University College, London.

Steele, H. (in press). The social matrix reloaded: An attachment perspective on Carpendale & Lewis. *Behavioral and Brain Sciences.*

Steele, H., & Steele, M. (1994). Intergenerational patterns of attachment. In K. Bartholomew & D. Perlman (Eds.), *Advances in personal relationships: Vol. 5. Attachment processes during adulthood* (pp. 93–120). London: Jessica Kingsley.

Steele, H., & Steele, M. (1998). Attachment and psychoanalysis: Time for a reunion. *Social Development. 7,* 92–119.

Steele, H., & Steele, M. (1999). Psychoanalytic views about development. In D. Messer & S. Millar (Eds.), *Exploring developmental psychology* (pp. 263–283). London: Francis Arnold.

Steele, H., & Steele, M. (2003). Clinical uses of the Adult Attachment Interview. In M. Marrone & M. Cortina (Eds.), *Attachment theory and the psychoanalytic process* (pp. 107–126). London: Whurr.

Steele, H., & Steele, M. (2004a). The construct of coherence as an indicator of attachment security in middle childhood: The Friends and Family Interview. In K. A. Kerns & R. A. Richardson (Eds.), *Attachment in middle childhood* (pp. 137–160). New York: Guilford Press.

Steele, H., & Steele, M. (2004b). *Friends and Family Interview protocol and scoring system.* Unpublished document, Department of Psychology, New School University, New York.

Steele, H., Steele, M., Croft, C., & Fonagy, P. (1999). Infant–mother attachment at one-year predicts children's understanding of mixed-emotions at six years. *Social Development, 8*, 161–178.

Steele, H., Steele, M., & Fonagy, P. (1996). Associations among attachment classification of mothers, fathers and their infants. *Child Development, 67*, 541–555.

Steele, H., Woods, R., & Phibbs, E. (2004). Coherence of mind in daughter caregivers of mothers with dementia: Links with their mothers' attachment security in a Strange Situation. *Attachment and Human Development, 6*.

Steele, M., & Baradon, T. (2004). The clinical use of the Adult Attachment Interview in parent–infant psychotherapy. *Infant Mental Health Journal, 25*, 284–299.

Steele, M., Hodges, J., Kaniuk, J., Hillman, S, & Henderson, K. (2003). Attachment representations in attachment: Associations between maternal states of mind and emotion narratives in previously maltreated children. *Journal of Child Psychotherapy, 29*, 187–205.

Steele, M., Steele, H., & Fonagy, P. (1992, May). Stability and change in maternal models of attachment across the transition to parenthood, and their association to the quality of the infant–mother attachment. In B. Vaughn (Chair), *Stability and change in maternal representations of attachment*, Symposium at the 8th International Conference of Infant Studies, Miami, FL.

Steele, M., Steele, H., & Johansson, M. (2002). Maternal predictors of children's social cognition: An attachment perspective. *Journal of Child Psychology and Psychiatry, 43*, 189–198.

Steele, M., Steele, H., Woolgar, M., Yabsley, S., Johnson, D., Fonagy, P., & Croft C. (2003). An attachment perspective on children's emotion narratives: Links across generations. In R. N. Emde, D. P. Wolf, & D. Oppenheim (Eds.), *Revealing the inner worlds of young children*. Oxford, UK: Oxford University Press.

Tompkins, S. S. (1963). *Affect, imagery, consciousness: Vol. 2. The negative affects.* New York: Springer.

Wallis, P., & Steele, H. (2001). Attachment representations in adolescence: Further evidence from psychiatric residential settings. *Attachment and Human Development, 3*, 259–268.

Winnicott, D. W. (1965). *The maturational processes and the facilitating environment.* London: Hogarth Press.

CHAPTER 7

Correlates of Attachment to Multiple Caregivers in Kibbutz Children from Birth to Emerging Adulthood

The Haifa Longitudinal Study

AVI SAGI-SCHWARTZ
ORA AVIEZER

In his depiction of personality development, Bowlby (1985) used the metaphor of railway tracks that start from a main station in a certain direction but soon branch into a variety of divergent routes. Initially, these routes are close together and continue in the general direction of the original track, but as they stretch further away from the main station they branch out more. By analogy, this metaphor can also be used to describe the multidimensionality of issues in attachment development and the inherent difficulties in its study. Thus, in line with Bowlby's metaphor and his notion of branching pathways, this chapter reports on one of the branching tracks in attachment research, joining a host of contributions that address issues of stability and continuity in attachment from infancy to adulthood. Though our research is based on a project with a unique population, namely, kibbutz-reared children, the various issues it has encountered are shared by all longitudinal studies of attachment. Let us begin with a brief description of our own research regarding how we became engaged in the study of attachment.

Both authors contributed equally to this chapter.

The origin of our research goes back to the late 1970s when Abraham ("Avi") Sagi-Schwartz visited his alma mater, the University of Michigan in Ann Arbor, where as a graduate student he focused on precursors of empathy under the guidance of Martin Hoffman and discrimination learning and language under the guidance of John Hagen and Alexander Z. Guiora. Avi met Michael Lamb there, and the two shared some data on fatherhood, an emerging topic in the field at that time. Their discussion eventually evolved to address the meaning of multiple caregiving and the roles of different caregiving figures in child development. The usefulness of the kibbutz setting (described in the next section) as a unique natural laboratory for examining these issues, including the formation of attachment relationships, became a central topic in their interaction. This collaboration brought about the first attachment study in Israel in which the Ainsworth Strange Situation procedure (SSP; Ainsworth, Blehar, Waters, & Wall, 1978) was employed. The primary inspiration for this study were the works of Fox (1977) and of Maccoby and Feldman (1972), who attempted to determine whether children formed attachment not only to their mothers, but also to their *metaplot* (Hebrew plural for professional caregivers; *metapelet* is the singular form).

The focus of our initial study was on the security of infant–mother, –father, and –*metapelet* attachment among kibbutz-reared Israeli children (Sagi, Lamb, Lewkowicz, et al., 1985). Although this study took place in the traditional kibbutz system, where infants slept at night away from their parents (see the section on collective sleeping, below), its main purpose was simply to describe the attachment relationships of infants who were raised in multiple-caregiver settings to their major caregiving figures, namely, mother, father, and *metapelet*. We were surprised to find so many insecurely attached infants, especially to their mothers and *metaplot*, but the absence of a control group of kibbutz-raised infants who were not separated from their parents at night did not allow us to draw clearcut conclusions about collective sleeping and its effects.

Moreover, the utilization of the SSP in cross-cultural settings and the extent to which this procedure could be conceived of as a valid measure to index early attachment relationships across cultures was a central issue of scientific discussion at the time. Subsequently, a major symposium entitled "The Strange Situation Procedure: Insights from an International Perspective" took place at the International Conference of Infant Studies (ICIS) in New York City in 1984, in which all the participants were non-American researchers conducting attachment studies in their countries, with Mary Ainsworth as a discussant. This was a memorable symposium, most notably for the moment when Jerome Kagan spoke from the floor and noted that although he had misgivings about whether the SSP indeed measured attachment, nevertheless in his mind such a symposium reflected the right way to conduct good science.

Scientific concerns about the cross-cultural validity of the SSP, coupled with a lack of a control group in the initial kibbutz study, led to our tentative suggestion that collective sleep might have had negative effects on infants. This suggestion was cautiously shared with the staff of the Institute of Research on Kibbutz Education, whose help with and support of our work was invaluable, particularly because at that time kibbutz people were heatedly debating the practice of collective sleeping for infants and children.

What is more, in this first study we already discovered some indications of attachment concordance for infants who were biologically unrelated. More specifically, we found concordant Strange Situation classifications with the *metapelet* for 12 out of 16 children whose *metapelet* took care of two or more different children participating in the study. We interpreted this finding to indicate that most caregivers behave in characteristic ways that potentiate either secure or insecure attachments for the infants in their care, thus suggesting tentative support for the concordance hypothesis (Sagi, Lamb, Lewkowicz, et al., 1985). This last finding, along with the indications that the practice of collective sleep had negative effects, served as an impetus for our new, more focused, and more controlled investigation that took place several years later and was published in the early 1990s, but not before we have already launched our longitudinal follow-up of the original kibbutz sample (in the early 1980s). The complexity of the research issues that are at the core of this chapter and the nonlinear evolution of our research dictate that our story line will not follow a rigid chronological order but will rather weave through the various questions, themes, and methodological issues that concerned us over the years.

We will proceed to the first follow-up phase of the longitudinal study, which took place in the early 1980s when the children were 4–5 years old and David Oppenheim, who was at that time an MA psychology student at the University of Haifa, joined the project for his MA thesis. Our previous description of the development of our research implies that the longitudinal follow-up evolved over time, but in fact it was not designed from the beginning as a long-term project. Furthermore, in our early conceptualizations of attachment and its consequential adaptations we adopted a broad rather than a narrow perspective and we used a variety of measures of adaptive functioning rather than focusing on assessments at the representational level, which were not yet very developed. Finding in this first follow-up phase that the infant–*metapelet* attachment relation was the best predictor of various outcome measures in kindergarten (Oppenheim, Sagi, & Lamb, 1988) led us to entertain the idea of a domain-specific realm of influence for early attachment relations. In other words, we hypothesized that in a multiple-caregiving setting like the kibbutz, where attachment figures played different and important roles in the daily routines of children (see more information in the following sections), the long-term influence of early attachment relations will be relevant to specific domains in the children's lives. This is when Marinus van IJzendoorn of Leiden University in the Netherlands joined our Israeli team.

In fact, the initial dialogue with van IJzendoorn had already started in the early 1980s, following the 1984 ICIS meeting in New York City when both van IJzendoorn and Sagi-Schwartz began addressing issues associated with the cross-cultural measurement of infant attachment. Their discussions were fueled by parallel dialogues between Sagi-Schwartz and Klaus and Karin Grossmann as he visited their lab in Regensburg. The focus on cross-cultural issues of attachment theory and research yielded secondary analyses of cross-cultural data on the primary appraisal of preseparation episodes in the Strange Situation (Sagi, van IJzendoorn, & Karie-Koren, 1991), and eventually a joint chapter on attachment and culture in the *Handbook of Attachment* (van IJzendoorn & Sagi, 1999). Moreover, the data from the first follow-up of the kibbutz longitudinal sample along with similar Dutch data also led to the notion of an attachment network as an approach for capturing the meaning of exposure to multiple attachment figures (Sagi & van IJzendoorn, 1996; van IJzendoorn, Sagi, & Lambermon, 1992).

Intrigued by opportunities provided by the kibbutz setting for the examination of the concordance hypothesis while avoiding the confounding of intergenerational transmission with biological relatedness lead us to design a new study and recruit a new kibbutz sample. Following discussions with Michael Nathan and Ora Aviezer, who was then at the Institute of Research on Kibbutz Education, a new and more controlled study that employed a quasi-experimental design was launched. At this time, Ora Aviezer joined the lab as a postdoctoral fellow after completing her graduate studies at the University of Chicago, where she had focused on nonverbal interaction between mothers and infants under the guidance of Starkey Duncan. We all became excited about the potential power of quasi-experimental designs in natural settings, such as the childrearing system of the kibbutz, which created its own "manipulations" by taking infants away from their parents for the night. It is clear that for obvious ethical reasons practices like collective sleep could not even be thought of as a viable option in designing true experimental manipulations. During this time we were also introduced to Mary Main's ideas about adult attachment representations, including Adult Attachment Interview (AAI; George, Kaplan, & Main, 1985) training in Charlottesville, Virginia, which allowed us to incorporate the AAI into our research endeavors within the Israeli context (Sagi, van IJzendoorn, Scharf, et al., 1994).

This is the place to call attention to the fact that contrary to what some colleagues in the field believe to be the case, the kibbutz per se has never been the focus of our research. Rather, it was the naturally occurring practices within the kibbutz childrearing system, such as multiple caregiving and the extended absence of attachment figures during the night, that offered us exceptional quasi-experimental conditions conducive for the examination of universal attachment-related issues and the validity of attachment theory. The upshot of this research was a number of publications that addressed several conceptual issues pertinent to the study of attachment: the effects of sleeping out of the home on infant–mother attachment (Sagi, van IJzendoorn, Aviezer, Donnell, & Mayseless, 1994); attachments in a multiple-caregiver and multiple-infant environment (Sagi et al., 1995); and ecological constraints for intergenerational transmission of attachment (Aviezer, Sagi, Joels, & Ziv, 1999; Sagi et al., 1997), all of which are discussed in greater detail later in this chapter.

Simultaneous to all this research effort we continued with our longitudinal project and collected more data when participants were 12, 17, and 21 years old. These follow-up data collection phases were directed by Aviezer and Sagi-Schwartz. In the future we plan to follow our participants as they start their own families and become parents themselves. Returning to Bowlby's metaphor of development, we believe this will be the next important developmental junction of branching tracks and a most interesting one to follow.

The growing body of work in assessments of attachment on the level of representation has influenced our own thinking. As can be seen in this chapter, our longitudinal work reflects some changing trends in attachment research and the complexity of conducting longitudinal research that evolved over time rather than was designed as such from the outset. This is one reason that we, as much as others in the field, needed to mature into realizing that though there are already some good answers with regard to longitudinal effects of early attachment relations, there still remain many good questions that we are currently better equipped to answer by planning carefully designed longitudinal research. Thus, we believe that our data mainly provide exploratory directions that might set a better ground for more refined longitudinal research and hypothesis testing in the future. We hope that we can shed some light on various major issues via our two decades and a half of studies with kibbutz-reared children, a unique childrearing setting that is described next.

THE ISRAELI KIBBUTZ

The Israeli kibbutz is a utopian experiment that successfully established a radically different way of living and raising children that has lasted for a period of 80–90 years. Kibbutzim are cooperative, multigenerational communities that are democratically governed. The average population of a kibbutz is 400–900 people. Currently kibbutzim constitute only a minority of about 1.5% of Israel's Jewish population. In the past, kibbutzim were fairly isolated agricultural communities in which living conditions were exceedingly hard. Nowadays kibbutz economies are based on industrial and agricultural diversity and most of them provide their members with satisfying standards of living. Each kibbutz is affiliated with the United Kibbutz Federation that was recently established in response to the fading of former ideological and political divisions. Finally, a major economic crisis in the 1980s led to substantial changes in all facets of kibbutz life (Ben-Rafael, 1999).

The pioneers who founded kibbutzim were idealistic young people seeking to create a new socialist-Zionist collective society that, in addition to production and physical labor, emphasized personal independence under conditions of perfect equality. The goals of this revolutionary and collectivist ideology were to discourage individualism, to abolish gender inequality, and to raise a new type of healthy and productive person who will be socialized for communal life (Gerson, 1978; Lewin, 1999). Tensions between the collective and the family were inherent to this collective society from the beginning because the family was viewed as a possible competing force of influence that might reduce identification with the collective and the effectiveness of its informal control over the members (Talmon, 1972).

Concordant with the collective ideology, the kibbutz community was regarded as a "collective parent" committed to satisfying the ordinary and special needs of children without the mediation of their families (Dar, 1998). These needs included material needs in the way of food, clothing, and medical care, as well as seeing to children's psychological well-being (Gerson, 1978). Children were regarded as being the "kibbutz's children," and hence an informal communal socialization network was created (Rabin & Beit-Hallahmi, 1982). However, it is important to note that in a psychological sense the family has always been present in the life of kibbutz members (Spiro, 1979) and that there was no preconceived ideology in favor of abolishing it altogether (Talmon, 1972).

Nonetheless, due to a distrust in parents' ability to raise their children well, especially for communal life, their caregiving roles were drastically limited by the collective. Psychoanalytical interpretations that emphasized parents' potential pathogenic impact on their children were utilized to justify the sharing of responsibility for child care and socialization tasks between parents and caregivers, as well as the separate group dwelling for children (Berman, 1988; Liban & Goldman, 2000). In fact, it was thought that two emotional centers for kibbutz children—the parental home and the children house—would protect them from their parents' shortcomings while preserving the benefits of parental love (Golan, 1959). Dividing parenting functions between parents who were *emotionally involved* and caregivers who were *instrumentally involved* was considered beneficial for children as it allowed them both parental love and caregivers' professional support for social learning and mastery of autonomous behavior. In addition, child-care duties and responsibilities were to be shared by men and women in order to promote gender equality (Gerson, 1978). Thus both parents were expected to spend time with their children even though child care was never viewed as men's primary responsibility.

Maintaining a balanced system of socialization based on the family and the community as two emotional centers for children and children's living with their peers, including sleeping away from their parents, constitute the most distinctive characteristics of kibbutz childrearing practices. Consequently, kibbutzim's children houses functioned as children's homes as well as their educational settings. It was in the children house with its home-like qualities that kibbutz children ate their meals, bathed, kept their personal belongings, played, and slept at night. Thus, typically, children houses consisted of a large space for play and learning, a dining area, showers, and bedrooms that were each shared by three or four children who had their own individual corners for their personal items. Family time was designated for afternoons and evenings (approximately 4:00–8:00 P.M.), when both parents made an effort to be available for the children in their home. Children returned to the children house for their night's sleep and were put to bed by their parents, but through the night they were looked after by two watchwomen who were responsible for all kibbutz children under the age of 12. Watchwomen were assigned based on weekly shifts and they monitored the children houses via intercom and by making rounds. Though such a system may have provided sufficient monitoring of the children's safety, it clearly allowed them only a precarious and limited sense of security, because sensitive responsiveness to children's needs was nearly impossible in the weekly rotation schedule (Aviezer, van IJzendoorn, Sagi, & Schuengel, 1994).

Though many cultures practice multiple caregiving (see, e.g., Konner, 1977; Morelli & Tronick, 1991), a worldwide sample of 183 societies showed that none of them employed a similar system in which infants and young children sleep away from their parents (Barry & Paxton, 1971). In fact, the issue of collective sleeping was debated from the early days of the kibbutz movement (1920–1930) and it became normative and an officially advocated practice only later when the interests of the collective were emphasized over the needs of individuals and families (Dror, 2001). In this context, children's sleeping away from their parents enhanced collectivist tendencies by significantly reducing the family's influence and its active participation in raising its children, with a particularly detrimental impact on maternal involvement (Dar, 1998).

Following a period of 20 years in which national and survival issues occupied center stage of public concern in kibbutzim in the 1930s–1950s, doubts about children's collective sleeping began to be loudly voiced along with a rise in familistic tendencies. Consequently, parents' participation in caring for their children gradually increased (Dar, 1998; Spiro, 1979) and growing numbers of kibbutzim changed to home sleeping (Dror, 2001; Tiger & Shepher, 1975). This process eventually peaked during the stressful period of the Gulf War of 1991 when practically all remaining kibbutzim that practiced collective sleeping voluntarily made the transition to home sleeping for children. Collective sleeping was an influential mechanism of the community. Thus the transition to home sleeping for children altered the balance of influence between the two socializing agents: the family and the community.

Despite ostentatious ideological convictions about gender equality in the kibbutz, the duties of early child care were primarily women's responsibility that was shared by mothers and caregivers. Although mothers' privileged status with their children had not been challenged, increased involvement in child care by nonmaternal others (caregivers and fathers) was regarded as beneficial to children. Both mothers and caregivers attributed to caregivers considerable influence over children's care and development, especially in their mastery of age-related tasks and social development (Feldman & Yirmiya, 1986; Kaffman, Elizur, & Rabinowitz, 1990). Furthermore, kibbutz culture placed a high value on paternal involvement (Shamai, 1992) and family time was organized such that both mothers and fathers were free to be with their children during the afternoons. Thus, in comparison to their non-kibbutz counterparts, kibbutz fathers tended to spend more time with their children. Indeed, kibbutz infants showed no preference for one parent over the other in a naturalistic home observation (Sagi, Lamb, Shoham, et al., 1985).

To summarize, the kibbutz philosophy valued children's intense involvement with peers and nonfamilial caregivers as a means for socialization to collective life and created a child-care environment that strongly supported children's relations with fathers in addition to their relations with mothers. Thus, it is natural to consider within such an ecology of child care the longitudinal correlates of children's attachment relations to both parents and to their professional caregiver, as well as their interrelations between these relations, as possible explanations for later development.

COLLECTIVE SLEEP FOR CHILDREN AND ITS EFFECTS ON INFANT ATTACHMENT RELATIONS

The focus of this section is on what we have described before, namely, the collective upbringing of children. Sleeping away from the parents at night was clearly a unique "experiment in nature" that had taken place for approximately 60–70 years in Israeli kibbutzim, and, as explained, its most distinctive characteristic was the practice of children sleeping together in children's houses away from their parents. Examining more closely this type of "experiment" is of special interest in the developmental sciences because this childrearing practice involved middle-class families consciously raising their normal children in institution-like conditions that are typically found in services for multiproblem families and low socioeconomic status (SES) populations. It thus offered a unique opportunity for quasi-experimental observations of the impact of unusual childrearing conditions, without confounding it with SES.

Over the past two decades we have been following the development of children who were sleeping together in children's houses away from their parents at night. We believe that data from this "experiment in nature" will contribute to our understanding of universal aspects of development and parenting by providing interesting information about the effects of naturally occurring childrearing practices that, though observed in kibbutzim, can be explained within a universal developmental framework. In this respect, it is interesting to note that the major milestones in the gradual process of abandoning collective sleeping were associated with life-threatening emergencies such as Israel's War of Independence (1948) and the 1991 Gulf War. Thus, clearly kibbutz parents felt that communal sleeping was no longer conducive to the protection of their children.

In our research we observed substantially higher rates of attachment insecurity among communally sleeping infants as compared to family-sleeping kibbutz infants, as well as to normative non-kibbutz samples in Israel and worldwide (van IJzendoorn & Sagi, 1999). It was concluded that the responsibility for the higher rate of insecurity was tied to the practice of communal sleeping because of the inconsistent responsiveness that was inherent in the day-to-day reality of communally sleeping infants. Clearly, these children's nighttime experiences were characterized by maternal inaccessibility and nonavailability, combined with exposure to numerous unfamiliar adults who were naturally unable to respond promptly and sensitively to the children's needs.

Moreover, if the childrearing ecology created by communal sleeping was problematic from an attachment perspective, then this should also be manifested in processes of attachment transmission from one generation to the next. Bowlby (1984) argued that parents' representations of their own past attachment experiences influence their parenting behaviors and the quality of their children's attachment to them. Several studies have demonstrated attachment transmission by showing correspondence between classifications of infants' attachment relationships and classifications of their parents' internal representations (e.g., Benoit & Parker, 1994; Fonagy, Steele, & Steele, 1991; H. Steele & M. Steele, Chapter 6, this volume). Sagi and colleagues (1997) found no difference in rates of autonomous attachment representations between mothers from collective-sleeping and home-sleeping kibbutzim. However, attachment transmission in dyads whose infants were sleeping communally was poorer compared to attachment transmission in dyads whose infants were sleeping at home. Thus, transmission of attachment across generations appears dependent upon specific childrearing arrangements and contextual factors, such as communal sleeping, and may override the influence of parents' attachment representations and their sensitive responsiveness. These findings highlight the limits of a context-free universal model of intergenerational transmission.

Though these findings supported the contention that communal sleeping constituted a difficult childrearing ecology, they did not explicate the possible moderating effects that were involved in this practice. It was therefore necessary to further explore the dynamic aspects of attachment formation, specifically, the interaction between mothers and their infants. Aviezer and colleagues (1999) found that the vast majority of kibbutz mothers were sensitive when interacting with their infants, and that the emotional availability displayed in the interaction of these kibbutz dyads was rather high. Second, it was found that both autonomous representations in mothers and secure attachment in infants were associated with higher emotional availability in dyadic interaction. These findings support the assumption that attachment representations of mothers and attachment classification of infants are associated with mothers' and infants' experiences in ordinary interactions with each other. However, distinctive differences were found between dyads from communal-sleeping and dyads from family-sleeping backgrounds, as only in family-sleeping samples was higher maternal sensitivity associated with infant attachment security. Similar results were found for infant–mother attachment in low-quality daycare. The expected associations between maternal sensitivity and infants' attachment security were only found when children were cared for at home, but were not found for children from low-quality daycare, despite absence of differences in maternal sensitivity between the two groups of mothers (Aviezer, Sagi-Schwartz, & Koren-Karie, 2003). Thus, these data indicate that interrelations between representations of attachment and actual behavioral processes might be conditional on the ecological context of child care (Hinde, 1988), and that environmental factors may interfere in the formation of attachment relationships.

However, as compelling as these findings and explanations appear to be, we cannot ignore another apparent fact in the above studies: about 50% of communally sleeping children were securely attached to their mothers in spite of the difficult circumstances created by communal sleeping. Apparently, despite the disruption, the surrounding support network provided a secure base, which was adequate for some children. Such discontinuity between unfavorable rearing conditions and positive outcomes certainly needs to be studied further. Nonetheless, naturally existing child-rearing practices, though setting-specific in their occurrence, may clarify further universal issues of parenting, as they represent an experiment in "nature" rather than in the lab. Communal sleeping is no longer practiced, but, so far as parenting is concerned, it is exactly the emergence of such extreme childrearing practices as well as their abandonment that make these processes universally important. It is clear that communal sleeping for infants and children presented kibbutz parents and children with obstacles to their relationships. It is also clear that overcoming these obstacles involved much strife, and was evidently insurmountable for some families, resulting in insecure attachment relationships for their infants. Although the only solution for families who were unhappy with communal sleeping in the early days of kibbutzim was to leave the kibbutz, such sentiments served as major motivations for social change that eventually resulted in the abandonment of this childrearing practice. It may be argued that communal sleep was perhaps doomed from the outset, because it represented ideologically motivated culture-level values that prevailed over individual-level values and ignored the psychological dynamics inherent in human nature and in universal aspects of social interaction. Hence the abandonment of collective sleeping as a normative childrearing practice in collective education was unavoidable. Indeed, it is surprising that it had not been abandoned sooner. The fall of communal sleep demonstrates the limits of the adaptability of parents and children to inappropriate child-care arrangements.

LONGITUDINAL EFFECT
OF ATTACHMENT RELATIONS: THE STUDY

With regards to the longitudinal effects of attachment relations, we considered two major issues: continuity and change in attachment representations and the contribution of early attachment quality to later adaptive functioning. Figure 7.1 presents a schema of data collection over the years from infancy to early adulthood.

First, we examined continuity and change in attachment representations from infancy to early and late adolescence, following Bowlby's (1982, 1988) argument that attachment patterns tend to resist dramatic changes, unless they get restructured in response to transformations in the caregiving environment. Previous research established continuity in mental representations from infancy to childhood (e.g., Main & Cassidy, 1988; Sroufe, Carlson, & Shulman, 1993; Wartner, Grossmann, Fremmer-Bombik, & Suess, 1994) and from infancy to young adulthood (Hamilton, 2000;

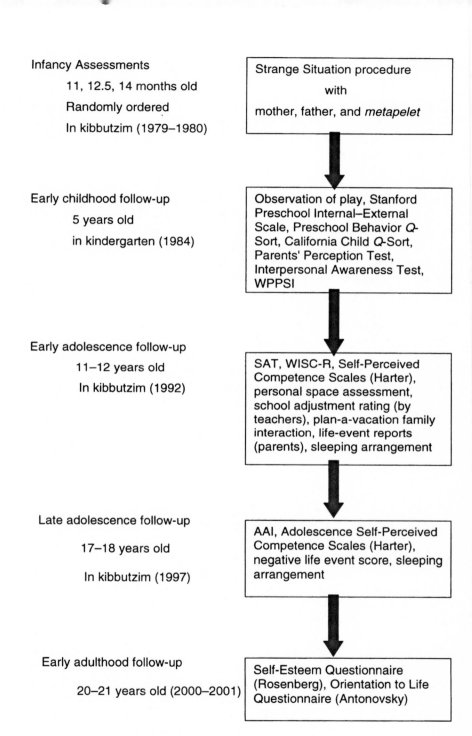

FIGURE 7.1. A schema of data collection.

Waters, Merrick, Treboux, Crowell, & Albersheim, 2000). However, discontinuities have also been observed and were attributed to characteristics of the caregiving environment (Erickson, Sroufe, & Egeland, 1985; K. Grossmann, K. E. Grossmann, & Kindler, Chapter 5, this volume; Grossmann, Grossmann, & Zimmermann, 1999; Sroufe, Egeland, & Kreutzer, 1990), or to more risks in the lives of children (Weinfield, Sroufe, & Egeland, 2000).

As summarized earlier, the practice of communal sleeping was a risk factor for the establishment of secure attachment relationships in infancy. Nonetheless, it is important to remember that the abandonment of children's communal sleep in favor of family sleeping influenced the life of the kibbutz family as a whole because of such factors as overcrowding and changes of daily parental responsibilities and duties (for reviews of the process, see Aviezer, Sagi, & van IJzendoorn, 2002; Maital & Bornstein, 2003). Thus, though home sleeping for children, which was preferred by the majority of kibbutz members in accordance with the wishes of most parents (Lavi, 1984), was intended to benefit children, it required families to reorganize and adjust to this radical change in their life. Given that attachment-related internal models are responsive to reorganizations in the environment, internal representations of kibbutz children could possibly have been affected by transformation in the caregiving environment that originated either in the microsystem of the family or in the mesosystem of the community—in this case, change in sleeping arrangements.

As part of the follow-up of the original cohort recruited by Sagi, Lamb, Lewkowicz, and colleagues (1985), attachment representations were examined in early adolescence and in late adolescence along with documentation of negative life events—such as a parent's death, parents' separation or divorce, and a major illness of child or parent—as well as ecology of sleeping arrangement, such as earlier or later abandonment of children's collective sleep in favor of transition to home sleep. This study involved 66 early adolescent children and 71 late adolescents that constituted a respective rate of 77 % and 83% of the original sample of 86 children recruited by Sagi and colleagues.

Attachment Representations in Early and Late Adolescence

In early adolescence, when participants were 11–12 years old, the Separation Anxiety Test (SAT; Hansburg, 1980) was used to assess individual differences in the representation of relationships in the context of imagined separations. Six pictures depicting mild and severe separations were chosen from Hansburg's original set and were presented to all participants in ascending order of separation distress. Participants' strategies of coping with separation from parents or familiar people, their ability to express openly feelings of vulnerability, and the clarity and organization of their responses were rated on three rating scales. Based on their responses, participants were classified as using an open strategy/secure, a minimizing strategy/insecure, or a heightening strategy/insecure.

In late adolescence, the AAI (George et al., 1985) was used to assess participants' state of mind with regard to their attachment experience in terms of emotional accessibility and openness to their past experience as well as the coherence in which these experiences were described. Based on their responses, participants' state of mind was classified as autonomous, dismissing of attachment, enmeshed with attachment, or unresolved (Main & Goldwyn, 1994).

Following Waters, Hamilton, and Weinfield (2000), we obtained a retrospective score of negative life events from participants' AAI transcripts. Of our early and late adolescents, 23% and 27%, respectively, reported the occurrence of a major negative life event, of which parental divorce was most frequent. In addition, children's longer or shorter exposure to communal sleeping was marked in terms of whether transformation to home sleeping took place before age 6 or afterward.

Regardless of the length of children's exposure to the arrangement of communal sleeping and their experiences of negative life events, no continuity in representations was found between infancy, as assessed by the SSP, and early adolescence with regard to infancy attachment to father and mother as well as to the network of attachment relations to both parents. However, examination of the associations between security of infancy attachment to father (SSP) and autonomy of state of mind in late adolescence (AAI) revealed the impact of negative life events on participants who were securely attached in infancy and changed early to home sleeping. If these participants experienced negative life events in their families, they tended to be nonautonomous in late adolescence, whereas their counterparts who did not experience negative life events tended to be autonomous.

With regard to continuity between infancy attachment to mother (SSP) and age-17 state-of-mind classifications (AAI), the interaction of negative life events and sleeping arrangement created an unexpected, almost counterintuitive effect. Significantly more participants who were securely attached as infants, who did not experience negative life events, but who were exposed to communal sleeping longer tended to be classified as autonomous compared to their securely attached counterparts who did not experience negative life events but had a shorter exposure to communal sleeping. In addition, fewer participants who were insecurely attached as infants tended to be classified as nonautonomous if they were exposed to communal sleeping longer with no experience of negative life events. Thus, both continuity from infancy security to adolescence autonomy and change from infancy insecurity to adolescence autonomy were contingent upon longer exposure to communal sleep and absence of negative life events. Lastly, when we categorized parental network of infancy attachment as at least secure with one parent versus insecure with both parents, no continuity in attachment representations from infancy to adolescence was found.

Finally, the continuity of attachment representations was assessed between early and late adolescence. Apparently, among participants who had a longer exposure to communal sleep and no negative life events, there was less continuity between early adolescence to late adolescence whether they were classified secure or insecure in early adolescence.

Overall, these findings provide additional support for the claim that continuity in attachment representations is influenced by transformations in the caregiving environment in the context of its personal, familial, and social supports and risks (Belsky, 1999). Such transformations include more specific proximal events such as a loss of a parent or of the intact family unit by divorce, life-threatening diseases to parents or child, and more general life changes such as the move to home sleeping. Finding that longer exposure to collective sleep was not always a disadvantage for children requires an evaluation of life events as a complex influence. Thus, a major change in the caregiving environment in and of itself, even if regarded as a positive event, may create considerable perturbations, may require adjustment, and may result in a negative effect on both children and parents. Although no significant interaction effect between sleeping arrangement and negative life events was observed, it is interesting to note that in both age groups more negative life events occurred for the home-sleeping group (27% vs. 18% and 33% vs. 21% for early and late adolescence, respectively).

Since divorce was the most frequent negative life event reported by our participants, it is conceivable that in some families children's home sleeping created unmanageable stress. Thus for some families change may be a stressor and a major challenge that could have interfered with their ability to preserve the family unit and attend to their children's needs. At the same time, the parents of collectively sleeping children were becoming well aware of the widespread practice of home sleeping and possibly more conscientious of their children's needs. Hence, they could have attempted to compensate for the nightly separations of their children and to buffer some of the difficulties inherent in collective sleeping (for some parental solutions during infancy, see Oppenheim, 1998). Since collective sleep is no longer in practice, these speculations would be hard to substantiate. Nonetheless, our data point to the need for studying continuity of attachment representations while considering diverse effects of the caregiving environment and particularly interactions between them.

Early Attachment Relations and Later Adaptations

The second longitudinal goal of our study was to explore the contribution of children's early attachment relations to the explanation of their later adaptive functioning. In other words, we asked whether children and adolescents whose infancy attachment relations were secure would conduct themselves differently from children and adolescents whose early attachments were insecure when coping with later age-related tasks. The initial phase of our research (see Figure 7.1) involved the use of the SSP (Ainsworth et al., 1978) for assessing attachment relationships of 86 infants to their mothers (n = 83), fathers (n = 83), and professional caregivers (n = 86). Though the classification included secure, insecure-ambivalent, and insecure-avoidant, the small frequency of the latter category and the relatively small sample size resulted in a secure–insecure dichotomy. Even though these multiple assessments probably provide a meaningful representation of children's attachment experiences in an environment of multiple caregivers, they present a theoretical challenge because to date there is no clear formulation about how several representations of individual relationships that are independently formed get organized into coherent internal working models.

This issue was addressed in the second data collection phase of the research when participants were in kindergarten (n = 59, 34 boys) and their socioemotional adjustment was evaluated with direct observations at school, a variety of individually administered tasks, and the descriptions and evaluations of their professional caregivers and teachers (Oppenheim et a., 1988; van IJzendoorn et al., 1992). According to van IJzendoorn and colleagues (1992), four organizational models of attachment relationships could possibly describe the associations of early multiple attachment relationships to children's later adaptive functioning.

The *monotropy* model (Bowlby, 1951) entails that only one caregiver, typically the mother, is the important attachment figure, and other caregivers' influence is marginal in terms of attachment. According to this model, only infant–mother attachment would be associated with later socioemotional functioning. The *hierarchy* model (Bowlby, 1984) suggests that one caregiver, again typically the mother, is the most important attachment figure, but that other caregivers may be considered secondary attachment figures that serve as a secure base when the principal attachment figure is not available. It derives from the hierarchy model that infant–mother attachment would be the most powerful determinant of later socioemotional functioning but other relationships would also be predictive in a weaker sense.

The *independence* model implies that although a child may be attached to several different caregivers, each caregiver serves as a secure base only in those certain life domains in which child and caregiver had experienced continuous and lengthy interactions. This model would then lead to the prediction that attachment relations with all three caregivers are equally important determinants of later socioemotional functioning, but different caregivers influence different developmental domains. Finally, the *integration* model suggests that secure attachments may compensate for insecure attachments in a network of multiple caregivers. Optimal functioning will be associated with a network of multiple secure relationships, whereas poorest functioning will be associated with a network of insecure relationships. Thus, a linear network effect on child's functioning is implied by the integration model, and the quality of the network as a whole would be the most powerful predictor of children's later development.

Data analysis of the second phase showed that children who were securely attached to their *metapelet* in infancy were more empathic, dominant, purposive, achievement-oriented, and independent, whereas quality of separate attachment relations to father and mother did not explain children's functioning. Note that the *metaplot* with whom attachment relations were initially assessed were no longer involved in the care of these children. Thus these surprising findings were interpreted as an indication of the independence model, suggestive of domain specificity because relations with caregivers explained children's adjustment as observed in the children's house rather than their adjustment in their family (Oppenheim et al., 1988).

Yet, when the contribution of a network of early extended attachment relations (EAN; mother, father, and caregiver) and a parental network of early attachment relations (mother and father) were examined, the former was associated with more independent behavior in kindergarten and higher IQ (van IJzendoorn et al., 1992). Children with secure infancy relations to more caregivers showed higher scores of ego resilience and field independence, as well as higher scores of empathy, dominance, and goal-directed behavior in kindergarten. Children with more secure relations in the family, on the other hand, received higher scores on several socioemotional variables, but were no different from children with less secure relations in the family on ego control, dominance, and empathy in kindergarten. Similar results were also found in a Dutch sample (van IJzendoorn et al., 1992).

Consequently, as the follow-up of our participants' development continued to adolescence and into young adulthood, we adopted an exploratory approach in studying the contribution of multiple attachment relationships to the explanation of children's later adjustments. In each developmental phase, separate relationships with each caregiver were considered, as well as the parental attachment network and an extended network of parents and *metapelet*. In constructing network scores, each attachment relationship received equal value and no hierarchical order was assumed. Thus a network score of 0 indicated no secure attachment, a network score of 1 indicated one secure attachment relation, a network score of 2 indicated two secure attachment relations (the highest possible score in the parental network), and a score of 3 indicated three secure attachment relations (the highest possible score in the extended attachment network). Missing data on early attachment with one of the parents disallowed network scores for either parental attachment network or extended attachment network, while missing data with the *metapelet* precluded a score for extended attachment network. As a result, parental attachment network (PAN) and extended attachment network (EAN) scores are available for only 81 participants out of the original infancy cohort. Recall also that in infancy all participants were sleeping collectively in the children's house. This report will focus on the connections of early attachment relations, either with individual caregivers or as part of networks of multiple relations, to later school adjustment; observation of interpersonal interaction with parents and regulation of personal space in early adolescence; the concept of self through adolescence; and the development of a sense of coherence in young adulthood.

School Adjustment in Early Adolescence

Home-room teachers reported on our participants' school adjustment in early adolescence (n=66, 33 boys). They rated children's attitude toward schoolwork, as well as their verbal skills and curiosity, social competence, emotional maturity, and behavioral difficulties. Results of hierarchical regression analyses showed that in early adolescence adjustment to school was concurrently linked to representations of relationships (SAT; Hansburg, 1980), as well as to IQ and self-perceived scholastic competence (Harter, 1982). However, beyond these concurrently assessed variables and life-event control variables (parental reports of marital relationships, extent of exposure to collective sleeping), infancy attachment to mother contributed a significant addition to the explained variance in verbal skills and curiosity as well as to the emotional maturity of our early adolescent participants (Aviezer, Sagi, Resnick, & Gini, 2002).

Interaction with Parents and Regulations of Personal Space in Early Adolescence

Another domain of adaptive functioning in the transitional stage of early adolescence is children's relations with parents. Participants' interaction with their parents was observed in a "plan-a-vacation" family interaction, a task of joint vacation planning. A *Q*-set of 43 items that was devised for this task was used to describe characteristic behaviors of child and parents while performing this task. A hierarchical cluster analysis was applied to the Q-set description and yielded four clusters: positive emotional atmosphere, negative emotional atmosphere, conflictual atmosphere and cooperative atmosphere. Intercorrelations between these four clusters suggest that they represent two orthogonal dimensions of "plan-a-vacation" family interaction: a dimension of emotional atmosphere and a dimension of negotiation style (Aviezer, Dolev, Dolev, & Scharf, 1998). Hierarchical linear regression analysis showed that current representations of relationships as assessed by the SAT contributed to the explained variance in the positive and negative emotional atmosphere clusters, but not to the negotiation style clusters. Furthermore, infancy attachment to mother contributed a significant addition to the explained variance in emotional atmosphere beyond the contribution of concurrently assessed representations, IQ, and parental reports on marital relationships. Parent–child interaction in families where the adolescent's infancy attachment to mother was secure was characterized by more positive and less negative atmosphere than the interaction in families where the adolescent's infancy attachment to mother was insecure. The clusters in the dimension of negotiation style were not associated with either concurrent representation of relationships or past attachment relations. Early attachment relations to father or *metapelet* were not associated with any of the interactive clusters. Also, neither PAN nor EAN contributed to the explained variance in either the emotional atmosphere of the interaction or its negotiation style (Aviezer, Dolev, & Dolev, 2004).

The personal space of individuals is thought to be a vital factor in their regulation of transactions with others in interpersonal contexts. "Regulation of personal space" refers to preferences in terms of optimal tolerance of interpersonal distance. We conducted a behavioral evaluation of its boundaries for our early adolescent participants (Bar-Haim, Aviezer, Berson, & Sagi, 2002). Results showed that young adolescents whose infancy attachment relations with mother and *metapelet* were secure tolerated less intrusions into their personal space compared to adolescents who were insecurely attached to mother and *metapelet* in infancy (Bar-Haim et al., 2002). Again infancy attachment to father did not have any effect on tolerance of interpersonal distance. Thus, the mother–*metapelet* network that effected personal space regulation was a new network that was not postulated in advance. Given that both personal space regulation and attachment relationships evolve early in life through interactions with caregivers, this is an interesting finding because in kibbutz child care mothers and *metapelet* shared the primary responsibility for everyday caretaking of children compared to fathers' less involved role.

Self-Concept in Adolescence

A major developmental task for adolescents is to construct a comprehensive, well-organized, and coherent self-concept that allows them to function adaptively in the context of daily tasks, in particular when social situations and relationships are involved. Children's self-concept tends to change with development. Such change is particularly noticeable in adolescence with its physical, cognitive, and social transformations. By late adolescence there is a considerable ability for self-reflection with regards to the self and its relations to others, which is significantly more developed than self-reflectivity in early adolescence (Harter, 1990). Parental support is necessary for adolescents' psychological development in general and for the development of the self in particular, and these efforts benefit from close enduring relationships with parents (Collins, 1990, 1997).

Within a lifespan perspective, longitudinal associations between early relations and later adjustments, such as developing a coherent and well-organized self-concept, are particularly congruent with the secure-base construct (Bowlby, 1988) that views parent–child relations as proceeding along a course that has already been set up in early childhood. Parent–child relationships serve as a basis for children's adjustment at all ages because internal representations that mediate developmental continuity are grounded in early attachment experiences (Bretherton, 1987).

In early adolescence, participants completed the Perceived Competence Scales (PC; Harter, 1985) (n = 66, 33 boys). When participants were seniors in high school (n = 71, 38 boys), they completed the Adolescent Perceived Competence Scales (APC; Harter, 1988) and the AAI (Main & Goldwyn, 1994). In young adulthood when our participants were at the end of their compulsory military service or had just been released from the service (n = 65, 34 men), they completed the Self Esteem Questionnaire (Rosenberg, 1989). The data indicated that there are similarities between the self-concept in early and late adolescence. Late self-perceptions of scholastic competence, appearance, and athletic competence were correlated significantly with their early counterparts, while the correlation between early and late perception of self-conduct was marginally significant. However, in this sample the overall self-concept in early adolescence was unrelated to the overall self-concept in late adolescence, which suggests that despite evident continuity in specific dimensions of the self-concept, its overall organization may be different in early and late adolescence.

In early adolescence, none of the self-perceived competence scales were associated with concurrently assessed representations of relationships (SAT; Hansburg, 1980) and only self-reported athletic competence was associated with early attachment relations. When a hierarchical linear regression model of analysis was applied to this scale in which concurrently measured variables were entered first and infancy attachment was entered last, the results showed that self-perceived appearance contributed most of the explained variance in athletic competence. However, when extended attachment network in infancy was entered last, this contributed a marginally significant additional portion to the explained variance. This finding indicates that individuals with more secure relations in their early attachment network reported higher perceived athletic competence. None of the separate infancy attachment relations contributed to the explained variance in any dimension of the self-concept in early adolescence.

In late adolescence, the associations of self-perceived competence to attachment representations were rather complex. A hierarchical linear regression model of analysis was applied to the APC Scales (Harter, 1988), such that concurrently measured control variables (e.g., IQ, gender, reports of life events, sleep) were entered first, followed by attachment representations that were entered in a backward chronological order so that AAI was entered first, followed by SAT, and then by infancy attachment. These analyses revealed that the variance in self-perceived conduct was only explained by concurrently assessed AAI representations, whereas the variance in academic competence was explained only by early adolescence representations of relationships (SAT) and IQ.

However, the variance in self-perceived appearance and social acceptance was explained by gender, AAI, and SAT. Yet infancy attachment to mother, which was entered last, added marginally significant contributions to the explained variance in these two self-perceived competences. Furthermore, infancy attachment to mother, when entered last, contributed significantly to the explained variance in self-perceived social relations with friends, while infancy attachment to father, when entered last, added a significant contribution to the explained variance in self-perceived romantic relations and overall self-esteem. Finally, the variance in self-esteem at age 20 was only explained by gender, with males having higher self-esteem than females. Our finding of only a few associations between participants' self-perceived competence in early and late adolescence supports Harter's (1991) claim that the concept of self undergoes major changes during adolescence. Furthermore, our finding of associations between infancy attachment relations and late adolescence concept of self, in the absence of such links to early adolescence concept of self, highlights the dynamic nature of development during adolescence. Finally, our finding that in late adolescence interpersonal aspects of self-perceived competence are linked to infancy attachment relations with mother and father strengthen the claim that early relations with parents support the development of the self-concept and that children's adjustment at all ages may be rooted in early parent–child relations.

Sense of Coherence

According to Antonovsky (1987, 1998), adaptive coping is contingent upon individuals' strong sense of coherence that facilitates successful dealing with the numerous stressors one confronts in the course of living. This sense of coherence stabilizes by the age of 30. A strong sense of coherence is a global orientation of confidence that inner and outer environments are comprehensible and meaningful and that one has resources available for their management. Early experiences in the family are crucial contexts within which the strength of individuals' sense of coherence is molded. Therefore we examined the longitudinal associations of early attachment relations and later attachment representations to participants' sense of coherence in young adulthood.

A hierarchical linear regression model of analysis was applied to the Orientation to Life Questionnaire (Antonovsky, 1987) such that concurrently measured control variables (e.g., gender, reports of life events, sleep) were entered first, followed by age-20 self-esteem (Rosenberg, 1989) and age-17 overall self-esteem (Harter, 1988). Attachment representations were entered next in a backward chronological order so that AAI was entered first and infancy attachment was entered last. This analysis revealed that the variance in age-20 sense of coherence was explained by age-20 self-esteem and age-17 overall self-esteem. However, though entered last, infancy attachment to mother added a significant contribution to the explained variance in sense of coherence at age 20, in addition to concurrently assessed self-esteem and age-17 overall self-esteem. Young adults who were securely attached to their mothers in infancy displayed a stronger sense of coherence compared to young adults whose infancy attachment to mother was insecure. This was particularly evident in a sense that one's environment is comprehensible and manageable. Furthermore, this finding is supportive of Antonovsky's (1998) claim that early experiences constitute a crucial context for the molding of one's inner strength when dealing with the challenges of life.

GENERAL DISCUSSION

As attachment theory became a central theoretical framework in developmental psychology, longitudinal correlates of early attachment relations began to occupy center stage in attachment research. However, available longitudinal studies of attachment were inconsistent in their predictions from infancy to adulthood (Fraley, 2002), and some reviews (e.g., Thompson, 1999, 2000; Waters et al., 2000) concluded that children vary considerably in the extent to which attachment security in infancy remains consistent over time. Hence, predicting later development based on early attachment experiences is a challenging and complex undertaking that requires consideration of major issues pertinent to both longitudinal research and attachment theory. In this chapter we used data on kibbutz-raised individuals that have been collected over a period of two decades in order to address, within the attachment perspective, some of the major issues involved in the study of individual differences beyond infancy.

A major issue that remains empirically unaddressed in most longitudinal studies is the interface between coherent developmental change across time and openness to environmental influences. In this regard, Thompson (1999, 2000) suggested that early experiences as well as contemporaneous events may influence developmental outcomes and that the joint effect of the two may vary for different children. Furthermore, continuity in attachment and its sequels would be more likely associated with somewhat more stable living conditions. Yet existing longitudinal research has hardly been designed to systematically examine the relations between stability in attachment representations and changes in attachment-related life circumstances.

In this regard, van IJzendoorn (1996) suggested that two competing hypotheses should be considered. The *prototype view of attachment* assumes that continuity in attachment representations reflects an internal model for later emotional and interpersonal developments that was molded by early attachment relationships. Alternatively, the *stable environment view of attachment* attributes continuity in attachment representations to stability in the caregiving environment. However, merely finding continuity in attachment representations in childrearing environments that are stable does not allow for a critical test between these two competing hypotheses. Hence van IJzendoorn argued for adopting a "weak version" of the prototype hypothesis which states that quality of early relationships will remain on the same developmental trajectory provided that changes in childrearing circumstances have been minor, whereas major changes would cause diversion into new trajectories. In order to evaluate a weak version of the prototype hypothesis, documentation of both minor and major changes in the childrearing environment is needed. However, though it is widely agreed what constitutes "major" changes, the definition of "minor" changes is not so evidently clear.

Our findings that attachment continuity was not only affected by the major changes in the family environment (e.g., divorce, illness, or death), but also by more minor change such as the move from collective sleeping to home sleeping, demonstrate the importance of adopting a multidimensional view of environmental influences on attachment relationships. Recall that based on our previous findings we hypothesized that an earlier move to home sleeping would be beneficial to children merely because infants and their parents seemed to suffer from the collective sleeping arrangement. However, this hypothesis assumed that by itself children's move to sleeping at home would entail improved parental care and overlooked the necessary adjustments that parents faced as a consequence of such change. As correctly remarked by Maital and Bornstein (2003), child-care arrangements are basically motivated by parents' needs, which are formulated within the context of cultural standards, and it is necessary to consider these needs because the ecology of parenting influences the quality of care children receive from parents (Belsky, 1999). The change to home sleeping affected the previous balance between the family and the community with regard to children's socialization such that parents' roles became more central and the role of the *metapelet* became more marginal. Furthermore, Plotnick (1998) reported that more hostile attitudes toward their children characterized parents (mainly fathers) who changed to home sleeping, particularly if they themselves were raised in collective sleeping, possibly because they lacked appropriate parenting models to guide them in their new roles. Thus, a change in the environment of child care, even if installed for the good of children, may still become a stressor for the family and stand in the way of parents' providing sensitive care while they are adjusting.

Another important issue is whether early attachment should be conceived as a grand theory-based construct (Waters et al., 2000) that predicts a broad spectrum of domains that can be seen as directly or indirectly related to the basic tenets of attachment theory, or whether predictions should be limited to a narrower view with a focus only on attachment-based constructs (K. E. Grossmann & K. Grossmann, 1990). Existing longitudinal studies have applied broad as well as narrow constructs (Goldberg, Grusec, & Jenkins, 1999; Pederson & Moran, 1999; Thompson, 1999), which may explain why we have so much variability in research findings across these studies, especially with the enormous number of later outcomes as discussed in Thompson's (1999) review.

Internal working models of attachment relations are constructed based on experienced interactions of individuals with their attachment figures and they include both representations of the self and of attachment figures. Secure relations entail that the self would be represented as valued and the attachment figures would be represented as emotionally available and supportive of exploration, whereas insecure relations bring about feelings of self-devaluation and incompetence and representations of attachment figures as rejecting, ignoring, or interfering with exploration (Bretherton & Munholland, 1999). This formulation of internal working models defines in general terms the territories to be explored by longitudinal research. Focusing on a sense of protection alone, as suggested by Goldberg and colleagues (1999), would nullify some important findings with regards to the contribution of early relationships to later adjustment. At the same time, it is important to avoid the pitfall of using attachment as a nonspecific general model in which all good things go together, as warned by Pederson and Moran (1999). Therefore, our findings speak to a midline position that remains within a broad definition of the balance between self-confidence with the accessibility of a supportive figure and willingness to explore the world and get involved with others.

More specifically, in our data evaluations of academic achievement in adolescence by self or by others (teacher) were not associated with early attachment relations. They are likely to reflect more concurrent experiences in the school context and factors such as IQ. However, beyond academic achievement, schools may be perceived as providing opportunities for age-appropriate exploration. Hence, our finding that young adolescents' curiosity, verbal abilities, and emotional maturity as evaluated by teachers were associated with infancy attachment is congruent with the broader definition of internal working models (K. E. Grossmann, K. Grossmann, & Zimmermann, 1999; K. Grossmann, K. E. Grossmann, & Kindler, Chapter 5, this volume). Similarly, our finding that the quality of the emotional atmosphere between parents and young adolescents in interaction and management of personal space are associated with infancy attachment is also congruent with the notion of internal working models guiding individuals in interpersonal relations. Furthermore, our finding that the quality of emotional atmosphere rather than the quality of a negotiation style in interaction with parents was associated with early security with mother is concordant with Berlin and Cassidy (1999), who argued for a closer connection between early attachment and later affectional bonds.

In addition, our finding that late adolescents' self-perceived competence in social relations with friends and in romantic relations were associated with infancy attachment whereas other self-perceived competences were not is congruent with the notion that internal working models include representations of the self in relations with others. Finally, our finding that a general sense of coherence (Antonovsky, 1998) in young adulthood, which reflects individuals' confidence in their ability to cope with normal life stresses, is associated with infancy attachment relations is compatible with the view of internal working models guiding self-adjustment as well as relations with others. All these later types of adaptive functioning can be easily viewed as age-appropriate manifestations of internal working models as defined by Bretherton and Munholland (1999). In particular, the sense-of-coherence construct in young adulthood (Antonovsky, 1998) represents individuals' ability to cope with stress in their lives based on their feelings that the world makes sense, that it is meaningful, and that they have at their disposal means to manage it.

Another insufficiently addressed issue in attachment research is the notion of a network of attachment relations, which was first introduced in two cross-cultural studies with Dutch and Israeli infants (Sagi & van

IJzendoorn, 1996; van IJzendoorn et al., 1992). These two studies raised issues regarding the nature of the joint effect of an attachment network. More specifically, it was proposed that we need to explore all existing early attachment relationships such that the cumulative effect of the attachment network may be a more powerful predictor of future development than each separate attachment relationship alone. Nonetheless, it is not always clear how individual relationships would be organized into a network of relationships. Should one attachment figure be regarded as primary in a hierarchy of relationships and have more noticeable influences on future personality development compared with the other attachment figures? Alternatively, should two or more primary attachment figures be regarded as having equal impact? Though it is as yet unclear how such potentially equal influences get internally organized into a more generalized personality construct, the conceptual and empirical meaning of generalized expectations about self, others, and the world may become more complex with the availability of more than one meaningful attachment figure.

Moreover, it is still unclear whether different attachment figures may exert differential and specialized effects on children, consisting of unique domain-specific ingredients in the course of personality development (K. Grossmann, K. E. Grossmann & Kindler, Chapter 5, this volume; Oppenheim et al., 1988). With regard to this issue our findings are inconclusive. Overall, infancy relations to mother contributed most to adaptive functioning at all ages (except in kindergarten), while the relations with father and the *metapelet* also contributed, but to a lesser degree. Beyond kindergarten, networks of infancy attachment relations did not contribute as much to the explanation of later behavior. Thus, our data provides relatively little support for the integration model (van IJzendoorn et al., 1992), where it is postulated that secure relations compensate for insecure relations in a network of attachment relations, and is more supportive of the hierarchy or the independence models. As supposed by the hierarchy model (Bowlby, 1984; van IJzendoorn et al., 1992), early relations with mother contributed most to later adaptive functioning, even in the kibbutz environment that deliberately introduced additional caregivers to be extensively involved in child care. Yet our findings argue against the monotropy model (Bowlby, 1951) that would contend that other caregivers are marginal. Our data is inconclusive with regard to the independence model (van IJzendoorn et al., 1992), we found that as attachment relations to father contributed to aspects of adaptive functioning that relations with mother did not contribute to. It is clear that more conceptual and empirical work is needed in order to explore the ways in which experiences with different attachment figures organize to form a coherent internal working model. It is now important to take into consideration multiple attachment relationships experienced within the family, as contended by Thompson (2000).

In all, the complexity of our findings suggests that the developmental trajectories from infancy to adulthood with regard to attachment are indeed multifaceted, that developmental outcomes are multidetermined, and that continuity is multidimensional. Various conceptual issues, some contradictory to each other, still compete in furthering our understanding with regard to issues of continuity/discontinuity and stability/instability. Recall that the groundbreaking Baltimore study of Ainsworth and colleagues (1978) generated hypotheses rather than tested them. It is exactly this kind of exploratory seminal work that has paved the way for extensive and fruitful forthcoming hypothesis-testing research on infant attachment worldwide. In a somewhat analogous way, some of the basic conceptual issues that are pertinent to longitudinal research have evolved in response to our study, which was already in motion, rather than serving as a guiding framework for the architecture of the research design. Therefore, we conceive our contribution as a comprehensive exploratory, hypothesis-generating study that poses more complex and better defined questions.

When pioneers in the field began their studies in the early 1970s they were mainly excited by the arrival of a procedure for assessing infant attachment (i.e., the Strange Situation), whereas longitudinal research at that time evolved really as a by-product of such exciting developments, and was not based on a priori conceptual or methodological planning. Although much of this research is based on hypothesis-generating models, nonetheless many of the issues discussed before have remained as yet unaddressed. We believe that our data too, with limitations similar to all existing longitudinal endeavors in the field, may provide a stronger foundation for more refined hypothesis testing and more complex longitudinal research paradigms that will take into consideration all available attachment networks and more ecologically based as well as attachment-based definitions of stable and changing life events in family life.

ACKNOWLEDGMENTS

These studies were supported by the Israel Science Foundation (Grant No. 336-93-2), the United States–Israel Bi-National Science Foundation (Grant No. 90-489), the Israel Foundations Trustees (Grant No. 60/2002), University of Haifa Research Authority grants, and an Oranim Academic Teachers College Research Authority grant. Many individuals have participated in and contributed to the work described in this chapter and most of them served as coauthors in the numerous publications cited in this chapter. In addition, we would like to thank Dr. Arza Avrahami and Dr. Michael Nathan, former directors of the Institute for Research in Kibbutz Education. Special thanks are due to our participants and their parents, who have cooperated with us again and again and shared their lives with us.

REFERENCES

Ainsworth, M. D. S., Blehar, M. C., Waters, E., & Wall, S. (1978). *Patterns of attachment: A psychological study of the Strange Situation.* Hillsdale, NJ: Erlbaum.

Antonovsky, A. (1987). *Unraveling the mystery of health.* San Francisco: Jossey-Bass.

Antonovsky, A. (1998). The sense of coherence: A historical and future perspective. In H. I. McCubbin, E. A. Thompson, A. I. Thompson, & J. E. Fromer (Eds.), *Stress, coping, and health in families: Sense of coherence and resiliency* (pp. 3–20). Thousand Oaks, CA: Sage.

Aviezer, O., Dolev, S., & Dolev, Y. (2004). *Emotional atmosphere between early adolescent children in interaction with parents: Associations to early attachment relationships.* Unpublished manuscript.

Aviezer, O., Dolev, S., Dolev, Y., & Scharf, M. (1998, July). *Attachment representations in early adolescence: Concurrent associations to behavior with parents.* Paper presented at the biennial meeting of the International Society for the Study of Behavioral Development, Bern, Switzerland.

Aviezer, O., Sagi, A., Joels, T., & Ziv, Y. (1999). Emotional availability and attachment representations in kibbutz infants and their mothers. *Developmental Psychology, 35,* 811–821.

Aviezer, O., Sagi-Schwartz, A., & Koren-Karie, N. (2003). Ecological constraints on the formation of infant–mother attachment relations: When maternal sensitivity becomes ineffective. *Infant Behavior and Development, 26,* 285–299.

Aviezer, O., Sagi, A., Resnick, G., & Gini, M. (2002). School competence in young adolescence: Links to early attachment relationships beyond concurrent self-perceived competence and representations of relationships. *International Journal of Behavioral Development, 26,* 397–409.

Aviezer, O., Sagi, A., & van IJzendoorn, M. H. (2002). Collective sleeping for kibbutz children: An experiment in nature predestined to fail. *Family Process, 41,* 435–454.

Aviezer, O., van IJzendoorn, M. H., Sagi, A., & Schuengel, C. (1994). "Children of the Dream" revisited: 70 years of collective child care in Israeli kibbutzim. *Psychological Bulletin, 116,* 99–116.

Bar-Haim, Y., Aviezer, O., Berson, Y., & Sagi, A. (2002). Attachment in infancy and personal space regulation in early adolescence. *Attachment and Human Development, 4,* 68–83.

Barry, H., & Paxton, L. M. (1971). Infancy and early childhood: Cross-cultural codes. *Ethnology, 10,* 466–508.

Belsky, J. (1999). Interactional and contextual determinants of attachment security. In J. Cassidy & P. R. Shaver (Eds.), *Handbook of attachment: Theory, research, and clinical applications* (pp. 249–264). New York: Guilford Press.

Benoit, D., & Parker, K. C. H. (1994). Stability and transmission of attachment across three generations. *Child Development, 65,* 1444–1456.

Ben–Rafael, E. (1999). The kibbutz beyond utopia. In W. Folling & M. Folling-Albers (Eds.), *The transformation of collective education in the kibbutz: The end of utopia?* (pp. 31–49). Frankfurt, Germany: Peter Lang.

Berlin, L. J., & Cassidy, J. (1999). Relations among relationships: Contributions from attachment theory and research. In J. Cassidy & P. R. Shaver (Eds.), *Handbook of attachment: Theory, research, and clinical applications* (pp. 688–712). New York: Guilford Press.

Berman, E. (1988). Communal upbringing in the kibbutz: The allure and risks of psychoanalytic utopianism. *Psychoanalytic Study of the Child, 43,* 319–335.

Bowlby, J. (1951). *Maternal care and mental health.* Geneva, Switzerland: World Health Organization.

Bowlby, J. (1982). *Attachment and loss: Vol. 1. Attachment* (2nd ed.). London: Hogarth Press.

Bowlby, J. (1984). *Attachment and Loss: Vol. 1. Attachment.* Harmondsworth, Middlesex, UK: Penguin Books.

Bowlby, J. (1985). *Attachment and Loss: Vol. II. Separation.* Harmondsworth, Middlesex, UK: Penguin Books.

Bowlby, J. (1988). *A secure base: Clinical applications of attachment theory.* London: Routledge.

Bretherton, I. (1987). New perspectives on attachment relations: Security, communication, and internal working models. In J. Osofsky (Ed.), *Handbook of infant development* (pp. 1061–1100). New York: Wiley.

Bretherton, I., & Munholland, K. A. (1999). Internal working models in attachment relationships: A construct revisited. In J. Cassidy & P. R. Shaver (Eds.), *Handbook of attachment: Theory, research, and clinical applications* (pp. 89–111). New York: Guilford Press.

Cassidy, J. (1999). The nature of the child's ties. In J. Cassidy & P. R. Shaver (Eds.), *Handbook of attachment: Theory, research, and clinical applications* (pp. 3–20). New York: Guilford Press.

Collins, W. A. (1990). Parent–child relationships in the transition to adolescence: Continuity and change in interaction, affect and cognition. In R. Montemayor, G. Adams, & T. Gullota (Eds.), *From childhood to adolescence: A transitional period?* (pp. 85–106). Beverly Hills, CA: Sage.

Collins, W. A. (1997). Relationships and development during adolescence: Interpersonal adaptation to individual change. *Personal Relationships, 4,* 1–14.

Dar, Y. (1998). The changing identity of kibbutz education. In Y. Dar (Ed.), *Education in the changing kibbutz: Sociological and psychological perspectives* (pp. 17–41). Jerusalem: Magnes.

Dror, Y. (2001). *History of kibbutz education: Practice into theory.* Frankfurt, Germany: Peter Lang.

Erickson, M. F., Sroufe, L. A., & Egeland, B. (1985). The relationship between quality of attachment and behavior problems in preschool in a high-risk sample. In I. Bretherton & E. Waters (Eds.), Growing points in attachment theory and research. *Monographs of the Society for Research in Child Development, 50*(1–2, Serial No. 209), 147–166.

Feldman, S. S., & Yirmiya, N. (1986). Perception of socialization roles: A study of Israeli mothers in town and kibbutz. *International Journal of Psychology, 21,* 153–165.

Fonagy, P., Steele, H., & Steele, M. (1991). Maternal representations of attachment during pregnancy predict the organization of infant–mother attachment at one year of age. *Child Development, 62,* 891–905.

Fox, N. A. (1977). Attachment of kibbutz infants to mother and metapelet. *Child Development, 48,* 1228–1239.

Fraley, R. C. (2002). Attachment stability from infancy to adulthood: Meta-analysis and dynamic modeling of developmental mechanisms. *Personality and Social Psychology Review, 6,* 123–151.

George, C., Kaplan, N., & Main, M. (1985). *Adult Attachment Interview.* Unpublished manuscript, University of California–Berkeley.

Gerson, M. (1978). *Family, women and socialization in the kibbutz.* Lexington, MA: D.C. Heath.

Golan, S. (1959). Collective education in the kibbutz. *Psychiatry, 22,* 167–177.

Goldberg, S., Grusec, J. E., & Jenkins, J. M. (1999). Confidence in protection: Arguments for a narrow definition of attachment. *Journal of Family Psychology, 13,* 475–483.

Grossmann, K. E., & Grossmann, K. (1990). The wider concept of attachment in cross-cultural research. *Human Development, 33,* 31–47.

Grossmann, K. E., Grossmann, K., & Zimmermann, P. (1999). A wider view of attachment and exploration: Stability and change during the years of immaturity. In J. Cassidy & P. R. Shaver (Eds.), *Handbook of attachment: Theory, research, and clinical applications* (pp. 760–786). New York: Guilford Press.

Hamilton, C. E. (2000). Continuity and discontinuity of attachment from infancy through adolescence. *Child Development, 71,* 690–694.

Hansburg, H. G. (1980). *Adolescent separation anxiety: A method for the study of adolescent separation problems.* Huntington, NY: Krieger.

Harter, S. (1982). The Perceived Competence Scale for Children. *Child Development, 53,* 87–97.

Harter, S. (1985). *Manual for the Self-Perception Profile for Children.* Denver, CO: University of Denver.

Harter, S. (1988). *Manual of the Self-Perception Profile for Adolescence.* Denver, CO: University of Denver.

Harter, S. (1990). Identity and self development. In S. S. Feldman & G. R. Elliot (Eds.), *At the threshold: The developing adolescent* (pp. 352–387). Cambridge, MA: Harvard University Press.

Hinde, R. A. (1988). Introduction. In R. A. Hinde & J. Steveson-Hinde (Eds.), *Relationships within families* (pp. 1–4). Oxford, UK: Clarendon Press.

Kaffman, M., Elizur, E., & Rabinowitz, M. (1990). Early childhood in the kibbutz: The 1980s. In Z. Lavi (Ed.), *Kibbutz members study kibbutz children* (pp. 17–33). New York: Greenwood Press.

Konner, M. (1977). Infancy among the Kalahari Desert Sam. In P.H. Liederman, S. R. Tulkin, & A. H. Rosenfeld (Eds.), *Culture and infancy* (pp. 287–328). San Diego, CA: Academic Press.

Lavi, Z. (1984, April). *Correlates of sleeping arrangements of infants in kibbutzim.* Paper presented at the International Conference for Infant Studies, New York.

Lewin, G. (1999). The success and failure of collective education in the kibbutz. In W. Folling & M. Folling-Albers (Eds.), *The transformation of collective education in the kibbutz: The end of utopia?* (pp. 136–144). Frankfurt, Germany: Peter Lang.

Liban, A., & Goldman, D. (2000). Freud comes to Palestine; A study of psychoanalysis in a cultural context. *International Journal of Psychoanalysis, 81,* 893–906.

Maccoby, E. E., & Feldman, S. S. (1972). Mother-attachment and stranger-reactions in the third year of life. *Monographs of the Society for Research in Child Development, 37* (1, Serial No. 146), 1–86.

Main, M., & Cassidy, J. (1988). Categories of response to reunion with the parent at age 6: Predictable from infant attachment classifications and stable over a one-month period. *Developmental Psychology, 24,* 415–426.

Main, M., & Goldwyn, R. (1994). *Adult attachment rating and classification system.* Unpublished manuscript, University of California–Berkeley.

Main, M., & Solomon, J. (1990). Procedures for identifying infants as disorganized/disoriented during the Ainsworth Strange Situation. In M. T. Greenberg, D. Cicchetti, & E. M. Cummings (Eds.), *Attachment in preschool years: Theory, research, and intervention* (pp. 121–160). Chicago: University of Chicago Press.

Maital, S. L., & Bornstein, M. H. (2003). The ecology of collaborative child rearing: A systems approach to child care on the kibbutz. *Ethos, 31,* 1–32.

Morelli, G. A., & Tronick, E. Z. (1991). Efe multiple caretaking and attachment. In J. L. Gewirtz & W. M. Kurtines (Eds.), *Intersections with attachment* (pp. 41–51). Hillsdale, NJ: Erlbaum.

Oppenheim, D. (1998). Perspectives on infant mental health from Israel: The case of changes in collective sleeping on the kibbutz. *Infant Mental Health Journal, 19,* 76–86.

Oppenheim, D., Sagi, A., & Lamb, M. E. (1988). Infant–adult attachments on the kibbutz and their relation to socioemotional development four years later. *Developmental Psychology, 24,* 427–433.

Pederson, D. R., & Moran, G. (1999). The relationship imperative: Arguments for a broad definition of attachment. *Journal of Family Psychology, 13,* 496–500.

Plotnick, R. (1998). In transition to home sleeping: How parents perceive their role and the role of the caregiver. In Y. Dar (Ed.), *Education in the changing kibbutz: Sociological and psychological perspectives* (pp. 84–95). Jerusalem: Magnes.

Rabin, A. I., & Beit-Hallahmi, B. (1982). *Twenty years later: Kibbutz children grown up.* New York: Springer.

Rosenberg, M. (1989). *Society and the adolescent self image.* Middletown, CT: Wesleyan University Press.

Sagi, A., Lamb, M. E., Lewkowicz, K. S., Shoham, R., Dvir, R., & Estes, D. (1985). Security of infant–mother, –father, and–metapelet attachment among kibbutz-reared Israeli children. In I. Bretherton & E. Waters (Eds.), Growing points of attachment theory and research. *Monographs of the Society for Research in Child Development, 50*(1–2, Serial No. 209), 257–275.

Sagi, A., Lamb, M. E., Shoham, R., Dvir, R., & Lewkowicz, K. (1985). Parent–infant interaction in families on Israeli kibbutzim. *International Journal of Behavioral Development, 8,* 273–284.

Sagi, A., & van IJzendoorn, M. H. (1996). Multiple caregiving environments: The kibbutz experience. In S. Harel & J. P. Shonkoff (Eds.), *Early childhood intervention and family support programs: Accomplishments and challenges* (pp. 143–162). Jerusalem: JDC-Brookdale Institute of Gerontology and Human Development.

Sagi, A., van IJzendoorn, M. H., Aviezer, O., Donnell, F., Karie-Koren, N., Joels, T., & Harel, Y. (1995). Attachments in a multiple-caregiver and multiple-infant environment: The case of the Israeli kibbutzim. In E. Waters, B. E. Vaughn, G. Posada, & K. Kondo-Ikemura (Eds.), Caregiving, cultural, and cognitive perspectives on secure-base behavior and working models: New growing points of attachment theory and research [Special issue]. *Monographs of the Society for Research on Child Development, 60*(2–3, Serial No. 244), 71–91.

Sagi, A., Van IJzendoorn, M. H., Aviezer, O., Donnell, F., & Mayseless, O. (1994). Sleeping out of home in a kibbutz communal arrangement: It makes a difference for infant–mother attachment. *Child Development, 65,* 992–1004.

Sagi, A., van IJzendoorn, M. H., & Karie-Koren, N. (1991). Primary appraisal of the Strange Situation: A cross-cultural analysis of preseparation episodes. *Developmental Psychology, 27,* 587–596.

Sagi, A., van IJzendoorn, M.H., Scharf, M., Joels, T., Koren-Karie, N., & Aviezer, O. (1997). Ecological constraints for intergenerational transmission of attachment. *International Journal of Behavioral Development, 20,* 287–299.

Sagi, A., van IJzendoorn, M. H., Scharf, M., Koren-Karie, N., Joels, T., & Mayseless, O. (1994). Stability and discriminant validity of the Adult Attachment Interview: A psychometric study. *Developmental Psychology, 30,* 771–777.

Shamai, S. (1992). *Patterns of paternal involvement in the kibbutz: The role of fathers in intact families in the education of their preadolescent children.* Unpublished master's thesis, University of Haifa, Haifa, Israel.

Spiro, M. E. (1979). *Gender and culture: Kibbutz women revisited.* Durham, NC: Duke University Press.

Sroufe, L. A., Carlson, E., & Shulman, S. (1993). Individuals in relationships: Development from infancy. In D.C. Funder, R. D. Parke, C. Tomlinson-Keasey, & K. Widaman (Eds.), *Studying lives through time: Personality and development* (pp. 315–342). Washington, DC: American Psychological Association.

Sroufe, L. A., Egeland, B., & Kreutzer, T. (1990). The fate of early experience following developmental change: Longitudinal approaches to individual adaptation in childhood. *Child Development, 61,* 1363–1373.

Talmon, Y. (1972). *Family and community in the kibbutz.* Cambridge, MA: Harvard University Press.

Thompson, R. A. (1999). Early attachment and later development. In J. Cassidy & P. R. Shaver (Eds.), *Handbook of attachment: Theory, research, and clinical applications* (pp. 265–286). New York: Guilford Press.

Thompson, R. A. (2000). The legacy of early attachments. *Child Development, 71,* 145–152.

Tiger, L., & Shepher, J. (1975). *Women on the kibbutz.* San Diego, CA: Harcourt Brace Jovanovich.

van IJzendoorn, M. H. (1996). Commentary. *Human Development, 39,* 224–231.

van IJzendoorn, M. H., Moran, G., Belsky, J., Pederson, D., Bakermans-Kranenburg, M.J., & Fisher, K. (2000). The similarity of siblings' attachments to their mother. *Child Development, 71,* 1086–1098.

van IJzendoorn, M. H., & Sagi, A. (1999). Cross-cultural patterns of attachment: Universal and contextual dimensions. In J. Cassidy & P.R. Shaver (Eds.), *Handbook of attachment: Theory, research, and clinical applications* (pp. 713–734). New York: Guilford Press.

van IJzendoorn, M. H., Sagi, A., & Lambermon, M. W. (1992). The multiple care-taker paradox: some data from Holland and Israel. *New Directions in Child Development, 57,* 5–24.

Wartner, U. G., Grossmann, K., Fremmer-Bombik, E., & Suess, G. (1994). Attach-ment patterns in south Germany: Predictability from infancy and implications for preschool behavior. *Child Development, 65,* 1014–1027.

Waters, E., Hamilton, C., & Weinfield, N. (2000). The stability of attachment security from infancy to adolescence and early adulthood: General discussion. *Child Development, 71,* 703–706.

Waters, E., Merrick, S., Treboux, D., Crowell, J., & Albersheim, L. (2000). Attach-ment security in infancy and early adulthood: A twenty-year longitudinal study. *Child Development, 71,* 684–689.

Weinfield, N. S., Sroufe, L. A., & Egeland, B. (2000). Attachment from infancy to early adulthood in a high-risk sample: Continuity, discontinuity, and their corre-lates. *Child Development, 71,* 695–702.

CHAPTER 8

The Interplay between Attachment, Temperament, and Maternal Style

A Madingley Perspective

JOAN STEVENSON-HINDE

INTANGIBLES: SOME PERSONAL RECOLLECTIONS

In the late 1950s and early 1960s, at least at Mount Holyoke College and Brown University where I studied, the psychology departments' strengths were in the experimental realm: perception, psychophysics, physiological psychology, and operant conditioning. My own research involved operant conditioning, namely, conditioned reinforcement in rats and discrimination learning in pigeons. But in a graduate seminar at Brown, I came across learning in naturally occurring contexts, including the work of William Thorpe on song learning in chaffinches. Here was a form of learning that involved complex patterns that could be quantitatively assessed, via sonograms. If Skinner was right, reinforcement should be involved. All this led to a postdoctoral fellowship in Professor Thorpe's thriving laboratory at Madingley, within the zoology department of Cambridge University—for a visit that was supposed to last 1 year. In fact, my work with birds took much longer than a year, and raised issues that continued into my later research. In using hand-reared or autumn-caught chaffinches and song as a reinforcer, I came to appreciate that unlike my laboratory-reared pigeons working for food, early experience and hormonal levels had to be taken into account, as well as individual differences. We also identified individual differences in the calls of Sandwich and Common terns as they returned to feed their young, who in turn responded to their own parents' calls but not to those of near neighbors.

Also at Madingley was the thriving rhesus monkey colony set up by Robert Hinde, with the encouragement of John Bowlby, to study the effects of separation on the mother–infant relationship. Over the years, my interest in this topic grew, particularly as I approached motherhood myself. I was fortunate in being able to switch to research with monkeys, and developed a personality scale for assessing individual differences in monkeys from 1 year of age onward. My first article in *Child Development* did not involve human subjects! The main personality component year after year was a "confident–fearful" dimension. On the one hand, Jerry Kagan took this result with monkeys to indicate the biological basis of fearfulness; on the other hand, our *Child Development* article focused on the relation between antecedent mother–infant interactions and the traits of the developing infants.

In the mid-1970s Robert Hinde and I carried out our first joint project, and also our first with *human* offspring. Whereas he observed peer–peer interactions in playgroups, I observed mother–child interactions at home, while also interviewing the mothers. Two things stood out for me, both of which reflected earlier observations with rhesus monkey mothers and infants: one was the differential sensitivity of the mothers; the other was the extreme shyness of a few of the children, as well as the concern of the mothers about this shyness, particularly if the shy child was a boy. In subsequent studies, I therefore assessed both attachment security and shyness in the laboratory, in addition to making observations at home. This involved setting up a Strange Situation in the laboratory, guided by Mary Main's example while we were on sabbatical at the University of California–Berkeley, plus visits to Madingley from Mary Main, Mary Ainsworth, and John Bowlby. Although the Strange Situation was therefore run properly, nevertheless a coding problem remained. My sample involved not infants, but 2.5-year-olds. Here, I must give enduring thanks to Mark Greenberg, who came by at just the right time and offered just the right solution. He invited me to join the MacArthur Working Group on Attachment in preschool children, which produced the Cassidy and Marvin Coding System for 2.5- to 4.5-year-olds. These Seattle meetings benefited from the supportive presence of Mary Ainsworth, who was secure enough to let her system be modified without herself remaining in the foreground. There I met Bob Marvin, who generously came over several times to keep our coding on track through reliability assessments, as well as to run a teaching workshop for others on this side of the Atlantic.

Lately my research has moved away from normative samples to selecting samples to contain a sufficiently large number of shy children, or, currently, of anxious mothers. In my view, it is time to focus in such a way on particular samples. Perhaps reflecting my own experimental upbringing, I think it is also time to aim for research designs that involve manipulation or intervention, so that we may test experimentally what the key variables are, rather than relying solely on complex statistical techniques.

What follows is not a comprehensive review of theoretical approaches and past disputes over the relation between temperament and attachment (see, e.g., Vaughn & Bost, 1999), but rather an interactionist view from the perspective of my own research. I have been particularly concerned with the interplay between fearfulness and attachment, while at the same time appreciating their distinctions. The chapter follows a logical order, starting with discussion of distinctions, then addressing common aspects, and finally examining the interplay that we see in practice.

DISTINCTIONS

Distinct Concepts

As Alan Sroufe (1985) so aptly argued some years ago, temperament and attachment are fundamentally different constructs, referring to different domains and operating at different levels of analysis. The term "temperament" refers *to early appearing individual differences* along a variety of dimensions, which vary according to particular theories. For example, Rothbart, who was concerned with infants' reactivity and self-regulation, assessed activity, duration of orienting, distress to limitations, smiling, soothability, and fear. The behavior geneticists Buss and Plomin defined temperament as inherited personality traits appearing early, namely, emotionality, activity, sociability, and shyness. However, as practicing psychiatrists dealing with families of children presenting problems, Thomas and Chess were concerned with the stylistic component of behavior reflected in nine dimensions: activity, initial approach–withdrawal, adaptability, intensity of reaction, quality of mood, rhythmicity, threshold of responsiveness, distractibility, and attention span/persistence (reviewed in Goldsmith et al., 1987). Note that all these theories contain a dimension related to fearfulness, a trait recognized over many years (e.g., Kagan, 1994), and in many species (Gosling & John, 1999), including other primates (Stevenson-Hinde, Stillwell-Barnes, & Zunz, 1980). Fearfulness is a particularly salient individual characteristic in early childhood, when increasing exploration beyond the family leads to encounters with unfamiliar people and events. Since temperament itself is not a trait, but rather a "rubric for a group of related traits" (Goldsmith et al., 1987, p. 506), fearfulness is used from here on as an exemplar of temperament.

In contrast with the above, "attachment" is defined as *an aspect of a relationship* with someone perceived as older/wiser, with the sensitivity of the caregiver playing a key causal role in the development of infant security. Powerful meta-analyses over many studies have shown significant associations between sensitivity and security (De Wolff & van IJzendoorn, 1997), even in non-Western cultures (van IJzendoorn & Sagi, 1999), as well as effects of intervention on sensitivity in promoting security (Bakermans-Kranenburg, van IJzendoorn, & Juffer, 2003). After systematically considering results concerning the role of temperament and maternal sensitivity in the formation of attachment, van IJzendoorn and Bakermans-Kranenburg (2004) conclude:

> In sum, the causal role of maternal sensitivity in the formation of the infant–mother attachment relationship is a strongly corroborated finding. Correlational, experimental, and cross-cultural studies have replicated the association between sensitivity and attachment numerous times, and through different measures and designs. In general, the maternal impact on the infant–mother attachment relationship has been shown to be much larger than the impact of child characteristics such as temperament. During the first few years after birth, parents are more powerful than their children in shaping the child–parent bond. (p. 208)

Distinct Origins

In accordance with the above definitions of temperament and attachment, significant genetic influences have been demonstrated for the former but not the latter. Both twin and adoption studies indicate that fearfulness is heritable, with genetic factors accounting for around 40–60% of the variance (reviewed in Schmidt, Polak, & Spooner, 2001). More recent molecular genetic studies have examined whether genes that code for the regulation and transportation of neurotransmitters are associated with complex human traits such as novelty seeking and shyness. Although results are inconsistent, possibly due to insufficient sample sizes to detect small effects, convincing associations are emerging (reviewed in Plomin & Rutter, 1998; Schmidt et al., 2001). For example, dopamine D4 receptor (DRD4) polymorphisms (long alleles) are associated with novelty seeking and related behaviors such as attention-deficit/hyperactivity disorder (ADHD). Since short alleles code for a receptor apparently more efficient in binding dopamine, "The theory is that individuals with the long-repeat DRD4 allele are dopamine deficient and seek novelty to increase dopamine release" (Plomin & Caspi, 1998, p. 393).

In addition, a polymorphism in the promoter region of the serotonin transporter gene (5-HTTLPR) has been associated with anxiety-related traits (Lesch et al., 1996). A short allele may contribute to reduced serotonin promotion and expression. Without the regulating effects of serotonin, the amygdala and the hypothalamic–pituitary–adrenal (HPA) system become overactive, leading to the physiological profile of fearful or anxious individuals (Schmidt et al., 2001). Lesch and colleagues (1996) conclude that approximately 10–15 genes might be involved in contributing to anxiety.

Such genetic evidence has *not* been found for patterns of attachment. In a carefully conducted behavioral genetic study involving two samples of twins (in Leiden and in London), the role of genetic factors in both attachment disorganization and attachment security was negligible, while genetic factors explained 77% of the variance in temperamental reactivity (Bokhorst et al., 2003). Turning to molecular genetics, a Budapest study found an association between DRD4 polymorphisms (long, exon III 7-repeat alleles, particularly in the presence of a specific allele in the promoter region of the DRD4 gene) and disorganized attachment in infancy (Lakatos et al., 2000, 2002). However, this does not imply a genetic basis for security versus insecurity of attachment, or indeed for any of the "organized" attachment patterns. That is, within the disorganized group of 17 infants (out of 95 in total), all of the main organized attachment patterns were found: eight were classified as secure, six as avoidant, and three as ambivalent (Lakatos et al., 2000, 2002). Furthermore, a recent study with a larger sample size (Leiden: n = 132; 26 in the D group) did not replicate the DRD4–disorganized association, even when the Leiden and Budapest samples were combined (Bakermans-Kranenburg & van IJzendoorn, 2004). This is not surprising in view of the key role played by frightened/frightening maternal behavior in the development of disorganization (see Main, Hesse, & Kaplan, Chapter 10, this volume). It is therefore clear that any genetic model of development of attachment patterns will not be a simple one (Gervai & Lakatos, 2004).

Distinct Behavior and Goals

Fearful behavior involves initial withdrawal from unfamiliar or challenging events, while *attachment behavior* involves gaining or maintaining proximity with a caregiver when stressed. While both may be viewed as "goal-directed" in the sense of having a predictable outcome (Hinde & Stevenson, 1970), the outcomes are very different. For fearful behavior, the goal is "withdrawal from threat." For attachment behavior, the goal is "proximity to the attachment figure," or Ainsworth's more psychological goal of "felt security."

In Bowlby's (1982) words,

> The simplest form in which the distinction can be stated is that, on the one hand, we try at times to withdraw or escape from a situation or object that we find alarming, and, on the other, we try to go towards or remain with some person or in some place that makes us feel secure. The first type of behaviour is commonly accompanied by a sense of fright or alarm, and is not far from what Freud had in mind when he spoke of "realistic fear." . . . The second type of behaviour is, of course, what is termed here attachment behaviour. So long as the required proximity to the attachment-figure can be maintained, no unpleasant feeling is experienced. When, however, proximity cannot be maintained . . . the consequent searching and striving are accompanied by a sense of disquiet, more or less acute; and the same is true when loss is threatened. In this disquiet at separation and at threat of separation Freud in his later work came to see "the key to an understanding of anxiety." (p. 330)

Distinct Motivational Systems

In line with the above distinctions, Bowlby postulated separate motivational systems for wary/fearful behavior and attachment behavior (e.g., Bowlby, 1982; see also Bischof, 1975), with both becoming organized into goal-corrected systems over the first year of life. Furthermore, according to Baerends (1976), "Differences in responsiveness of one individual at different times can be understood on the basis of variations in the balance between different motivational systems" (p. 733). For example, Bretherton and Ainsworth (1974) and Greenberg and Marvin (1982) found coherence in apparently diverse sequences of behavior by referring to the organization of four distinct but interacting behavior systems: wary/fear, attachment, exploration, and sociable. Within this framework, an unfamiliar stimulus would involve activation of both the fear and attachment behavior systems, with corresponding deactivation of the exploratory and sociable systems (for further discussion, see Stevenson-Hinde, 1991).

COMMON ASPECTS

In keeping with John Bowlby's reliance on ethology, common aspects are discussed within the framework of Niko Tinbergen's *four why's* of behavior: development *(What are the developmental pathways?)*, causation *(How does it work?)*, function *(What is the use upon which natural selection acts?)*, and evolution *(Evolutionary origins?)* (see, e.g., Hinde, 1987, pp. 15–18, and Chapter 1, this volume). Until recently, questions concerning function and evolution tended to be overlooked by psychologists, so these are considered first.

Function and Evolution

Bowlby postulated that both fear behavior and attachment behavior share a common evolutionary function: protection from harm (Bowlby, 1982; see also Ainsworth, Blehar, Waters, & Wall, 1978; Sroufe, 1977; Stevenson-Hinde, 2000). Both fear of the unfamiliar and fear of being left alone would have been essential for survival in the environments in which we evolved. The argument is that individuals who exhibited fear of the unfamiliar would have been more apt to survive and leave offspring who in turn reproduce—that is, to have increased their inclusive fitness—compared with those who did not. In harmony with this view, Stevenson, Batten, and Cherner (1992) have shown that fears concerning harm possibly relevant during the course of evolution (e.g., fear of the unknown, fear of animals, fear of danger) have significant heritability estimates, while modern-day fears not involving risk of life (e.g., fear of criticism, fear of medical procedures) do not.

In a similar way, attachment behavior and its complement, caregiving behavior, would have been selected for during the course of evolution (Bowlby, 1982). However, the particular pattern of attachment behavior that develops is flexible, depending not upon genetic factors (as we have seen), but rather on environmental circumstances. And here a functional argument may be applied. For example, Belsky (1999) argues that "patterns of attachment represent nascent facultative reproductive strategies that evolved to promote reproductive fitness in particular ecological niches" (p. 150). At the same time, we must recognize that a pattern required for the above "biological desiderata" of increasing inclusive fitness need not be the same as a pattern fitting "cultural desiderata" (e.g., in Bielefeld, where an avoidant pattern was the norm, vs. Regensburg, where a secure pattern predominated; see K. Grossmann, Fremer-Bombik, Rudolph, & K. E. Grossmann, 1988). Additionally, it was the secure pattern that Bowlby, as a practicing psychiatrist, saw as absolutely basic for "psychological well-being." These three desiderata—biological, cultural, and psychological—while influencing each other, may differ, especially in modern industrialized societies (Hinde & Stevenson-Hinde, 1991).

One advantage of the functional/evolutionary view is that what had been termed "the irrational fears of childhood" become not so irrational after all. Bowlby (1973) argued that our tendency to fear what had been dangers in the environments in which we evolved is to be regarded as a natural disposition of man . . . that stays with him in some degree from infancy to old age. . . . Thus it is not the presence of this tendency in childhood or later life that is pathological; pathology is indicated either when the tendency is apparently absent or when fear is aroused with unusual readiness and intensity. (p. 84)

Similarly, attachment behavior in times of stress should not be viewed as a sign of weakness at any age. Long before research began on the role of attachment in adulthood, Bowlby (1973) wrote:

Such tendencies . . . are present not only during childhood but throughout the whole span of life. Approached in this way, fear of being separated unwillingly from an attachment figure at any phase of the life-cycle ceases to be a puzzle, and instead, becomes classifiable as an instinctive response to one of the naturally occurring clues to an increased risk of danger. (p. 86)

In one of his final contributions Bowlby (1991) maintained this view:

Once we postulate the presence within the organism of an attachment behavioural system regarded as the product of evolution and having protection as its biological function, many of the puzzles that have perplexed students of human relationships are found to be soluble. . . . An urge to keep proximity or accessibility to someone seen as stronger or wiser, and who if responsive is deeply loved, comes to be recognised as an integral part of human nature and as having a vital role to play in life. Not only does its effective operation bring with it a strong feeling of security and contentment, but its temporary or long-term frustration causes acute or chronic anxiety and discontent. When seen in this light, the urge to keep proximity is to be respected, valued, and nurtured as making for potential strength, instead of being looked down upon, as so often hitherto, as a sign of inherent weakness. (p. 293)

Development

Behavior patterns serving as attachment behavior, such as sucking, clinging, smiling, and crying, are present from birth, and so too are components of fearful behavior, such as crying or startle responses. Furthermore, individual differences in attachment behavior and fearful behavior show significant stability during the course of development. Evidence for behavioral stability relies on indices such as directly observed patterns of attachment or – "behavioral inhibition" (BI). BI is defined by Kagan (e.g., 1989, 1994) as a child's initial withdrawal from unfamiliar or challenging events. Longitudinal studies have demonstrated BI to be moderately stable from infancy into childhood (e.g., Fordham & Stevenson-Hinde, 1999; Kagan, Reznick,

Snidman, Gibbons, & Johnson, 1988; Kagan, Snidman, & Arcus, 1998; Kerr, Lambert, Stattin, & Klackenberg-Larsson, 1994; Stevenson-Hinde & Shouldice, 1995a). Similarly, patterns of attachment have shown high stability from infancy to age 6 years, both in a sample from Berkeley (84% concordance for avoidant, secure, and disorganized patterns; Main & Cassidy, 1988) and in a sample from Regensburg (82% concordance for avoidant, secure, ambivalent, and disorganized patterns; Wartner, Grossmann, Fremmer-Bombik, & Suess, 1994). As may be expected from attachment theory itself, stability is dependent upon family context and life experiences, which are particularly open to change as one passes from childhood into adolescence and then into early adulthood (see, e.g., Waters, Hamilton, & Weinfield, 2000, and Sroufe et al., Chapter 3, in this volume).

Causation: How Does It Work?

Since similar stimuli, namely, unfamiliar or challenging events, elicit both attachment behavior and fearful behavior, it is possible that similar mediating mechanisms might be involved. Behavioral inhibition has been associated with a high and steady heart rate, elevated cortisol, and right frontal EEG asymmetry. Current models focus on variation in the excitability of neural circuits in the limbic system with the amygdala playing a central role (reviewed in Davidson & Rickman, 1999; Marshall & Stevenson-Hinde, 2001; Schmidt et al., 2001). Schwartz, Wright, Shin, Kagan, and Rauch (2003) have recently found that adults who had been categorized in the second year of life as inhibited, compared with an uninhibited group, showed greater functional MRI signal response within the amygdala to novel versus familiar faces.

It is tempting to predict that, like behavioral inhibition, insecure attachment should also be associated with high amygdalar responsiveness, high heart rate, and elevated cortisol. However, cardiac evidence is either lacking or mixed (critically reviewed in Fox & Card, 1999). For example, comparing heart rate over three patterns of attachment in 12-month-olds (secure, avoidant, and disorganized), Spangler and K. Grossmann (1993) found no main effect for attachment, although the disorganized infants' heart rate increased significantly when left alone in the Strange Situation (see also Willemsen-Swinkels, Bakermans-Kranenburg, Buitelaar, van IJzendoorn, & van Engeland, 2000). Similarly, in 4.5-year-olds, when cardiac functioning (heart period and respiratory sinus arrhythmia) was compared over the three main "organized" patterns of attachment (avoidant, secure, and ambivalent), no significant effects occurred (Stevenson-Hinde & Marshall, 1999).

High cortisol levels have been associated with insecurity, with some intriguing differences across studies (Spangler, personal communication,

September 2, 2003). For example, Spangler and K. Grossmann (1993) found higher cortisol levels in traditionally insecure infants as well as in disorganized ones, while Hertsgaard, Gunnar, Erickson, and Nachmias (1995) found elevated cortisol only in disorganized infants, and Spangler and Schieche (1998) found highest levels in ambivalent infants. What is common to all these studies is that no study found elevated cortisol levels in secure infants. But why do cortisol elevations vary inconsistently across the insecure patterns? The answer may lie in the need to take BI into account, as well as insecurity. Indeed, when both BI and attachment were assessed, cortisol levels were highest in those infants who were both inhibited and insecure (Nachmias, Gunnar, Mangelsdorf, Porritz, & Buss, 1996; Spangler & Schieche, 1998). As Gunnar (1994) has suggested, adrenocortical activity may not map neatly onto fear-related constructs, but rather cortisol levels may be also be related to the maintenance or failure of coping strategies. To the extent that security is associated with good coping strategies, protection is offered, even to inhibited children (Marshall & Stevenson-Hinde, 2001).

A CONTINUOUS INTERPLAY

If we accept the above distinctions between fear and attachment as well as their common aspects, then it follows that in practice there must be interplay between the two. Before turning to data focusing on our own studies, consideration of some general issues will pave the way toward building a diagram of interacting effects.

Other Influences

Results from a variety of studies indicate an influence of relationships and culture on fearfulness; conversely, with patterns of attachment, we may infer some influence of temperament. That is, with behavioral inhibition, correlations across time (see above references), across measures (e.g., Reznick, Gibbons, Johnson, & McDonough, 1989; Stevenson-Hinde & Glover, 1996), and particularly across different contexts (Stevenson-Hinde, 1989, 1998) are far from perfect, leaving room for environmental influences. Social influences are suggested by the findings that moderate shyness is more acceptable in girls than in boys (e.g., Mills & Rubin, 1993; Stevenson-Hinde & Hinde, 1986), at least in Western cultures. Furthermore, cross-cultural differences are evident. Thus, observed behavioral inhibition was greater in China than in Canada, where it was associated with low maternal acceptance, low encouragement of achievement, and high punishment. The opposite held in China (Chen et al., 1998).

Turning to attachment, we too often overlook the fact that Bowlby himself allowed for a range of influences on patterns of attachment, including temperament. He wrote: "It is evident that the particular pattern taken by any one child's attachment behaviour turns partly on the initial biases that infant and mother each bring to their partnership and partly on the way that each affects the other during the course of it" (1982, p. 340). After presenting data, Bowlby continues: "By the time the first birthday is reached both mother and infant have commonly made so many adjustments in response to one another that the resulting pattern of interaction has already become highly characteristic" (p. 348). In addition to the immediate characteristics of the infant, the behavior of the caregiver is determined by "the particular sequence of environments, from infancy onwards, within which development takes place" (p. 378).

Limits on Attachment Patterns

The rare co-occurrence of the avoidant (A) and the ambivalent (C) pattern of attachment for any one child suggests some limitation on what patterns may develop. Indeed, the exemplars for each pattern suggest two quite different, possibly incompatible, strategies. Whereas the avoidant pattern involves physical and conversational avoidance of calling attention to the relationship, minimal but polite responses, and maintenance of neutrality upon reunion, the ambivalent pattern involves angry, whiny resistance directed to caregiver and/or immature, coy behavior, often with ambivalence to physical proximity, and an emphasis on dependence (Cassidy & Marvin, 1992).

One set of evidence for the incompatibility of the two patterns comes from assessments across time. For example, when we assessed stability from 2.5 to 4.5 years using the Cassidy and Marvin (1992) coding system, we found reasonable consistency, in spite of the fact that entering preschool intervened. Across four categories consisting of avoidant, secure, ambivalent, and other (controlling, disorganized, and insecure-other), 62% (48/78) of the children remained in the same category. However, no child was avoidant at one time and ambivalent at the other. That is, of the nine children who were A at Time 1, none became C at Time 2; of the 13 who were C at Time 1, none became A at Time 2 (Stevenson-Hinde & Shouldice, 1993).

Another set of evidence comes from assessing the same child with two different caregivers. If by definition an attachment pattern reflects an aspect of a particular relationship, then for any given child patterns across different relationships should be independent of each other. In a meta-analysis of 14 studies on 950 families, the infant–mother versus infant–father attachment correlation was indeed low (phi = .17; van IJzendoorn & De Wolff, 1997). Furthermore, even that low correlation could be partially explained by the significant correspondence between husbands' and wives' attachment representations (van IJzendoorn & Bakermans-Kranenburg, 1996). What is of particular interest here, however, is that for any given child, A and C patterns were highly unlikely to co-occur (e.g., Belsky & Rovine, 1987; Fox, Kimmerly, & Schafer, 1991, Fig. 2, p. 218). For example, in the first two studies to confirm independence of classifications, one in Bielefeld (K. E. Grossmann, Grossmann, Huber, & Wartner, 1981) and the other in Berkeley (Main & Weston, 1981), only one child was A with one parent and C with the other.

A Continuum of Characteristics
Rather Than a Simple Dichotomy

We are thus moving away from a simple "temperament versus relationship dichotomy." As I wrote some years ago, we need to

> postulate a continuum, which is personological at one end, and relational at the other [see Figure 8.1]. Temperament would lie toward the person end, but different dimensions of temperament might lie at different places on the continuum. For example, activity might be more independent of relationships than negative mood. (Stevenson-Hinde, 1986, p. 97)

Furthermore, the position of any given characteristic on such a continuum may change with age. For example, behavioral inhibition "may be relatively independent of relationships from 0–6 months, then modified by attachment relationships and social reinforcement, and finally relatively fixed" (Stevenson-Hinde, 1988, p. 75). Finally, the placement of characteristics may be different for different individuals, depending upon "phenotypically inflexible" versus "phenotypically plastic" genotypes (Stevenson-Hinde, 2000; Wilson, Clark, Coleman, & Dearstyne, 1994; Wilson, Coleman, Clark, & Biederman, 1993).

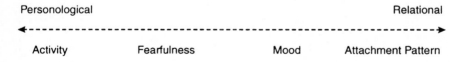

FIGURE 8.1. Against a simple genetic–environmental dichotomy: A postulated continuum of bidirectional influences, with individual characteristics lying along it.

TOWARD AN INTERACTIONIST MODEL

The above sets the stage for an interactionist model, with mutual influences between aspects of temperament and attachment during the course of development. This is basically a systems perspective, in which there are cycles of interaction among elements (e.g., Minuchin, 1985). With this approach, the "chicken or egg" question of priority fades away (Stevenson-Hinde, 1991). After considering interactions at the physiological level, we shall move on to construct a diagram of associations at the behavioral level.

A Methodological Preface

First, in keeping with the ethological tradition of our laboratory, our studies focus on direct observations. In addition to the obvious point that questionnaires that rely on the same observer carry the risk of cross-temporal and cross-situational bias, parents may introduce particular individual biases. For example, insensitive mothers might read their children's behavior in a more dismissive way than sensitive mothers do. Indeed, we found that mothers of securely attached children tended to overestimate their children's shyness as compared with our direct observations, while mothers of insecurely attached children did the opposite (Stevenson-Hinde & Shouldice, 1990; see also Kemp, 1987; Sameroff, Seifer, & Elias, 1982; Stevenson-Hinde & Shouldice, 1995b; Vaughn, Taraldson, Crichton, & Egeland, 1981). Similarly, when given an attachment Q-sort, mothers of children observed in the Strange Situation as secure underestimated their children's security compared with our security ratings from the Strange Situation, while mothers of insecure children, particularly the avoidant group, overestimated security (Stevenson-Hinde & Shouldice, 1990; see also van IJzendoorn & Bakermans-Kranenburg, 2004). Finally, while a recent meta-analysis involving 27 samples showed significant relations between an *observer*-rated attachment Q-sort and indices of validity, including security in the Strange Situation ($r = .31$, $n = 1,070$), the relations did not hold for *maternal* ratings of security. These correlated with Strange Situation security at only $r = .14$ ($n = 911$). Furthermore, mothers overestimated security in comparison with observers (van IJzendoorn, Vereijken, Bakermans-Kranenburg, & Riksen-Walraven, 2004).

Second, in keeping with Mary Ainsworth's lead in assessments of attachment, our observations of behavioral inhibition are expressed in terms of *quality* as opposed to *quantity*. That is, instead of measuring BI by indices reflecting the frequency of responses or latency to first occurrence of a particular response, we apply rating scales to both verbal and nonverbal behavior, thereby indexing a child's behavioral style along the lines of temperament theorists such as Thomas and Chess mentioned above. The ratings may be made in the home or in the lab (see Fordham & Stevenson-Hinde, 1999). We repeatedly view a videotaped sequence: first, to get an overview, then for rating verbal behavior, next for rating nonverbal behavior, and finally to determine a global rating, with 4 as the "norm for age." Such coding can be applied over a wide age range, and we have used it at 2.5 years (Stevenson-Hinde & Shouldice, 1990), 4.5 and 7 years (Marshall & Stevenson-Hinde, 1998), and 10 years (Fordham & Stevenson-Hinde, 1999). What does change with age is the nature of the challenge—with older children not simply being invited to approach the stranger "to see what is in my hand," but rather being asked conversational questions, ending with a request to stand up and "sing your favorite song."

Interacting Influences between Behavioral Inhibition and Security of Attachment on Cardiac Functioning

As indicated above, Kagan and coworkers have extensively studied BI. They proposed that differences in reaction to novelty between inhibited and uninhibited children arise from variation in the excitability of neural circuits in the limbic system, which in turn affect cardiac pacemaker activity and provide a rationale that inhibited children should show consistently higher heart rates than uninhibited children. This finding has been supported by some studies, but not all (see Stevenson-Hinde & Marshall, 1999).

We suggest that those studies that do support the predicted relation between BI and autonomic functioning may have a high proportion of children who are securely attached to their mothers. Within our own sample of children selected for low, medium, or high BI we showed that it was only the secure children who showed the predicted relations—with the high BI group having significantly lower heart period (or higher heart rate) than the low BI group. A characteristic of secure children is that, through interactions with a sensitively responsive caregiver, they are able to express their emotions in a relaxed and open manner, without the need to develop any particular strategy. With such "emotional coherence" (K. E. Grossmann & K. Grossmann, 1991, p. 108), secure children should exhibit a more direct relation between autonomic functioning and behavior to strangers than should insecure children. Indeed, our insecure children did not show any significant relations between BI and heart period (Stevenson-Hinde & Marshall, 1999).

Behavioral Inhibition and Ambivalent Attachment

High BI ←—→Ambivalent (& Insecure-other) attachment
Low BI ←—→Secure and Avoidant attachment

Consideration of attachment-related differences in the expression of emotions leads to the expectation that the ambivalent pattern might be particularly associated with high BI. Suppose we have three children with similar underlying predispositions to BI. In practice, the secure (B) child who expresses emotions openly may receive a higher BI rating than the avoidant (A) child who tries very hard to appear neutral, thereby hiding his emotions. However, the ambivalent (C) child, with the strategy of overemphasizing emotions and dependence, might "overplay" emotions and be observed to be the most fearful.

Indeed, with both infants and young children, assessed respectively with the Ainsworth infancy coding system or the Cassidy and Marvin preschool system (Cassidy & Marvin, 1992; see also Stevenson-Hinde & Verschueren, 2002, for a review of validation studies), significant associations have been found between high BI and the ambivalent (C) pattern, and between low BI and the secure or avoidant patterns. That is, in two different samples BI for ambivalent infants was significantly greater than BI for avoidant infants (Calkins & Fox, 1992; Kochanska, 1998).

In a sample of 2.5-year-olds, the very secure (B3) children were observed to be the least fearful, and the ambivalent children the most fearful, at a highly significant level ($p < .001$; Stevenson-Hinde & Shouldice, 1990). Further studies suggest that relations between BI and attachment are more apt to appear in samples including a good proportion of high BI children. That is, whereas in the above-mentioned "normal" sample the relations found at 2.5 years disappeared at 4.5 years (Stevenson-Hinde & Shouldice, 1993), significant relations at 4.5 years did occur within a sample selected to contain a sufficient proportion of children with high BI. Here, BI in ambivalent children was significantly greater than BI in avoidant children (Stevenson-Hinde & Marshall, 1999), and this significant difference also held at 7 years (Stevenson-Hinde, 2000). As expected over the whole of this selected sample, BI significantly decreased with age (Marshall & Stevenson-Hinde, 1998).

In addition to the three main patterns of attachment identified in Ainsworth's original study (Ainsworth et al., 1978), our selected sample also included more recently identified insecure patterns: controlling, characterized by the child rather than the mother structuring the reunion episode; and insecure-other, reflecting insecurity but with no particular pattern or a mixture of patterns. At both 4.5 and 7 years, avoidant children showed the lowest BI of all five attachment groups (avoidant, secure, ambivalent, controlling, and insecure-other). The highest BI ratings of all at each age occurred in children classed as insecure-other, with ambivalent children coming next. The insecure-other pattern, as well as the disorganized pattern (not considered here since only one child in the sample showed it), have been particularly associated with disorder (see Cassidy & Shaver, 1999). The association between high BI, an ambivalent pattern, an insecure-other pattern, and the development of anxiety disorder warrants further study.

Similar Mother–Child Interactions for Both Behavioral Inhibition and Ambivalent Attachment

Mothers of both fearful and ambivalent children may be characterized as overprotective, and their children as excessively in need of comfort. For example, BI has been associated with parental overprotection, especially with girls (Kagan, Reznick, & Snidman, 1987), overcontrol (Rapee, 1997; Rubin & Mills, 1991), and less allowance of psychological autonomy and failure to encourage independent opinions (Siqueland, Kendall, & Steinberg, 1996). Such maternal interactions are similar to those associated with the development of an ambivalent pattern of attachment: close protection (George & Solomon, 1999), as well as interfering, inconsistent, and unpredictable interactions (reviewed in Cassidy & Berlin, 1994). With an unpredictable caregiver, "infants live with the constant fear of being left vulnerable and alone. . . . The anxiety associated with this fear of separation lasts beyond infancy as well" (Weinfield, Sroufe, Egeland, & Carlson, 1999, p. 78). Furthermore, both fearful and ambivalent children excessively demand soothing and comfort (Ainsworth et al., 1978; Dadds & Roth, 2001; Fox & Calkins, 1993). The child's upset behavior may in turn increase maternal overprotection, thereby setting up a positive feedback loop between mother and child interactions, particularly in stressful situations, as indicated in Figure 8.2.

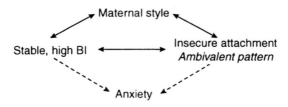

FIGURE 8.2. A model of mutual influences between distinct domains.

Behavioral Inhibition and Ambivalent Attachment as Precursors to Anxiety

Within our own sample of 4.5-year-olds selected to contain children with low, medium, or high BI (as observed both at home and in the lab), the high BI children had significantly higher worries and fears, negative mood (both reported by mothers and observed), and problem behavior in playgroup. The latter was especially high for boys, who showed acting-out behavior as well as social withdrawal (Stevenson-Hinde & Glover, 1996). Moreover, stable high BI has been shown to be a risk factor for later anxiety, particularly social anxiety (Turner, Beidel, & Wolff, 1996). Social anxiety may be viewed as a spectrum, with no empirically derived threshold clearly demarcating normal from clinically significant social anxiety (Schneier, Blanco, Antia, & Liebowitz, 2002). Recently, two of Kagan's longitudinal samples have associated high BI in early childhood (21 months and 31 months) specifically with social anxiety at 13 years. While 61% of inhibited toddlers went on to show social anxiety, only 27% of the uninhibited children did so (Schwartz, Snidman, & Kagan, 1999; see also Biederman et al., 2001). Yet, as the above authors point out, high BI is neither a necessary nor a sufficient condition for the development of anxiety, with other factors playing a role in risk and resilience.

A likely factor is attachment, since anxiety concerning attachment figures could be particularly devastating to a behaviorally inhibited child. As indicated earlier, loss or threat of loss of an attachment figure is a key to understanding anxiety (Bowlby, 1982). Furthermore, "Such anxiety should be particularly characteristic of individuals with resistant attachment history, because these relationships are characterized by an unpredictable, erratic responsiveness that can prove particularly anxiety-provoking" (Weinfield et al., 1999, p. 78). In the Minnesota longitudinal sample, an ambivalent pattern of attachment at 12 months was specifically and uniquely related to anxiety disorder at 17.5 years. That is, an ambivalent pattern did not predict externalizing disorders, and other insecure patterns did not predict anxiety disorder. Furthermore, the ambivalent–anxiety disorder relation remained significant even when Brazelton measures (e.g., slow to habituate) were taken into account (Warren, Huston, Egeland, & Sroufe, 1997). Thus, both stable, high BI and an ambivalent attachment pattern may be precursors to anxiety, as indicated in Figure 8.2.

CONCLUSION

Behavioral inhibition and attachment are distinct, key constructs in child development (Section 1) which nevertheless have important properties in common (Section 2). Given the interplay between high BI and ambivalent attachment (Section 3), their co-occurrence may result in a web of mutual influences (Section 4 and Figure 8.2), particularly when supported by the family context (e.g., Berlin & Cassidy, 1999; Cowan, Cohn, Cowan, & Pearson, 1996; Dadds & Roth, 2001; Scher & Mayseless, 2000). The route to anxiety via stable, high BI suggests a possible overestimation of threat, while an ambivalent pattern of attachment suggests an underestimation of self-worth and poor coping strategies, with different routes indicating different interventions (Dadds & Barrett, 2001; Juffer, Bakermans-Kranenburg, & van IJzendoorn, 2004).

ACKNOWLEDGMENTS

As the discussant to my Regensburg presentation, Gottfried Spangler made valuable contributions to the sections involving physiological results. I am especially grateful to Marinus van IJzendoorn for his generosity in sharing prepublication manuscripts and for his thoughtful and constructive comments. This is a stronger chapter thanks to him.

REFERENCES

Ainsworth, M. D. A., Blehar, M. C., Waters, E., & Wall, S. (1978). *Patterns of attachment*. Hillsdale, NJ: Erlbaum.

Baerends, G. P. (1976). The functional organization of behaviour. *Animal Behaviour, 24*, 726–738.

Bakermans-Kranenburg, M. J., & van IJzendoorn, M. H. (2004). No association of the dopamine D4 receptor (DRD4) and -521 C/T promoter polymorphisms with infant attachment disorganization. *Attachment and Human Development, 6*, 211–218.

Bakermans-Kranenburg, M. J., van IJzendoorn, M. H., & Juffer, F. (2003). Less is more: Meta-analyses of sensitivity and attachment interventions in early childhood. *Psychological Bulletin, 129*, 195–215.

Belsky, J. (1999). Modern evolutionary theory and patterns of attachment. In J. Cassidy & P. R. Shaver (Eds.), *Handbook of attachment: Theory, research, and clinical applications* (pp. 141–161). New York: Guilford Press.

Belsky J., & Rovine, M. (1987). Temperament and attachment security in the Strange Situation: An empirical rapprochement. *Child Development, 58*, 787–795.

Berlin, L. J., & Cassidy, J. (1999). Relations among relationships: Contributions from attachment theory and research. In J. Cassidy & P. R. Shaver (Eds.), *Handbook of attachment: Theory, research, and clinical applications* (pp. 688–712). New York: Guilford Press.

Biederman, J., Hirshfeld-Becker, D.R., Rosenbaum, J. F., Herot, C., Friedman, D., Snidman, N., Kagan, J., & Faraone, S. V. (2001). Further evidence of association between behavioral inhibition and social anxiety in children. *American Journal of Psychiatry, 158*, 1673–1679.

Bischof, N. (1975). A systems approach toward the functional connections of fear and attachment. *Child Development, 46*, 801–817.

Bokhorst, C. L., Bakermans-Kranenburg, M. J., Fearon, R. M. P., van IJzendoorn, M. H., Fonagy, P., & Schuengel, C. (2003). The importance of shared environment in mother–infant attachment security: A behavioral genetic study. *Child Development, 74*, 1769–1782.

Bowlby, J. (1973). *Attachment and loss: Vol 2. Separation, anxiety and anger.* London: Hogarth Press.

Bowlby, J. (1982). *Attachment and loss: Vol 1. Attachment* (2nd ed.). London: Hogarth Press.

Bowlby, J. (1991). Postscript. In C. M. Parkes, J. Stevenson-Hinde, & P. Marris (Eds.), *Attachment across the life cycle* (pp. 293–297). London: Routledge.

Bretherton, I., & Ainsworth, M. D. A. (1974). Responses of one-year-olds to a stranger in a Strange Situation. In M. Lewis & L. A. Rosenblum (Eds.), *The origins of fear* (pp. 131–164). New York: Wiley.

Calkins, S. D., & Fox, N. A. (1992). The relations among infant temperament, security of attachment, and behavioral inhibition at twenty-four months. *Child Development, 63*, 1456–1472.

Cassidy, J., & Berlin, L. J. (1994). The insecure/ambivalent pattern of attachment: Theory and research. *Child Development, 65*, 971–991.

Cassidy, J., & Marvin, R. S. (1992). *Attachment organization in preschool children: Procedures and coding manual.* Seattle, WA: MacArthur Working Group on Attachment.

Cassidy, J., & Shaver, P. R. (Eds.). (1999). *Handbook of attachment: Theory, research, and clinical applications.* New York: Guilford Press.

Chen, X., Hastings, P. D., Rubin, K. H., Chen, H., Cen, G., & Stewart, S. L. (1998). Child-rearing attitudes and behavioral inhibition in Chinese and Canadian toddlers: A cross-cultural study. *Developmental Psychology, 34*, 677–686.

Cowan, P. A., Cohn, D. A., Cowan, C. P., & Pearson, J. L. (1996). Parents' attachment histories and children's externalizing and internalizing behaviors: Exploring family systems models of linkages. *Journal of Consulting and Clinical Psychology, 64*, 53–63.

Dadds, M. R., & Barrett, P. M. (2001). Practitioner review: Psychological management of anxiety disorders in childhood. *Journal Child Psychology and Psychiatry, 42*, 999–1011.

Dadds, M. R., & Roth, J. H. (2001). Family processes in the development of anxiety problems. In M. Vasey & M. R. Dadds (Eds.), *The developmental psychopathology of anxiety.* Oxford, UK: Oxford University Press.

Davidson, R. J., & Rickman, M. (1999). Behavioral inhibition and the emotional circuitry of the brain. In L.A. Schmidt & J. Schulkin (Eds.), *Extreme fear, shyness, and social phobia* (pp. 67–87). Oxford, UK: Oxford University Press.

De Wolff, M. S., & van IJzendoorn, M. H. (1997). Sensitivity and attachment: A meta-analysis on parental antecedents of infant attachment. *Child Development, 68*, 571–591.

Fordham, K., & Stevenson-Hinde, J. (1999). Shyness, friendship quality, and adjustment during middle childhood. *Journal of Child Psychology and Psychiatry, 40*, 757–768.

Fox, N. A., & Calkins, S. D. (1993). Social withdrawal: Interactions among temperament, attachment, and regulation. In K. H. Rubin & J. B. Asendorf (Eds.), *Social withdrawal, inhibition and shyness in childhood* (pp. 81–100). Hillsdale, NJ: Erlbaum.

Fox, N. A., & Card, J. A. (1999). Psychophysiological measures in the study of attachment. In J. Cassidy & P. R. Shaver (Eds.), *Handbook of attachment: Theory, research, and clinical applications* (pp. 226–245). New York: Guilford Press.

Fox, N. A., Kimmerly, N. L., & Schafer, W. D. (1991). Attachment to mother/attachment to father: A meta-analysis. *Child Development, 62,* 210–225.

George, C., & Solomon, J. (1999). Attachment and caregiving: The caregiving behavioral system. In J. Cassidy & P. R. Shaver (Eds.), *Handbook of attachment: Theory, research, and clinical applications* (pp. 649–670). New York: Guilford Press.

Gervai, J., & Lakatos, K. (2004). Comment on "No association of dopamine D4 receptor (DRD4 and -521 C/T promoter polymorphisms with infant attachment disorganization" by M. J. Bakermans-Kranenburg and M. H. van Ijzendoorn. *Attachment and Human Development, 6,* 219–222.

Goldsmith, H. H., Buss, A. H., Plomin, R., Rothbart, M. K., Thomas, A., Chess, S., Hinde, R. A., & McCall, R. B. (1987). Roundtable: What is temperament? *Child Development, 58,* 505–529.

Gosling, S. D., & John, O. P. (1999). Personality dimensions in nonhuman animals: A cross-species review. *Current Directions in Psychological Science, 8,* 69–75.

Greenberg, M. T., & Marvin, R. S. (1982). Reactions of preschool children to an adult stranger: A behavioral systems approach. *Child Development, 53,* 481–490.

Grossmann, K., Fremer-Bombik, E., Rudolph, J., & Grossmann, K. E. (1988). Maternal attachment representation as related to patterns of infant–mother attachment and maternal care during the first year. In R.A. Hinde & J. Stevenson-Hinde (Eds.), *Relationships within families* (pp. 241–262). Oxford, UK: Clarendon Press.

Grossmann, K. E., & Grossmann, K. (1991). Attachment quality as an organizer of emotional and behavioral responses in a longitudinal perspective. In C. M. Parkes, J. Stevenson-Hinde, & P. Marris (Eds.), *Attachment across the life cycle* (pp. 93–114). London: Routledge.

Grossman, K. E., Grossmann, K., Huber, F., & Wartner, U. (1981). German children's behavior towards their mothers at 12 months and their fathers at 18 months in Ainsworth's Strange Situation. *International Journal of Behavioral Development, 4,* 157–181.

Gunnar, M. (1994). Psychoendocrine studies of temperament and stress in early childhood: Expanding current models. In J.E. Bates & T.H. Wachs (Eds.), *Temperament: Individual differences at the interface of biology and behavior* (pp. 175–198). Washington, DC: American Psychological Association.

Hertsgaard, L., Gunnar, M., Erickson, M. F., & Nachmias, M. (1995). Adrenocortical responses to the Strange Situation in infants with disorganized/disoriented attachment relationships. *Child Development, 66,* 1100–1106.

Hinde, R. A. (1987). *Individuals, relationships and culture: Links between Ethology and the Social Sciences.* Cambridge, UK: Cambridge University Press.

Hinde, R. A., & Stevenson, J. G. (1970). Goals and response control. In L. R.

Aronson, E. Tobach, D. S. Lehrman, & J. S. Rosenblatt (Eds.), *Development and evolution of behavior: Essays in memory of T. C. Schneirla* (pp. 216–237). San Francisco: Freeman.

Hinde, R. A., & Stevenson-Hinde, J. (1991). Perspectives on attachment. In C. M. Parkes, J. Stevenson-Hinde, & P. Marris (Eds.), *Attachment across the life cycle* (pp. 52–65). London: Routledge.

Juffer, F., Bakermans-Kranenburg, M. J., & van IJzendoorn, M. H. (2004). Enhancing children's socio-emotional development: A review of intervention studies. In D. M. Teti (Ed.), *Handbook of research methods in developmental psychology.* Cambridge, MA: Blackwell.

Kagan, J. (1989). The concept of behavioral inhibition to the unfamiliar. In J. S. Reznick (Ed.), *Perspectives on behavioral inhibition* (pp. 1–23). Chicago: University of Chicago Press.

Kagan, J. (1994). *Galen's prophecy.* New York: Basic Books.

Kagan, J., Reznick, J. S., & Snidman, N. (1987). The physiology and psychology of behavioral inhibition in children. *Child Development, 58,* 1459–1473.

Kagan, J., Reznick, J. S., Snidman, N., Gibbons, J., & Johnson, M. O. (1988). Childhood derivatives of inhibition and lack of inhibition to the unfamiliar. *Child Development, 59,* 1580–1589.

Kagan, J., Snidman, N., & Arcus, D. (1998). The value of extreme groups. In R. B. Cairns, L. R. Bergman, & J. Kagan (Eds.), *Methods and models for studying the individual: Essays in honor of Marian Radke-Yarrow* (pp. 65–80). Thousand Oaks, CA: Sage.

Kemp, V. (1987). Mothers' perception of children's temperament and mother–child attachment. *Scholarly Inquiry for Nursing Practice, 1,* 51–68.

Kerr, M., Lambert, W. W., Stattin, H., & Klackenberg-Larsson, I. (1994). Stability of inhibition in a Swedish longitudinal sample. *Child Development, 65,* 138–146.

Kochanska, G. (1998). Mother–child relationship, child fearfulness, and emerging attachment: A short-term longitudinal study. *Developmental Psychology, 34,* 480–490.

Lakatos, K., Nemoda, Z., Toth, I., Ronai, Z., Ney, K., Sasvari-Szekely, M., & Gervai, J. (2002). Further evidence for the role of the dopamine D4 receptor (DRD4) gene in attachment disorganization: Interaction of the exon III 48-bp repeat and the -521 C/T promoter polymorphisms. *Molecular Psychiatry, 7,* 27–31.

Lakatos, K., Toth, I., Nemoda, Z., Ney, K., Sasvari-Szekely, M., & Gervai, J. (2000). Dopamine D4 receptor (DRD4) gene polymorphism is associated with attachment disorganization in infants. *Molecular Psychiatry, 5,* 633–637.

Lesch, K.-P., Bengel, D., Heils, A., Sabol, S. Z., Greenberg, B.D., Petri, S., Benjamin, J., Müller, C. R., Hamer, D. H., & Murphy, D. L. (1996) Association of anxiety-related traits with a polymorphism in the serotonin transporter gene regulatory region. *Science, 274,* 1527–1531.

Main, M., & Cassidy, J. (1988). Categories of response to reunion with the parent at age 6: Predictable from infant attachment classifications and stable over a 1-month period. *Developmental Psychology, 24,* 1–12.

Main, M., & Weston, D. (1981). Security of attachment to mother and father: Related to conflict behavior and the readiness to establish new relationships. *Child Development, 52,* 932–940.

Marshall, P. J., & Stevenson-Hinde, J. (1998). Behavioral inhibition, heart period, and respiratory sinus arrhythmia in young children. *Developmental Psychobiology, 33*, 283–292.

Marshall, P. J., & Stevenson-Hinde, J. (2001). Behavioral inhibition: Physiological correlates. In W. R. Crozier & L. E. Alden (Eds.), *International handbook of social anxiety* (pp. 53–76). Chichester, UK: Wiley.

Mills, R. S. L., & Rubin, K. H. (1993). Socialization factors in the development of social withdrawal. In K. H. Rubin & J. Asendorpf (Eds.), *Social withdrawal, inhibition, and shyness in childhood* (pp. 117–148). Hillsdale, NJ: Erlbaum.

Minuchin, P. (1985). Families and individual development: Provocations from the field of family therapy. *Child Development, 56*, 289–302.

Nachmias, M., Gunnar, M., Mangelsdorf, S., Parritz, R., & Buss, K. (1996). Behavioral inhibition and stress reactivity: The moderating role of attachment security. *Child Development, 67*, 508–522.

Plomin, R., & Caspi, A. (1998). DNA and personality. *European Journal of Personality, 12*, 387–407.

Plomin, R., & Rutter, M. (1998). Child development, molecular genetics, and what to do with genes once they are found. *Child Development, 69*, 1223–1242.

Rapee, R. M. (1997). The potential role of child-rearing practices in the development of anxiety and depression. *Clinical Psychology Review, 17*, 47–67.

Reznick, J. S., Gibbons, J. L., Johnson, M. O., & McDonough, P. M. (1989) Behavioral inhibition in a normative sample. In J. S. Reznick (Ed.), *Perspectives on behavioral inhibition* (pp. 25–49). Chicago: University of Chicago Press.

Rubin, K. H., & Mills, R. S. L. (1991). Conceptualising developmental pathways to internalizing disorders in childhood. *Canadian Journal of Behavioural Science, 23*, 300–317.

Sameroff, A. J., Seifer, R., & Elias, P. K. (1982). Sociocultural variability in infant temperament ratings. *Child Development, 53*, 164–173.

Scher, A., & Mayseless, O. (2000). Mothers of anxious/ambivalent infants: Maternal characteristics and child-care context. *Child Development, 71*, 1629–1639.

Schmidt, L., Polak, C. P., & Spooner, A.L. (2001). Biological and environmental contributions to childhood shyness: A diathesis–stress model. In W. R. Crozier & L. E. Alden (Eds.), *International handbook of social anxiety* (pp. 29–51). Chichester, UK: Wiley.

Schneier, F. R., Blanco, C., Antia, S. X., & Liebowitz, M. R. (2002). The social anxiety spectrum. *Psychiatric Clinics of North America, 25*, 757–774.

Schwartz, C. E., Snidman, N., & Kagan, J. (1999). Adolescent social anxiety as an outcome of inhibited temperament in childhood. *Journal of the American Academy of Child and Adolescent Psychiatry, 38*, 1008–1015.

Schwartz, C. E., Wright, C. I., Shin, L. M., Kagan, J., & Rauch, S. L. (2003). Inhibited and uninhibited infants "grown up": Adult amygdalar response to novelty. *Science, 300*, 1952–1953.

Siqueland, L., Kendall, P. C., & Steinberg, L. (1996). Anxiety in children: Perceived family environments and observed family interaction. *Journal of Clinical Child Psychology, 25*, 225–237.

Spangler, G., & Grossmann, K. (1999). Individual and physiological correlates of attachment disorganization in infancy. In J. Solomon & C. C. George (Eds.), *Attachment disorganization* (pp. 95–124). New York: Guilford Press.

Spangler, G., & Grossmann, K. E. (1993). Biobehavioral organization in securely and insecurely attached infants. *Child Development, 64,* 1439–1450.

Spangler, G., & Schieche, M. (1998). Emotional and adrenocortical responses of infants to the Strange Situation: The differential function of emotional expression. *International Journal of Behavioral Development, 22,* 681–706.

Sroufe, L. A. (1977). Wariness of strangers and the study of infant development. *Child Development, 48,* 731–746.

Sroufe, L. A. (1985). Attachment classification from the perspective of infant–caregiver relationships and infant temperament. *Child Development, 56,* 1–14.

Stevenson, J., Batten, N., & Cherner, M. (1992). Fears and fearfulness in children and adolescents: A genetic analysis of twin data. *Journal of Child Psychology and Psychiatry, 33,* 977–985.

Stevenson-Hinde, J. (1986). Towards a more open construct. In G. A. Kohnstamm (Ed.), *Temperament discussed: Temperament and development in infancy and childhood* (pp. 97–106). Lisse, Holland: Swets & Zeitlinger.

Stevenson-Hinde, J. (1988). Individuals in relationships. In R. A. Hinde & J. Stevenson-Hinde (Eds.), *Relationships within families: Mutual influences* (pp. 68–80). Oxford, UK: Clarendon Press.

Stevenson-Hinde, J. (1989). Behavioral inhibition: Issues of context. In J. S. Reznick (Ed.), *Perspectives on behavioral inhibition* (pp. 125–138). Chicago: University of Chicago Press.

Stevenson-Hinde, J. (1991). Temperament and attachment: An eclectic approach. In P. Bateson (Ed.), *Development and integration of behaviour* (pp. 315–329). Cambridge, UK: Cambridge University Press.

Stevenson-Hinde, J. (1998). The individual in context. In R. B. Cairns, L. R. Bergman, & J. Kagan (Eds.), *Methods and models for studying the individual: Essays in honor of Marian Radke-Yarrow* (pp. 123–132). Thousand Oaks, CA: Sage.

Stevenson-Hinde, J. (2000). Shyness in the context of close relationships. In W. R. Crozier (Ed.), *Shyness: Development, consolidation, and change* (pp. 88–102). London: Routledge.

Stevenson-Hinde, J., & Glover, A. (1996). Shy girls and boys: A new look. *Journal of Child Psychology and Psychiatry, 37,* 181–187.

Stevenson-Hinde, J., & Hinde, R. A. (1986). Changes in associations between characteristics and interactions. In R. Plomin & J. Dunn (Eds.), *The study of temperament: Changes, continuities, and challenges* (pp. 115–129). Hillsdale, NJ: Erlbaum.

Stevenson-Hinde, J., & Marshall, P. J. (1999). Behavioral inhibition, heart period, and respiratory sinus arrhythmia: An attachment perspective. *Child Development, 70,* 805–816.

Stevenson-Hinde, J., & Shouldice, A. (1990). Fear and attachment in 2.5-year-olds. *British Journal of Developmental Psychology, 8,* 319–333.

Stevenson-Hinde, J., & Shouldice, A. (1993). Wariness to strangers: A behavior systems perspective revisited. In K. H. Rubin & J. Asendorpf (Eds.), *Social withdrawal, inhibition, and shyness in childhood* (pp. 101–116). Hillsdale, NJ: Erlbaum.

Stevenson-Hinde, J., & Shouldice, A. (1995a). 4.5 to 7 years: Fearful behaviour, fears and worries. *Journal of Child Psychology and Psychiatry*, 36, 1027–1038.

Stevenson-Hinde, J., & Shouldice, A. (1995b). Maternal interactions and self-reports related to attachment classifications at 4.5 years. *Child Development*, 66, 583–596.

Stevenson-Hinde, J., Stillwell-Barnes, R., & Zunz, M. (1980). Subjective assessment of rhesus monkeys over four successive years. *Primates*, 21, 66–82.

Stevenson-Hinde, J., & Verschueren, K. (2002). Attachment in childhood. In P. K. Smith & C. H. Hart (Eds.), *Blackwell handbook of social development* (pp. 182–204). Oxford, UK: Blackwell.

Turner, S. M., Beidel, D. C., & Wolff, P. L. (1996). Is behavioral inhibition related to the anxiety disorders? *Clinical Psychology Review*, 16, 157–172.

van IJzendoorn, M. H., & Bakermans-Kranenburg, M. J. (1996). Attachment representations in mothers, fathers, adolescents, and clinical groups: A meta-analytic search for normative data. *Journal of Consulting and Clinical Psychology*, 64, 8–21.

van IJzendoorn, M. H., & Bakermans-Kranenburg, M. J. (2004). Maternal sensitivity and infant temperament in the formation of attachment. In G. Bremner & A. Slater (Eds.), *Theories of infant development* (pp. 233–258). London: Blackwell.

van IJzendoorn, M. H., & De Wolff, M. S. (1997). In search of the absent father: Meta-analyses on infant–father attachment: A rejoinder to our discussants. *Child Development*, 68, 604–609.

van IJzendoorn, M. H., & Sagi, A. (1999). Cross-cultural patterns of attachment: Universal and contextual dimensions. In J. Cassidy & P. R. Shaver (Eds.), *Handbook of attachment: Theory, research, and clinical applications* (pp. 713–734). New York: Guilford Press.

van IJzendoorn, M. H., Vereijken, C. M. J. L., Bakermans-Kranenburg, M. J., & Riksen-Walraven, J. M. (2004). Assessing attachment security with the Attachment Q-Sort: Meta-analytic evidence for the validity of the Observer AQS. *Child Development*, 75, 1188–1213.

Vaughn, B. E., & Bost, K. K. (1999). Attachment and temperament: Redundant, independent, or interacting influences on interpersonal adaptation and personality development? In J. Cassidy & P. R. Shaver (Eds.), *Handbook of attachment: Theory, research, and clinical applications* (pp. 198–225). New York: Guilford Press.

Vaughn, B. E., Taraldson, B. J., Crichton, L., & Egeland, B. (1981). The assessment of infant temperament: A critique of the Carey Infant Temperament Questionnaire. *Infant Behavior and Development*, 4, 1–17.

Warren, S. L., Huston, L., Egeland, B., & Sroufe, L. A. (1997). Child and adolescent anxiety disorders and early attachment. *Journal of the American Academy of Child and Adolescent Psychiatry*, 36, 637–644.

Wartner, U. G., Grossmann, K., Fremmer-Bombik, E., & Suess, G. (1994). Attachment patterns at age six in south Germany: Predictability from infancy and implications for preschool behavior. *Child Development*, 65, 1010–1023.

Waters, E., Hamilton, C. E., & Weinfeld, N. S. (2000). The stability of attachment security from infancy to adolescence and early adulthood: General introduction. *Child Development*, 71, 678–683.

Weinfield, N. S., Sroufe, L. A., Egeland, B., & Carlson, E. A. (1999). The nature of individual differences in infant–caregiver attachment. In J. Cassidy & P. R. Shaver (Eds.), *Handbook of attachment: Theory, research, and clinical applications* (pp. 68–88). New York: Guilford Press.

Willemsen-Swinkels, S., Bakermans-Kranenburg, M.J., Buitelaar, J. K., van IJzendoorn, M. H., & van Engeland, H. (2000). Insecure and disorganized attachment in children with a pervasive developmental disorder: Relationship with social interaction and heart rate. *Journal of Child Psychiatry and Psychology, 41,* 759–767.

Wilson, D. S., Clark, A. B., Coleman, K., & Dearstyne, T. (1994). Shyness and boldness in humans and other animals. *Trends in Ecology and Evolution, 9,* 442–446.

Wilson, D. S., Coleman, K., Clark, A. B., & Biederman, L. (1993). Shy–bold continuum in pumpkinseed sunfish (*Lepomis gibbosus*): An ecological study of a psychological trait. *Journal of Comparative Psychology, 107,* 250–260.

CHAPTER 9

Attachment Representations, Secure-Base Behavior, and the Evolution of Adult Relationships

The Stony Brook Adult Relationship Project

JUDITH CROWELL
EVERETT WATERS

The Stony Brook Relationship Project illustrates how the complementarity of diverse training and backgrounds can be knit together to enrich a decade of developmental research. In our case these include (1) attachment theory and ethological methods as taught in Mary Ainsworth's laboratory at Johns Hopkins University; (2) the Minnesota traditions of developmental analysis, construct validation, and thinking carefully about psychology; (3) the emphasis on development, careful diagnosis, and knowing individuals in detail that is central to clinical training in child psychiatry; and (4) a developmental perspective on mental representations.

From 1978 to 1987, Everett Waters's attachment research at Stony Brook primarily involved observational studies of secure-base behavior and secure-base support in infancy and toddlerhood. A primary goal was to replicate the links Mary Ainsworth had established between secure-base behavior at home and in the Strange Situation. This seemed critical to securing Ainsworth's interpretation of the procedure and establishing an important line of defense against her critics. At the same time, a series of studies and theoretical articles highlighted the continuing role of secure-base support beyond infancy. These addressed the perception that, for attachment theorists, experience in infancy is destiny.

Judith Crowell became interested in attachment theory while holding a child psychiatry fellowship at Stanford University. The opportunity to present one of her clinical cases to John Bowlby during a visit he made to the Bay Area helped consolidate her interest and encouraged her to participate, during a 1984–1987 postdoctoral fellowship at Stanford, in Mary Main's first Adult Attachment Interview (AAI; George, Kaplan, & Main, 1985) training class. In addition to learning the AAI, she met Mary Ainsworth, Karin Grossmann, Inge Bretherton, and others at that time.

Planning for the Stony Brook Relationship Project began in 1987, when Judy joined Stony Brook's faculty in child psychiatry and proposed a collaborative study of the newly developed AAI. The initial research proposal to the National Institute of Mental Health (NIMH) was simple. It proposed to examine discriminant and construct validity of the AAI, including examination of stability and couples' relationships. A narrative measure as complex as the AAI lends itself to a variety of alternative interpretations. We would administer the AAI and evaluate potential discriminant validity issues. Discriminant validity had been a perennial problem in self-report and interview assessment. We believed it was better to discover any problems ourselves and to address them constructively than to leave them for critics to discover and attack. Grand theories and new measures are always tempting targets.

There were few genuine attachment enthusiasts at the time. But there was kind soul on our NIMH review panel who proposed an expansion of the adult relationship component of the study. We promptly resubmitted, proposing, this time, 5 years of longitudinal research at substantially more than five times the cost. Our planned study, Adult Attachment Models: Development after Marriage?, was approved in 1989 and, after some disconcerting delays in the release of funds, our longitudinal study began in 1990. Our colleague Dominique Treboux joined us, first as a postdoctoral fellow and then as a co-investigator. Her training in adolescent and adult development, measurement, and data analysis was a mainstay of the project for the next 10 years. Six years into the project, Harriet Waters joined to help us investigate the cognitive architecture of adult attachment representations.

The design, of course, was framed by the ages and phases of assessment outlined in our initial award and in our renewal. These addressed important issues of measurement, stability, and change, and links between attachment and marriage. But the real innovations from the project were developed as the project progressed and were only reflected in annual reports and renewal applications after the fact. These included our adaptation of the AAI for assessing working models of the marital relationship, an observational approach to assessing secure-base use and support from videotaped marital interactions, the prompt-word method for assessing knowledge of the secure-base script from short narratives, and an observational approach to assessing parental secure-base support in preschoolers. The project's ultimate scope and design (outlined in Figure 9.1) were as much a product of the ongoing research as any of our results.

This reflects one of the great advantages of the approach to funding longitudinal research. Rather than treating the research proposal as a con-

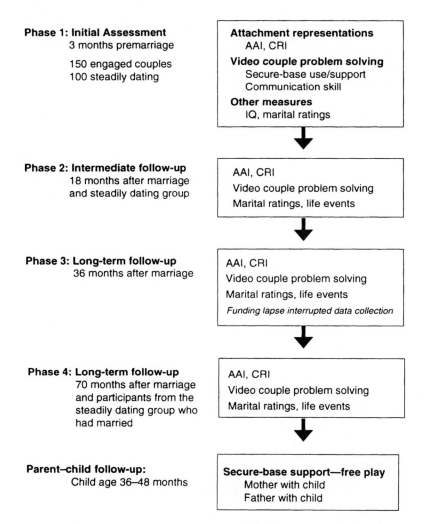

Phase 1: Initial Assessment
3 months premarriage

150 engaged couples
100 steadily dating

Attachment representations
AAI, CRI
Video couple problem solving
Secure-base use/support
Communication skill
Other measures
IQ, marital ratings

Phase 2: Intermediate follow-up
18 months after marriage
and steadily dating group

AAI, CRI
Video couple problem solving
Marital ratings, life events

Phase 3: Long-term follow-up
36 months after marriage

AAI, CRI
Video couple problem solving
Marital ratings, life events
Funding lapse interrupted data collection

Phase 4: Long-term follow-up
70 months after marriage
and participants from the
steadily dating group who
had married

AAI, CRI
Video couple problem solving
Marital ratings, life events

Parent–child follow-up:
Child age 36–48 months

Secure-base support—free play
Mother with child
Father with child

FIGURE 9.1. Overview of the Stony Brook Relationship Project.

tract that binds researchers to goals outlined in advance, NIMH has always encouraged and accepted longitudinal researchers going well beyond what was anticipated in their formal applications. NIMH does not issue a blank check, but it does offer the encouragement and freedom to stay alert, take some chances, and capitalize on ideas, observations, and opportunities that can only arise from knowing individual subjects and mapping data over long intervals. Of course, a project has to stay on course and there has to be some way to set priorities and to distinguish between significant opportunities and mere empirical curiosities. In our case, this was provided by our understanding of Bowlby–Ainsworth attachment theory and our unflagging sense that the secure-base concept is its core concept from infancy to adulthood.

Although our prior research experiences, background in measurement, developmental theory, and cognitive psychology gave the project a certain coherence and focus across the transitions from engagement to marriage, from early marriage to established marriage, and from them (in most cases) to parenthood, the key ingredient was the breadth and coherence of attachment theory. It guided every phase of the project, inspired every innovation, and fueled our eagerness to see if adult relationships really operate as Bowlby proposed. The breadth of the theory also fueled our desire to secure it by giving it the chance to pass dangerous tests of core hypotheses, especially regarding the organizing role of the secure base.

THEORETICAL ISSUES

The *prototype hypothesis*, the notion that the infant–mother relationship is the prototype of later love relationships, is central to Bowlby's attachment theory. We first addressed this hypothesis by examining the stability of attachment security from infancy to young adulthood (in a concurrent 20-year follow-up of infants seen in the Strange Situation) and across two developmental transitions in young adult life: the transition to marriage and the transition to parenthood. A second theoretical focus reflected Judy Crowell's clinical interests: What helps people recover from the negative effects of a difficult childhood? We proposed to address this question by examining the flip side of the stability question, that is, what factors were associated with change in attachment representations, especially movement toward security? Our longitudinal study of young couples began with these core ideas.

Several other themes and theoretical issues emerged as we pursued these questions, both in designing and executing the studies. Bowlby (1969/1982) hypothesized that attachment is a vital process across the lifespan. In adult life, partners join or even replace parents as attachment figures. Mary

Ainsworth (1991) wrote about the hypothesized benefits of a secure attachment in adult life. According to Ainsworth, there is "a seeking to obtain an experience of security and comfort in the relationship with the partner. If and when such security and comfort are available, the individual is able to move off from the secure base provided by the partner, with the confidence to engage in other activities" (p. 38).

Based on this description, we hypothesized that adult attachment behavior should be similar in its structure to parent–child secure-base behavior with the exception that adult partners manifest reciprocal secure-base behavior. That is, both partners seek and provide support, and one role is not inherently more "powerful" for adult partners as is true between parents and children. Since we believe that the core of the attachment system is the secure-base phenomenon (Waters & Cummings, 2000), we wanted to observe adult secure-base behavior and assess how it related to adult attachment representations. A link between a stable attachment representation and adult secure-base behavior would provide further support for the hypothesis that the parent–infant relationship is a prototype of later love relationships.

We also sought to understand how the attachment system fits within the larger construct of the marital relationship. Are there specific as well as generalized attachment representations? How does an attachment relationship develop within the context of the marital relationship? van IJzendoorn and Bakermans-Kranenburg's (1996) meta-analysis and our own work indicate that young adults do not select partners based on attachment status. That is, there is minimal assortative mating with respect to attachment (Crowell, Treboux, & Waters, 2002). This led us to consider the possibility that the attachment relationship between adult partners would show development and that part of this process might include the development of a specific cognitive representation of the adult relationship that would in some way either replace or be assimilated into a more general attachment representation that developed across childhood and adolescence in the family of origin. These were primary research goals from the beginning of the project and were of special interest to Judy Crowell and Dominique Treboux.

When the couples began to have children, Everett Waters also pursued the parenting aspects of secure-base behavior, and explored how parental attachment representations impacted parental secure-base support. In addition, Harriet Waters applied her expertise in cognitive psychology and the development of prose-processing skills to the task of clarifying the cognitive architecture of adult attachment representations. This has helped clarify what the AAI measures and pointed us toward economical alternative assessment strategies that better distinguish between generalized versus relationship-specific and child–adult versus adult–adult representations.

THE PROBLEM OF MEASUREMENT

As we approached these hypotheses and questions, we were aware that our ability to study them was highly dependent upon the quality of the measures. The AAI (George, Kaplan, & Main, 1985; Main & Goldwyn, 1985/1994) was a relatively new measure when we began writing our proposal in late 1987, and very little work had been done to examine questions concerning its discriminant validity or correlates, especially in samples other than parents of young children. The proposal therefore included specific aims to address the discriminant and construct validity of this core measure of the project, with a particular interest in possible relations between the AAI and self-report assessments of attachment.

In addition, we were aware that we would need to develop several new measures to investigate our questions. Using the AAI as a model, Gretchen Owens and Judy Crowell developed the Current Relationship Interview (CRI; Crowell & Owens, 1996) as an assessment of a relationship-specific attachment representation, that is, the representation of the current attachment relationship with the partner. Under the assumption that secure-base behavior between adults should parallel that between parent and child, we drew upon Mary Ainsworth's ideas of mother and child behavior to develop a coding system of adult secure-base behavior (Crowell et al., 1998).

These three measures of adult attachment, the AAI, the CRI, and the secure-base coding system, are at the heart of our longitudinal study, and are central to the description of the study and its findings. These are summarized below. Several other measures deserve mention but will not be described in detail. For example, Harriet Waters developed a narrative production task designed to assess knowledge and also to access script-like representations of early secure-base experience (Waters & Rodrigues, 2001). Drawing upon concepts from Craik (1943) and Piaget, Bowlby hypothesized that attachment experiences are represented in the mind as an internal working model (see Bretherton, Chapter 2, this volume). Bretherton (1985) and Main (Main, Kaplan, & Cassidy, 1985) had suggested that the internal working model or attachment representation is script-like in nature. Using a methodology that she had employed to examine the development of scripts and narratives on other topics, Harriet Waters and colleagues developed a method that captures a secure-base script (Waters & Rodrigues-Doolabh, 2001).

The secure-base script is a temporal-causal cognitive structure that summarizes key elements in often-repeated secure-base interactions. Following up on a suggestion by Inge Bretherton, we were interested in the possibility that such cognitive structures are actively coconstructed during childhood with the help of primary attachment figures (Guttman-

Steinmetz, Elliott, Steiner, & Waters, 2003) and play important roles in recalling secure-base experiences, organizing later secure-base behavior, and anticipating partners' behavior in secure-base contexts.

UNDERSTANDING THE ADULT ATTACHMENT INTERVIEW

The first study we conducted upon receiving funding for the longitudinal study was an investigation of the discriminant and construct validity of the AAI. This was a vital first step before embarking on the longitudinal study, in which we planned to recruit 500 participants and to administer repeated AAIs to them. We conducted a cross-sectional study of 54 mothers of preschool children (Crowell et al., 1996). In addition to the AAI, they completed assessments of IQ, social adjustment, discourse style, and social desirability, as well as a variety of attachment self-reports that were in use at the time (see Table 9.1). There were moderate correlations between AAI coherence and intelligence and social adjustment in this sample of women, who had a wide range of IQ scores (range of raw scores = 20–85, median = 50), but a restricted range in social adjustment (all the women scored in the top two out of seven categories of adjustment). Correlations between AAI

TABLE 9.1. Correlates of AAI Coherence and Discriminant and Construct Validity variables

	AAI coherence Pearson r =
Discriminant validity variables[a]	
Raw IQ scores	.42**
Social Adjustment Scale	.46**
Education and Employment Interview	.10
Social desirability	.10
Construct validity variables	
Self-report attachment scales for partner—sum[b]	.21
Experiences in Close Relationships[c]	
Avoidance of closeness	−.23*
Anxiety about abandonment	−.03
Secure-base behavior: mother–child[d]	.54***
Secure-base script: mother–child and adult–adult combined[e]	.58***

Note. The discriminant validity measures and self-reports of partners were administered in the cross-sectional study of mothers of preschool children ([a]Crowell et al., 1995; [b]Crowell et al., 1999). The ECR, secure-base behavior, and script assessments were administered in the longitudinal study ([c]Treboux et al., 2004; [d]Elliott et al., 2001; [e]Waters & Rodrigues, 2001).
*$p \leq .05$; **$p \leq .01$; ***$p \leq .001$.

coherence, social desirability, and discourse style on the topic of education and jobs were low and nonsignificant.

Examining construct validity of the AAI in this study (Crowell, Treboux, & Waters, 1999) and later in the couples' longitudinal study (Treboux, Crowell, & Waters, 2004), we found few meaningful correlations between the AAI and attachment self-reports (see Table 9.1 and Table 9.3, below). In contrast, we found moderate to high correlations between maternal secure-base behaviors directed toward preschool children (Elliott, Crowell, Gao, & Waters, 2003), and secure-base behavior between adults (see Table 9.1 and Table 9.3, below) (Crowell, Treboux, Gao, Fyffe, Pan, & Waters, 2002). AAI coherence was also highly correlated with secure-base scripts produced from prompt-word outlines of both mother–child and adult–adult attachment scenarios (Waters, Crowell, Elliott, Corcoran, & Treboux, 2002; Waters & Rodrigues-Doolabh, 2001). Thus from our initial study of mothers and subsequent work in the longitudinal study, the AAI behaves as an attachment-specific assessment, and in addition as a generalized representation of attachment. Although the script assessment outlined below can be an economical alternative in research that focuses only on the security-coherence dimension and does not require detailed biographical information or information about defensive processes.

THE STONY BROOK RELATIONSHIP PROJECT

Feeling confident about the core measure of the study, we then embarked on a longitudinal study of young couples. One hundred fifty-seven engaged couples participated in the study, as did 101 steadily dating couples that matched them on a variety of demographic variables. The sample was representative of the population of young adults in Suffolk County, Long Island, New York. Participants were 95% white. At the time of recruitment, the average age of the women was 23.5 years and of the men 24.5 years. To be eligible for participation, the individuals could not have a child nor could they have been married before.

The engaged couples were assessed initially within 3 months of their weddings, and twice more at 18 months and 6 years of marriage. Although we had planned a 3-year follow-up, only a subset of the couples were seen at that point due to a funding interruption. The dating sample was seen initially and 21 months later. Those who married were assessed at the 6-year follow-up.

Across the years of the study, we had 73% retention of participants (Treboux et al., 2004). Dropping out of the study was associated with separation or divorce from the original partner, although we followed those who were willing to come back alone or with a new partner. At the time of the 6-year assessment, 22% of the original engaged couples had separated, divorced, or never married. Forty-three percent of the original steadily dating sample had married. Most of the analyses presented here use the original engaged sample and follow them through the early years of marriage.

At the initial assessment and at each subsequent assessment, we administered the AAI, the CRI, a couple's interaction task (scored with the secure-base scoring system), and various self-report measures of the relationship, including the Family Behavior Survey developed by German Posada and Everett Waters (1988), which assesses frequency of discord and conflict tactics, and Sternberg's (1988) Triangular Theory of Love Scale, which assesses feelings of intimacy, commitment, and passion. At the first assessment, we gave the Henmon–Nelson Test of Mental Ability (Lamke & Nelson, 1973), a questionnaire IQ test. At subsequent assessments, we added Spanier's Dyadic Adjustment Scale (Spanier, 1976), the Sarason Life Events Survey (Sarason, Johnson, & Siegel, 1978), the Self-Esteem Inventory (O'Brien & Epstein, 1988), and the Beck Depression Inventory (Beck, Ward, Mendelson, Mock, & Erbaugh, 1961). At 6 years, we gave the Experiences in Close Relationships, a self-report attachment measure developed by Brennan, Clark, and Shaver (1997), which has scales of Avoidance of Closeness and Anxiety about Abandonment.

THE PROTOTYPE HYPOTHESIS AND OPPORTUNITIES FOR CHANGE

Stability of Attachment Representation from Infancy to Adulthood

Returning to the core theoretical questions and hypotheses, a primary interest was the prototype hypothesis, the idea that the parent–infant relationship is a prototype for later love relationships. One aspect of examining this hypothesis involved investigation of the stability of attachment representations. Around the midway point of the longitudinal study, Everett Waters arranged a 20-year follow-up of the infants who had participated in his dissertation study of the stability of the Strange Situation classifications (Waters, 1979). Susan Merrick and Leah Albersheim in Minnesota found and recruited 50 of the original 60 infants, now 21–22 years old, who were interviewed with the AAI. We found a 64% correspondence (kappa = .40, p ≤.01) across 20 years between three-way classifications of the Strange Situation and of the AAI, and a 72% correspondence (kappa = .44, p ≤.01) when a secure versus insecure dichotomy was used (Waters, Merrick, Treboux, Crowell, & Albersheim, 2000).

Change in attachment status appeared to be lawful, being associated with significant change in the caregiving environment over the 20-year interval due to events such as parental divorce, parental death, and serious illness in the parent or child. Only one-third of the secure infants who had experienced one or more such events remained secure, whereas if no such events occurred 85% of those classified as secure in infancy were also classified as secure in adulthood (Waters et al., 2000). Of course, these challenging life events most often led to secure infants being classified as insecure young adults, but this was not always the case. There were two cases in which the life event clearly improved the quality of the attachment relationship between parent and child, leading to an insecure infant being classified as a secure young adult. Thus we found quite remarkable support for the continuity of attachment patterns across this 20-year interval from infancy to young adult life, and a solid first step for demonstrating that the parent–infant relationship may be a prototype for later love relationships.

Stability of Attachment Representation in Adulthood: The Transition to Marriage

We assessed the stability of attachment representations in the couples study. We were particularly interested in what would allow individuals with insecure attachment representations to develop secure representations.

We found that across the transition to marriage—that is, the 21-month interval from 3 months before to 18 months after marriage—78% of the participants (kappa = .62, $p \leq .001$) were given the same AAI classification at both times using the three primary classifications, and 83% had the same classification (kappa = .70, $p \leq .001$) when a secure versus insecure dichotomy was used (Crowell, Treboux, & Waters, 2002). This did not include the unresolved classification, which we examined separately from the major classifications, and which was much less stable (46%).

Examination of the stability of secure versus insecure classifications revealed that stability of the secure AAI classification was 96% across the transition to marriage (Crowell, Treboux, & Waters, 2002). Thus individuals who had a secure representation were extremely unlikely to "lose" it. In contrast, the insecure classification was 76% stable. Although still very stable, it appeared that most of the people who changed classification across this transition "became secure" or more coherent. Comparison of these "newly secure" individuals with those who did not change, that is, who were classified as insecure at both assessments, revealed the group who "became secure" was more likely to have secure specific attachment representations assessed with the CRI and more positive feelings about their relationships. Higher education and living away from parents prior to marriage also appeared to create opportunities for change.

Correlates of stability of the unresolved classification were very different from those associated with the major classifications (Crowell, Treboux,

& Waters, 2002). Maintenance of the unresolved classification was associated with experiencing a greater number of negative life events and physical aggression in the relationship (characteristic of unresolved for trauma but not loss). These findings have led us to view the unresolved classification of the AAI as being conceptually distinct from the major classifications, and therefore requiring distinct data-analytic strategies.

Stability of Attachment Representation in Adulthood: The Transition to Parenthood

From 18 months of marriage to 6 years of marriage, approximately two-thirds of the participants became parents. There was 83% correspondence (kappa = .59, $p \leq .001$) of three-way classifications of the AAI across the 4.5 years between the two phases (Crowell, Treboux, & Waters, 2004). Across this interval, there was no difference in the stability of secure versus insecure classifications. Therefore, movement toward security was not prominent across this developmental phase in the marriage. Examining the transition to parenthood, we also looked at possible gender differences. There was no significant difference in the stability of classification for men and women who did not become parents (78% and 86%, respectively). However, there was a significant difference in the stability of AAI classifications between men and women who did become parents. Women who became mothers across this interval had 94% stability of AAI classification, and men who became fathers, had 71% stability. These men were as likely to "become secure" as to "become insecure." No factor other than the transition to parenthood was found to be associated with change. Thus parenthood for women appeared to "set" the attachment representation, whereas for some men this was an opportunity for change.

THE SECURE-BASE PHENOMENON IN ADULT PARTNERSHIPS

Do Adults Engage in Secure-Base Behavior, and How Can We Assess It?

Using Ainsworth's concepts of mother and child secure-base behavior, we developed ratings of secure-base support and secure-base use (see Table 9.2) (Crowell et al., 1996). We scored adult secure-base behavior from standard 15-minute couples' interactions in which a topic of disagreement was selected from the partners' individually generated descriptions of what they most frequently disagreed on or argued about.

The secure-base scoring system differs from communication/emotion-based coding systems of couples' interactions in two important ways. The

TABLE 9.2. Secure-Base Scoring System for Adult Partnerships

Secure-base use	Secure-base support
Quality of initial signal	Interest (availability)
Maintenance of signal as needed	Recognition of signal/distress (sensitivity)
Approach (proximity seeking)	Interpretation (cooperation)
"Contact" is comforting	Responsiveness

Note. Corresponding parent–child concepts all in parentheses.

context is critical, so the quality of a behavior is judged within the context of the seriousness of the topic from an attachment perspective. Thus the demands and significance of a situation involving trust between partners are considered greater than those for prioritizing household tasks. In addition, emotional expression is not judged to have the same meaning as in communication-based systems. Communication/emotion scoring systems often nest or aggregate conceptually related behaviors under a single code. As a result, they rate negative affect, anger, sadness, and hostility as being negative, and more predictive of marital outcome than positive elements of an interaction. Problem-solving behavior that has minimal affective tone is considered neutral and relatively unimportant. Within the secure-base coding system, negative affect is not necessarily problematic because it may represent appropriate distress, and use of humor is not necessarily positive because it may represent avoidance. Problem solving can be very important, especially depending upon the nature of the problem.

Using this system, we found that the quality of secure-base behavior of both men and women was related to their AAI coherence (see Tables 9.3 and 9.4, below) (Crowell, Treboux, Gao, et al., 2002). In addition, it was not accounting for the same variance as the communication-based coding, which was not strongly associated with AAI coherence. Furthermore, the secure-base coding was as good a predictor of marital variables as the communication coding in this normative sample, especially for women.

What Aspects of Marital Relationships Are Attachment-Related?

We never felt that attachment assessments in adulthood would or should relate to all aspects of an adult partnership. Just as the parent–child relationship is broader than the domain of attachment, we assumed that not all good things go together in adult relationships. Indeed, Mary Ainsworth (1991) clearly differentiated between attachment and other important aspects of close relationships, such as common interests, sexual compatibility, feeling needed, and companionship.

TABLE 9.3. Correlations among Measures at 6 Years of Marriage

	AAI coherence r =	CRI coherence r =	Secure-base behavior r =	Experiences in close relationships	
				Avoidance r =	Anxiety r =
AAI coherence	—	.47***	.48***	−.23*	−.03
CRI coherence	—	—	.41**	−.25*	−.15
Secure-base behavior	—	—	—	−.16	.01
Negative behavior/R-MICS (communication-based)	−.21*	−.24*	−.35**	Not available	Not available
Negative life events	−.01	−.09	.02	.11	.35**
Relationship conflict	−.05	−.18*	−.17*	.41**	.44**
Feelings re relationship	.11	.24*	−.02	−.61***	−.46***
Feelings re self	.21*	.19*	.27*	−.37**	−.48***

*p ≤ .05; **p ≤.01; ***p ≤.001.

Table 9.3 presents the correlations among the key variables in married couples at the 6-year assessment (Treboux et al., 2004). Most significant on this table are the strong correlations among the attachment-related measures, the AAI, Current Relationship Interview (CRI), and secure-base behavior. There are also strong correlations among the various self-report measures, the two Experiences in Close Relationships (ECR) self-report scales, and composite scales of relationship conflict behaviors, positive relationship feelings, and positive feelings about the self. The avoidance scale of the ECR shows low-level correlations with the AAI and the CRI, but there was no significant relation between ECR anxiety and other attachment measures. AAI coherence showed little association with self-report variables, but, not surprisingly, the more relationship-specific attachment measures of secure-base behavior and CRI show significant, but low-level, correlations with self-report relationship variables.

GENERALIZED VERSUS SPECIFIC REPRESENTATIONS OF ATTACHMENT

One of the early questions that developed into an important area of investigation involves the issue of generalized versus specific representations of attachment. In childhood, early representations are relationship-specific, and, over time, they are believed to generalize, providing a guide for attachment-related thoughts, feelings, and behaviors in relationships beyond the parent–infant relationship. Bowlby (1969/1982) proposed this as a mechanism by which early experience would influence later relationships, and indeed the stability studies described earlier support this hypothesis. The AAI itself was developed as an assessment of the generalized representation rather than as a representation of any specific individual or relationship (Main et al., 1985).

However, the formation of an adult partnership involves two partners who each bring a generalized representation to the relationship. About 55% of individuals match on representational security status of their partner—that is, both are secure or both are insecure (Crowell, Treboux, & Waters, 2002; van IJzendoorn & Bakermans-Kranenburg, 1996). Therefore, each partner should respond to the attachment ideas, reactions, and behaviors of the other, the "new" attachment figure. At least early on in the relationship, we anticipated that this would lead to a relatively specific representation of the adult partnership (Owens et al., 1995). There were competing hypotheses about the relation between the generalized and the specific representation over time, and their significance. The "new" and more specific representation might become the more predictive and significant representation, a finding that would be consistent with Julian Rotter's (1982) suggestion that the influence of generalized expectations diminishes as a person gains specific experience with a situation or relationship. Alternatively, attachment theory would suggest that over time the specific representation would be integrated into, or become more similar to, the generalized representation.

The CRI was developed to assess a more specific representation of attachment (Crowell & Owens, 1996). It is a parallel measure to the AAI, but with questions that refer to the current relationship. Correspondence between coherence scales of the AAI and CRI before marriage was significant ($r = .51$, $p = .001$). Thus it appeared that the specific representation is indeed informed by the generalized representation, but was also influenced by experiences in the current relationship (Owens et al., 1995).

DEVELOPMENT OF ATTACHMENT REPRESENTATIONS IN ADULT PARTNERSHIPS

We were interested in evidence suggesting that attachment representations would show development across the early years of the marital relationship, and how links among generalized representations, specific representations, secure-base behavior, and reports of the marriage might change over time.

Table 9.4 shows these findings at the three phases of our study (Crowell, 2003; Crowell et al., 2004). The results of Furman's and col-

TABLE 9.4. Development of Relations among Attachment Variables in Adults

	Dating[*] HS seniors +18 yr old	Engaged 3 mo prewedding 24 yr old	Married	
			18 mo marriage 26 yr old	6 yr marriage 30 yr old
AAI and CRI Three-way correspondence	46% kappa = .14	58% kappa = .35*	64% kappa = .39*	58% kappa = .35*
Predicting CRI coherence with AAI coherence	2%			
Women		4%	17%	19%
Men		15%	5%	23%
AAI and SB behavior r =	—			
Women		.42***	.50***	.46***
Men		.35**	.47***	.49***

[*]Furman, Simon, Shaffer, and Bouchey (2002).
*$p \leq .05$; **$p \leq .01$; ***$p \leq .001$.

leagues study of late adolescents and their partners are included as well (Furman, Simon, Shaffer, & Bouchey, 2002). This study used the AAI and a CRI adapted for use with adolescents, and provides related information about an earlier phase of relationship development. In late adolescents who were in dating relationships, the links between the AAI and the CRI were not significant. This finding contrasts with the young adults engaged to be married, in whom correspondence between the AAI's and the CRI's three primary classifications is significant. The correspondence remains significant across the first 6 years of marriage. Predicting CRI coherence using AAI coherence, the percent of variance predicted by the AAI increased over the 6-year interval, with a possible developmental difference between women and men in the transition-to-marriage phase. The AAI was also consistently related to secure-base behavior. These findings suggest that the developmental stage of the relationship may be a significant factor in the meaning of the assessments vis-à-vis one another, and that adults in different developmental stages of relationships should be assessed separately just as is the case when examining developmental questions in childhood. It also suggests that the two representations become more similar over time, and that the specific representation becomes more informed by the generalized representation.

IMPLICATIONS FOR MARITAL FUNCTIONING

Most recently we have investigated Ainsworth's important idea that there should be benefits to having a secure attachment relationship in adult life. This means more than having a secure generalized representation; it means that one must also have confidence or belief in *one's partner's* availability and responsiveness. For this reason, we began to investigate what we call "attachment configurations."

The configurations are derived from the security status of both the AAI and the CRI, and are based on the idea that cognitions about the current relationship are referenced against the generalized representation of attachment (See Table 9.6). Within this framework, the generalized representation reflects the individual's ability to present a coherent, organized, scripted knowledge base about attachment with respect to his or her past experiences, that is, if he or she is secure. Or if he or she cannot do this, he or she is insecure. The specific representation, assessed with the CRI, can also be either secure or insecure. The individual can present a coherent, organized, scripted knowledge base about attachment with respect to this particular relationship, or he or she cannot. Table 9.7 provides examples of coherent and incoherent personal secure base scripts from the AAI and the CRI. There are four possible configurations based on the coherence of the general and the specific representations: $Secure_{AAI}/Secure_{CRI}$, $Insecure_{AAI}/Insecure_{CRI}$, $Secure_{AAI}/Insecure_{CRI}$, and $Insecure_{AAI}/Secure_{CRI}$.

Our work indicates that each of these configurations has implications for relationship functioning and response to stressful events (Treboux et al., 2004). The distribution of the configurations 3 months before marriage was $Secure_{AAI}/Secure_{CRI}$ ($n = 77$), $Insecure_{AAI}/Insecure_{CRI}$ ($n = 122$), $Secure_{AAI}/Insecure_{CRI}$ ($n = 47$), and $Insecure_{AAI}/Secure_{CRI}$ ($n = 44$) when overall participants reported very high relationship satisfaction. Findings revealed that premarital configurations predicted relationship breakup. Thirty couples separated, divorced, or never married. The individuals who were $Secure_{AAI}/Insecure_{CRI}$ were most likely to leave their partners, and such individuals were found in almost 50% of the failed relationships. We take this to mean that those individuals who have a secure generalized representation, and who are incoherent about their partner's availability, find this very distressing, and it appears that in many cases they will leave the relationship early. Indeed, this was the least satisfied group before marriage.

We then focused on how the configurations were associated with marital functioning and stressful events in individuals who were married (Treboux et al., 2004). We examined four variables: secure-base behavior, reported conflict in the relationship, feelings about the relationship, and feelings about the self, using z-scores for each component so that variables would be comparably scaled. The conflict domain included frequency of discord and negative conflict tactics. The positive feelings about the relationship combined marital satisfaction and feelings of intimacy, commitment, and passion. The positive feelings about the self combined the self-esteem inventory scales of global self-esteem, lovability, and likeability, and the depression inventory reverse-coded. Nonmarital negative life events were used to assess stress.

Not surprisingly, the Secure$_{AAI}$/Secure$_{CRI}$ group in the low-stress condition was the best functioning overall; they had the most effective secure-base behavior, and they reported high positive feelings about their relationships. Relationship conflict was low and conflict strategies are not as maladaptive as, for example, physical or psychological aggression would be. They felt positively about themselves. Although those who experienced high stressful life events did report frequent conflict with their partners, secure-base behavior and positive feelings about the self and the relationship were high relative to other groups.

Each of the groups with an insecure representation has a particular pattern of relationship vulnerability. The Insecure$_{AAI}$/Insecure$_{CRI}$ group had the least effective secure-base behavior and exhibited negative feelings about the self and the relationship in the low-stress condition. Under conditions of high stress, conflict (especially aggression) increased and feelings about the self and the relationship were even more negative.

The Secure$_{AAI}$/Insecure$_{CRI}$ group's behavior and feelings cluster around the mean under low-stress conditions. However, when stressed by high life events, individuals with this configuration reported high relationship conflict and negative feelings about the relationship. Their feelings about themselves were not different.

The Insecure$_{AAI}$/Secure$_{CRI}$ group has relatively weak secure-base behavior, but in the low-stress condition had the highest scores for positive feelings about the relationship and reported the lowest relationship conflict. This pattern differed dramatically when they experience multiple negative life events, and they were very unhappy about their relationships and relationship aggression was high.

SCRIPT-LIKE REPRESENTATION OF EARLY SECURE-BASE EXPERIENCE

The AAI does not directly measure attachment representations or attachment working models. Instead, it provides a narrative that is more or less coherent and allows us to make inferences about the "goodness" of underlying representations. Our cross-sectional work on the secure-base script is an effort to learn more about the architecture and development of the underlying cognitive representation. The key elements of the secure-base script are (1) parent and child or adult partners are interacting or otherwise constructively engaged, (2) an interruption or obstacle arises, (3) the child or one of the adult partners is upset, (4) there is a signal or request for help, (5) help is offered, (6) the help is effective in resolving the problem, (7) the help is comforting to the person who requested it, (8) they return to comfortable constructive interaction or activity.

Subjects are presented with a set of 12–14 words arranged in three columns. The words suggest a story organized around the secure-base script. For example, the words "mother," "baby play," "blanket," "story," "teddy bear," "lost," "find," "smile," and so on suggest a story about a mother and baby playing together on a blanket; they are acting out a story with toys when they notice that the baby's teddy bear is missing. The baby gets upset, and mother searches and searches. They find the teddy bear, the baby is happy, and they carry on, make lunch, nap, and so on. Adults who have summarized their own secure-base experience in terms of this script see that it is implied in the prompt words and tell a story clearly organized around the secure-base script. If they are not familiar with (or don't have access to) the secure base script, they ordinarily tell an equally coherent story with a different story line.

We are currently preparing a monograph-length report from our project and related studies suggesting that mother–child and adult–adult relations tap a single secure-base script, that script knowledge captures most of the valid variance of the AAI coherence scale (and thus the secure–insecure distinction), and that script knowledge parallels AAI coherence in its links to infant Strange Situation and adult secure-base use and support. We have also found that script knowledge is significantly related to mothers' ability to help preschool age children organize their secure-base experience into script-like representations (Guttmann-Steinmetz et al., 2003). But these are more recent dividends rather than primary goals of our project, which involved understanding the AAI and the development of attachment representations within marriages.

In conclusion, the key findings of the longitudinal study can be summarized as follows. Elements of the attachment control system can be assessed in adults. Generalized representations of attachment are very stable, and if there was change it was lawful because it related to challenging life events. In particular, movement toward security is associated with positive feelings and coherent cognitions about the attachment elements of the current relationship, as well as exposure to alternatives and opportunities represented by education and living away from the family of origin. Parenthood appears to "solidify" the attachment representation in women, but may be an impetus for revision in some men. Generalized representations inform representations of the current relationship, which are also influenced by the quality of the current relationship. Thus the attachment components of an adult relationship appear to develop with time and experience. The notion that attachment status that incorporates both generalized and specific representations has important implications for relationship functioning and reactions to stressful life events deserves high priority in future research.

The Stony Brook Adult Relationships Project was, in many respects, interdisciplinary. Much of our success (and few of our difficulties) arose from the investigators' very different backgrounds, strengths, and interests. But unlike many interdisciplinary projects, it was not a patchwork of experts. We shared a detailed understanding of Bowlby–Ainsworth attachment theory and an enduring interest in developmental analysis. This was critical to our day-to-day interactions, our planning, and our ability to identify opportunities for innovation and to set priorities as our couples' marriages and families unfolded.

Long-term longitudinal research is methodologically important. It is also an important crucible for innovation and for training the next generation of developmental theorists and researchers. Yes, there was pressure to publish prolifically before we had reached key outcomes. And there were funding delays and interruptions, management headaches, and other difficulties attendant to any project this size. Yet as we look back on the project, foremost in our minds is the fact that society would allocate significant resources to better understand and help our families and children. We have tried hard to hold up our end of the bargain.

ACKNOWLEDGMENTS

This research was supported by a grant from the National Institute of Mental Health (No. MH44935, 1990–2001), *Adult Attachment Models: Development after Marriage*.

REFERENCES

Ainsworth, M. D. S. (1991). Attachment and other affectional bonds across the life cycle. In C. M. Parkes, J. Stevenson-Hinde, & P. Marris (Eds.), *Attachment across the life cycle* (pp. 33–51). London: Routledge.

Beck, A. T., Ward, C. H., Mendelson, M., Mock, J., & Erbaugh, J. (1961). An index

Bowlby, J. (1969/1982). *Attachment and loss: Vol. 1. Attachment.* New York: Basic Books.

Brennan, K.A., Clark, C. L., & Shaver, P. (1997). Self-report measurement of adult attachment: An integrative overview. In J.A. Simpson & W.S. Rholes (Eds.), *Attachment theory and close relationships* (pp. 46–76). New York: Guilford Press.

Bretherton, I. (1985). Attachment theory: Retrospect and prospect. In I. Bretherton & E. Waters (Eds.), Growing points in attachment theory and research. *Monographs of the Society for Research in Child Development, 50*(1–2, Serial No. 209), 3–35.

Craik, K. (1943). *The nature of explanation.* Cambridge, UK: Cambridge University Press.

Crowell, J. A. (2003, July). *The Stony Brook Relationship Project: Understanding adult attachment.* Paper presented at the annual meeting of ATICA, Regensburg, Germany.

Crowell, J. A., & Owens, G. (1996). *The Current Relationship Interview and scoring system.* Unpublished manuscript, State University of New York at Stony Brook.

Crowell, J. A., Pan, H. S., Gao, Y., Treboux, D., O'Connor, E., & Waters, E. (1996). *The secure base scoring system for adults.* Unpublished manuscript, State University of New York at Stony Brook.

Crowell, J. A., Treboux, D., Gao, Y., Fyffe, C., Pan, H., & Waters, E. (2002). Assessing secure base behavior in adulthood: Development of a measure, links to attachment representations, and relations to couples' communication and reports of relationships. *Developmental Psychology, 38,* 679–693.

Crowell, J. A., Treboux, D., & Waters, E. (1999). The Adult Attachment Interview and the Relationship Questionnaire: Relations to reports of mothers and partners. *Personal Relationships, 6,* 1–18.

Crowell, J. A., Treboux, D., & Waters, E. (2002). Stability of attachment representations: The transition to marriage. *Developmental Psychology, 38,* 467–479.

Crowell, J. A., Treboux, D., & Waters, E. (2004). *Understanding relationship-specific attachment representations: The early years of marriage and parenting.* Manuscript submitted for publication.

Crowell, J. A., Waters, E., Treboux, D., O'Connor, E., Colon-Downs, C., Feider, O., Posada, G., & Golby, B. (1995). The discriminant validity of the Adult Attachment Interview. *Child Development, 67,* 2584–2599.

Elliott, M., Crowell, J. A., Gao, Y., & Waters, E. (2003). *Mothers, fathers, and marriage: Sources of secure base support in the preschool years.* Unpublished manuscript, State University of New York at Stony Brook.

Furman, W., Simon, V. A., Shaffer, L., & Bouchey, H. A. (2002). Adolescents' working models and styles for relationships with parents, friends, and romantic partners. *Child Development, 73,* 241–255.

George, C., Kaplan, N., & Main, M. (1985). *The Adult Attachment Interview.* Unpublished manuscript, University of California–Berkeley.

Guttmann-Steinmetz, S., Elliott, M., Steiner, M., & Waters, H. (2003, April). *Co-constructing script-like attachment representations.* Paper presented at the biennial meeting of the Society for Research in Child Development, Tampa, FL.

Lamke, T. A., & Nelson, M. J. (1973). *The Henmon–Nelson Test of Mental Ability.* Boston: Houghton Mifflin.

Main, M., & Goldwyn, R. (1985/1994). *The Adult Attachment Interview Scoring System.* Unpublished manuscript, University of California–Berkeley.

Main, M., Kaplan, N., & Cassidy, J. (1985). Security in infancy, childhood and adulthood: A move to the level of representation. In I. Bretherton & E. Waters (Eds.), Growing points in attachment theory and research. *Monographs of the Society for Research in Child Development, 50*(1–2, Serial No. 209), 3–35.

O'Brien, E. J., & Epstein, S. (1988). *The Multi-Dimensional Self-Esteem Inventory.* Odessa, FL: Psychological Assessment Resources, Inc.

Owens, G., Crowell, J. A., Pan, H. S., Treboux, D., O'Connor, E., & Waters, E. (1995). The prototype hypothesis and the origins of attachment working models: Parent–child relationships and adult–adult romantic relationships. In E. Waters, B. Vaughn, G. Posada, & K. Kondo-Ikemura (Eds.), Culture, caregiving and cognition: Perspectives on secure base phenomena and attachment working models. *Monographs of the Society for Research in Child Development, 60* (2–3, Serial No. 244), 216–233.

Posada, G., & Waters, E. (1988). *The Family Behavior Survey.* Unpublished manuscript, State University of New York at Stony Brook.

Rogger, J. B. (1982). *The development and application of social learning theory.* New York: Praeger.

Sarason, B. R., Johnson, J. H., & Siegel, J. M. (1978). Assessing the impact of life changes: Development of the Life Experiences Survey. *Journal of Clinical and Consulting Psychology, 46,* 932–946.

Spanier, G. B. (1976). Measuring dyadic adjustment: New scales for assessing the quality of marriage and similar dyads. *Journal of Marriage and the Family, 38,* 15–28.

Sternberg, R. (1988). *Triangular Theory of Love Scale.* Unpublished manuscript, Yale University.

Treboux, D., Crowell, J. A., & Waters, E. (2004). When "new" meets "old": Configurations of adult attachment representations and their implications for marital functioning. *Developmental Psychology. 40,* 295–314.

van IJzendoorn, M. H., & Bakermans-Kranenburg, M. (1996). Attachment representations in mothers, fathers, adolescents, and clinical groups: A meta-analytic search for normative data. *Journal of Clinical and Consulting Psychology, 64,* 8–21.

Waters, E. (1979). The reliability and stability of individual differences in infant–mother attachment. *Child Development, 49,* 483196494.

Waters, E., Crowell, J. A., Elliott, M., Corcoran, D., & Treboux, D. (2002). Bowlby's secure base theory and the social/personality psychology of attachment styles: Work(s) in progress. *Attachment and Human Development, 4,* 230–242.

Waters, E., & Cummings, M. (2000). A secure base from which to explore relationships. *Child Development, 71,* 164–172.

Waters, E., Merrick, S., Treboux, D., Crowell, J., & Albersheim, L. (2000). Attachment security in infancy and early adulthood: A 20-year longitudinal study. *Child Development, 71*, 684–689.

Waters, H. S., & Rodrigues-Doolabh, L. M. (2001). *Are attachment scripts the building blocks of attachment representations?: Narrative assessment of representations and the AAI*. Paper presented at the biannual meeting of the Society for Research in Child Development, Minneapolis, MN.

CHAPTER 10

Predictability of Attachment Behavior and Representational Processes at 1, 6, and 19 Years of Age

The Berkeley Longitudinal Study

MARY MAIN
ERIK HESSE
NANCY KAPLAN

This chapter summarizes the current findings from the Berkeley longitudinal study of attachment. Here we describe what we have learned to date regarding the attachment-related trajectories taken by 42 participants in our sample, and report striking overall predictability of behavioral, representational, and linguistic processes from infancy to 6 years, and then to 19 years of age. We trace these developments separately via initial infant 'attachment category' ("secure," "insecure-avoidant," or "insecure-disorganized"[1]; see category descriptors below), and when possible, we refer as well to the continuous scales associated with the Strange Situation and the Adult Attachment Interview (AAI). At the time of this writing, a handful of cases have yet to be analyzed, and therefore only the simplest of tests have been conducted, and no exact statistics can yet be given.

Our longitudinal study began with the assessment of attachment in infancy, utilizing Mary Ainsworth's Strange Situation procedure. Although laboratory-based, this procedure had its origins in Ainsworth's early adherence to the traditions of ethology, which focus upon the behavior of organisms in their natural environments. Thus, well prior to devising the Strange

Situation procedure, Ainsworth undertook extensive observations of both Ugandan and American infant–mother dyads in the home. As her work progressed, Ainsworth drew increasingly upon her intimate understanding of attachment theory as a conceptual backdrop for formulating and testing hypotheses. For example, she was well aware of John Bowlby's (1969/ 1982) point that for primate infants, maintaining proximity to the attachment figure (usually, but not necessarily, the biological parent) in situations of danger is critical for survival. Moreover, Bowlby had proposed that for infant primates there are "natural clues to danger"—including, for example, unfamiliar settings, darkness, separation from the attachment figure, and (often) the approach of strangers. Propensities to seek the attachment figure (the infant's "haven of safety") may be aroused by any of these clues, but are especially expectable when more than one is present (Bowlby, 1969/ 1982).

Ainsworth devised the Strange Situation after she completed her extensive home observations of infant–mother interactions in Baltimore across the first year of life. The Strange Situation is a naturalistic procedure intended to permit the observation of attachment (and its complement, exploratory behavior) in the face of singular and combined natural clues to danger. Here, an infant and an attachment figure are observed as they respond to an unfamiliar setting, to the approach of a stranger, and to two separations and reunions between the infant and the attachment figure (in Ainsworth's studies and most others, the infant's mother). Somewhat surprisingly, Ainsworth found that infant responses to separation and reunion in this procedure fell into three distinct, coherently organized patterns of attachment ("secure," "insecure-avoidant," and "insecure-ambivalent"—later termed the "organized" patterns of attachment; see Main, 1990, and below). These three central behavioral responses to the Strange Situation procedure were detailed by Ainsworth for identification by later researchers (Ainsworth, Blehar, Waters, & Wall, 1978). Ainsworth regarded this set of three categories as exhaustive, and—based on her previous home observations—as originating in differences in maternal sensitivity and responsiveness to infant signals and communications. Specifically, secure infants had mothers who were judged sensitively responsive[2] on her 9-point rating scales, while mothers of insecure-avoidant and insecure-ambivalent infants were markedly less sensitive. However, in none of Ainsworth's original observations was the possibility considered that some mothers, whether sensitive or insensitive, could also be frightening.

Later—in conjunction with the discovery of a fourth Strange Situation attachment category, "insecure-disorganized/disoriented" (or "D") (Main & Solomon, 1990)—we began to extend attachment theory to include the potential import of infant exposure to anomalous fear-arousing parental behaviors, instead of or in addition to the external fear-arousing conditions examined by Bowlby (Main & Hesse, 1990). We proposed that fear of the parent could account for many instances of disorganized behavior, since the infant's natural haven of safety will have simultaneously and paradoxically become the source of its alarm (Hesse & Main, 1999, 2000).

Aided by this expanded outlook, and beginning with the Strange Situation procedure as our "ethological" or "naturalistic" base, we then observed the continuing development of our sample in other contexts, using both behavioral and representational methods we had designed for assessing attachment at 6 years and in later life. We interpreted the prediction from early Strange Situation responses found in our sample as the product of each participant's early—and, in our stable, low-risk sample, quite likely enduring—experiences involving the primary attachment figure(s). Later, we suggested that these early experiences may initially operate by influencing infant attentional processes related to attachment (Main, 1990, 1999)—yielding, respectively, unrestricted or flexible attention (sensitively responsive parenting); inflexibility of attention (insensitive but not frightening parenting, whether involving rejection or unpredictable responsiveness); and collapse of attention caused by excesses of fear or stress (frightening parenting). At present, our study has progressed to 18 years following the Strange Situation, at which time an attachment-focused life history interview (the AAI; see below) has been conducted with each former infant (George, Kaplan, & Main, 1984, 1985, 1996). This interview is intended by means of its structure to "surprise the unconscious" and, via examination of exact language usages, to elucidate critical aspects of mind (Main & Goldwyn, 1984–1998; Main, Goldwyn, & Hesse, 2003). In all four U.S. samples examined to date, individual differences in coherence during this interview have been found to be systematically related to early attachment status with the mother.

Throughout this chapter, then, we refer to the import of recurring interactions as a factor in constructing social mind. A consideration of the role of early interactions in the development of mind is far from new; indeed, Grossmann (1995) has drawn attention to Plato's (see Plato, 1953) view that character is shaped by the caregiver's responses to the infant within the first 3 years of life. The import of interaction in the development of social mind is also underscored in Stern's (1985) RIGS theory ("representations of interactions that have been generalized"); script theory (see Bretherton, 1985); and the recent focus upon the import of implicit (procedural) memories, especially when these are constructed early and relate to attachment (see, e.g., Amini, Lewis, Lannon, & Louie, 1996).

This presentation is intended for both those new to and those familiar with the field. Persons already familiar with attachment research and procedures (e.g., the Strange Situation and its background, early British work concerning parent–child separations, and the AAI) can of course skip lightly over these parts. Given the length and complexity of this chapter, however, we suggest that individuals who are busy or less familiar with this topic divide their reading across several time periods related to its three central corresponding parts (secure attachment, pp. 261–273; avoidant attachment, pp. 273–279; and disorganized attachment, pp. 279–288).

PRELUDE

Together with The Guilford Press, the editors have requested that the first authors of presentations in this volume provide personal biographical discussions of their backgrounds with respect to their eventual decisions to undertake their particular studies. Although all three authors have contributed equally to this presentation, the Berkeley study was initiated by Mary Main. This prelude is therefore written by Main in the first person.

I completed my secondary education at a Quaker school in Philadelphia (Friends' Select), where my best subjects were physics and chemistry, while in contrast my favorite subjects were literature, music, and art. Unwilling to narrow my interests to a single "major" as most universities require, I next attended St. John's College in Annapolis, Maryland, which uses no textbooks, instead providing its students only with original works. St. John's requires each student to undertake 4 years of mathematics; 4 years of literature and philosophy (philosophy was much admired by my parents, who had introduced me to Plato, Kant, and several Eastern philosophies by age 10); 2 years of languages; and 4 years of the natural or "hard" sciences (which continued to be my best subjects). Because I had married one of my professors, the late Alvin Nye Main (whose doctoral training at UCLA had been in linguistic philosophy, a branch of philosophy that—short of Wittgenstein for his work and character, and Moore for his character—he did not much admire), I needed to find a graduate school nearby. After considering applying to the Peabody Conservatory to study piano, and The Johns Hopkins University for the graduate study of history, I read Noam Chomsky's work and—fascinated and persuaded by his assertions regarding the implications of the often unique, creative, and yet grammatical nature of many speakers' sentences—applied to Hopkins (whose doctoral program relied upon the apprentice system) to study psycholinguistics with James Deese. However, I was accepted instead by Mary Ainsworth (then at Stanford University for her sabbatical) as her prospective student in the field of infant–mother attachment.

I was doubtful about the advisability of taking up Ainsworth's offer, since my interest in linguistics had been sincere. Just as some children are drawn to music or mathematics in their earliest years, I had been drawn from the age of 2 to language in the form of natural speech and speech usages, and wrote down some especially interesting sentences I had heard as soon as I was able. I had, however, found verbal metaphors torturous, since they frequently violated my tentatively developing sense of what a particular word actually indicated, as well as of what to expect in terms of space–time relations and causality. As I often ran about in circles of now-humorous linguistic complaint ("I am a *little girl*! I know what *pills* are, and a little girl *cannot also be a pill*!"[3]), my parents learned to calm me with the phrase "It's just a 'spression"[4] when they were using metaphors. This phrase was intended to indicate that they were using language in ways set apart from those I understood at the time, and hence that I need not presently be worried about them.

Ainsworth's offer for me to enter Hopkins as a student of attachment continued to trouble me, and I complained that babies and individual differences in parent–child relationships had no connection to language. My philosopher husband argued, however, that a given field can be approached from many angles, and that learning to recognize variations in emotional relationships in children too young to speak could still eventually bring me back to language—perhaps enriched by this seemingly unpromising vantage point. Less than 10 years later, this had become true, with the advent in our laboratory of a method for scoring and classifying exact speech usages in life history transcripts (the AAI; see below) and the power of this methodology to predict the quality of the infant's highly emotional attachment to the speaker.

Johns Hopkins did not permit specialization until its students had spent 2 years establishing a broad initial knowledge base in psychology, ranging from personality to vision and psychophysiology. My favorite three books, each read repeatedly, were Hinde's (1966) *Animal Behaviour*, Underwood's (1966) *Experimental Psychology*, and Bowlby's (1969/1982) *Attachment*. As a professor, Mary Ainsworth also encouraged breadth, and I took several extracurricular courses in evolution. At the time I entered Hopkins, Ainsworth had just developed the Strange Situation procedure. To satisfy her that I could use it in my own work, she required that I reach a high level of agreement with her across 100 transcribed procedures (videotape had yet to be utilized) in her three major classifications and eight subclassifications. I did, and was then ready to undertake my doctoral dissertation.

For my dissertation at Johns Hopkins (Main, 1973), I watched 50 children seen in the Strange Situation at 12 months as they responded to opportunities for both free and structured play at 21 months. The toddlers were observed in their mothers' presence in a playroom that my friend Everett Waters and I had made very comfortable and attractive (besides filming all the play sessions, Everett cut and re-sewed the carpet to better fit the playroom). I found that infants secure with their mothers were the most intensely and lengthily engaged in exploration, and showed the most "game-like" spirit when playing with another close friend, Inge Bretherton.

I also presented each toddler with what are now called "story stems." Here Inge was asked to pick up a toy dog and, barking and growling vivaciously, to make it approach a small baby doll placed in a toy carriage. She was then to return to human status and cry out, "Oh, don't let the doggy bite the baby!" Although my findings were in the predicted directions (dogs in the grasp of secure infants protected the baby, while dogs in the grasp of some avoidant infants attacked), they seemed too minor to publish.

Looking at speech, Everett and I could see how intensely many of these 21-month-olds seemed to believe that their incomprehensible utterances were understandable language (e.g., one child said, with incisive gestures and a sincere expression, "Ho-lee-gah-ho-lee-ho-gey—ho*kee*!!"). I found no relation between security of attachment and overall level of either early language development or symbolic play. We did find, however, that children who were insecure with their mothers were as fascinating, intelligent, and likable to us as were secure children. This was exemplified by our affection for the highly talkative but insecure toddler just mentioned, who greatly hoped to be comprehended, but was not.

Using Ainsworth's three-part classification system (secure, avoidant, and resistant/ambivalent), I found that at least five infants in my sample could not be classified. These were informally called "A-C" or "avoidant/resistant" infants; however, following a practice Ainsworth had already established for a single earlier case, she and I force-classified them into what seemed to us to be the best-fitting category. I had visited most of the mothers in my sample earlier in their homes to discuss the forthcoming Strange Situation procedure,[5] and I knew that at least three of the five mothers of the unclassifiable infants had behaved most peculiarly with their offspring: One— frighteningly, to me—had treated her toddler as an animal. Observing especially those five as well as some other infants, and greatly influenced by Hinde's (1966) *Animal Behaviour*, I counted the occurrences of any anomalous-appearing conflict behaviors[6] in the play session. By 1979, in a scale developed for use with similar laboratory-based free-play observations in Regensburg, I would come to call these behaviors "disorganized/ disordered" (later "disorganized/disoriented"; Main & Solomon, 1990).

A related and influential observation took place in my office as I discussed the forthcoming play session with the mother of an avoidant infant, during a typically sudden and violent Baltimore thunderstorm. A very close clap of thunder startled all of us, and the toddler ran unpredictably to me rather than to her mother, burying her head in my lap. This provided my first strong illustration that infant insecurity can be associated with disorientation under stress.

I completed my graduate work in 4 years, and presented my findings very soon afterward in Germany at Klaus Grossmann's invitation (see Main, 1977). From Hopkins I went directly to take a faculty position at Berkeley, where I spent my first 2 years trying to replicate many of the findings uncovered earlier within Ainsworth's narrative records. Replicability is one of the principles distinguishing the "hard" sciences (Hinde, 1983), and from that time forward, publication of my findings would often await one (and sometimes two), replications.

At Berkeley, many of the themes I have mentioned above would be repeated. First, via the AAI developed with Carol George and Nancy Kaplan (George et al., 1984, 1985, 1996) I would at last return to my original interest in spoken language usage or discourse. More specifically, the rules that Ruth Goldwyn and I (1984) developed for identifying the speech characteristics of the parents of secure, insecure-ambivalent, and insecure-avoidant infants would several years later be partly expressed in terms of adherence to as opposed to violations of Grice's maxims for achieving cooperative, rational discourse (Grice, 1975, 1989).

I would also have the opportunity to study individual differences in the "creativity" of speakers' sentences, an interest derived from my early reading of Chomsky. Although Chomsky had been referring to our universal human capacity to speak sentences never before said or heard, this now seems to me to appear most often in the fresh, yet coherent, sentences seen most frequently in the parents of secure infants. Second, I would expand my interest in children's responses to story stems, by acting as Nancy Kaplan's dissertation advisor in her work with transcripts of 6-year-olds' responses to questions concerning pictured child–parent separations (Kaplan, 1987). Third, I would become highly focused on the problem of "unclassifiable" or "A-C" infants. The frightening behavior originally observed in the Baltimore homes of a few such infants (now "disorganized" or "D" infants) would turn out to be the distinguishing feature of the mothers of D infants in several samples studied in later years (Hesse & Main, 2000). And I would continue to believe, with Mary Ainsworth, that a great deal can be revealed even in very short intervals—as shown in a 6-year-old's reunion behavior towards a parent observed for 3–5 minutes following an hour-long separation (Main & Cassidy, 1988; see below).

My interests in animal behavior and evolutionary theory, encouraged early by Mary Ainsworth and John Bowlby, would continue as well. These were extended and amplified during a year-long visit in 1977 to the Center for Interdisciplinary Research in Bielefeld, Germany, at the invitation of the Grossmanns. There I spent much time learning from various biologists, evolutionary theorists, and ethologists, including especially John Crook, Richard Dawkins, and Robert Hinde. These new friends had a strong impact upon my thinking by making me aware of (1) the import of the ecology of the immediate environment in producing differing "conditional strategies" for reproductive success (e.g., Crook & Gartlan, 1966; Trivers, 1974); (2) the rigorous yet changing nature of Darwinian theory following the "evolutionary synthesis" with genetics in the 1930s, and the emergence of kin selection theory (e.g., Dawkins, 1976/1989); and (3) theories of motivation and, relatedly, the analysis of the outcomes of conflicting behavioral propensities (e.g., Hinde, 1966).

ATTACHMENT THEORY

This chapter now returns to triple authorship, and will shortly begin to focus upon our longitudinal findings regarding the sequelae to early individual differences in attachment. However, because this work is written for those new to the field as well as others more familiar with it, we start with a brief review of Bowlby's (1969/1982) "ethological–evolutionary" theory of attachment, which focuses upon the *universals* of attachment (for a complete overview, see Hinde, Chapter 1, this volume). We then discuss the two pathways that have generally been considered most plausible by those attempting to account for the origins of *individual differences* in patterns of attachment. Although these pathways can ultimately interact, here we will put the matter simply—that is, as taking their origins either (1) via "heritable"[7] genetic differences between individuals (an aspect of "behavior genetics"), or (2) via "nonheritable" types of conditional strategies (alternatively, "contingent decision rules"; see Daly, 1996) of the type utilized when individuals who are equipped with the same behavioral programs respond in systematically differing ways to differing rearing environments.

Bowlby's Theory of Attachment: A Species-Wide "Behavioral System" and Its Operation

Attachment theory represented a radical departure from previous conceptualizations of the nature of the child's tie to the mother, and took Bowlby over 30 years to formulate. The most fundamental distinction between Bowlby's thinking regarding parent–child ties and that of his predecessors was his requirement that his formulations conform to the paradigm of natural selection. This was due to his introduction in the early 1950s to recent developments in the field of ethology. Guided in large part by Robert Hinde (see Bretherton, 1992), Bowlby was taken with the reasoning that species-specific behavior patterns, like species morphology, are the products of selection pressures that assist in individual survival and ultimately in reproductive success. Eventually, following an extensive review of the human and nonhuman primate literature, Bowlby was led to the conclusion that crying, calling, following, clinging, and other behaviors that become focused on one or two selected caregivers during the first year of life have come over evolutionary time to be virtually universal among primates (including, of course, humans). Because of their species-wide nature, Bowlby ultimately attributed these characteristics to the working of an instinctively guided "attachment behavioral system."

Bowlby further proposed that the infant primate's focus upon the attachment figure (usually, but not necessarily, the biological mother) has been rendered all the more emotional and insistent because—due to the fact that many primates are seminomadic—it is inevitably closely intertwined with fear. The substantial distances traveled by most primates means that they cannot establish a fixed location for protection of the young, such as a burrow or den. In contrast to those mammals for whom a special *place* provides the infant's haven of safety, then, for the primate infant *the attachment figure is the single location that must be sought under conditions of alarm* (Bowlby, 1969/1982; Hesse & Main, 1999).

Bowlby suggested that the specific environmental pressure accounting for infant proximity maintenance has been attacks from predators, and that protection from predation has served as the biological or adaptive function leading to the incorporation of attachment behavior into the species-wide repertoire. Because predation is a constant and pervasive danger to primate infants, he maintained that attachment behavior is of equal import to feeding and mating. Later, informed by John Crook (personal communication, 1977), Main (e.g., 1979) suggested that the biological or adaptive functions served by proximity-keeping to caregivers could be broadened to include protection from starvation, unfavorable temperature changes, natural disasters, attacks by conspecifics, and the risk of separation from the troop. This extension was ultimately endorsed by Bowlby (1988), and maintenance of proximity to attachment figures is now believed to serve multiple survival-related functions. And for young primates currently living in the wild, as well as humans living in their "environments of evolutionary adaptedness" (Bowlby, 1969/1982), it is now widely agreed that even brief separations can threaten infant survival in minutes, and certainly within hours (Hinde, 1974; Hrdy, 1999).

Attachment has therefore come to be viewed as the central "external" or "behavioral" mechanism regulating infant safety, and maintenance of proximity to attachment figures is understood to be the sine qua non of primate infant survival (Hinde, 1974; Hrdy, 1999). Of necessity, then, the attachment system must remain continually responsive; hence the infant will at some level continually "track" the physical and psychological accessibility of the primary attachment figure(s), whether or not attachment behavior is explicitly displayed at any given time.

Bowlby's theory of attachment thus refers to a universal or species-wide characteristic: the genetically channeled propensity for all young, so long as they are given even very minimal[8] environmental input during the earliest years of life, to form a highly emotional bond to at least one older individual and thereafter to seek, monitor, and attempt to maintain proximity to that individual(s).[9] The developing child's proclivity to learn the language of his or her immediate surroundings—again, so long as even minimal input is available during the earliest years of life—also provides a good example of what is meant by a "universal" or "species-wide" characteristic. Like the proclivity to form an attachment, language acquisition is also considered a matter of population-wide genetics (a term that is used as well, with somewhat different meanings, in other contexts). These in-built, species-wide propensities are often referred to as "behavioral programs" or "behavioral systems" (formerly "instinctive behaviors"; see Hinde, Chapter 1, this volume).

Individual Differences in Attachment-Related Behavior

Since this chapter focuses upon individual differences in attachment and their sequelae, we begin with the following: Attachments are formed virtually universally, and thereafter are expected to arouse *propensities* to seek proximity to attachment figures in the face of "natural clues to danger." At the same time, primates have associated propensities to decrease attachment behavior in the service of exploration and play in "safe" conditions, (see especially Grossmann, Grossmann, & Zimmermann, 1999). How then could a substantial minority of infants presented with clues to danger and safety in the Strange Situation violate the outcomes that would be anticipated, given our understanding of this species-wide "behavioral program"?

One example is the insecure-avoidant Strange Situation response, which is exhibited by a substantial minority of infants worldwide. These infants, who show virtually no distress but instead explore throughout the Strange Situation, not only fail to greet their mothers on the mothers' return but also actively turn away, ignore, and/or move away from them. The attachment behavior of these infants has been repeatedly observed to be rejected by their mothers in the home; however, interestingly, many of these infants show overt distress and anxiety as their mothers move from room to room in this familiar setting. Main (1981) has proposed that in the unfamiliar (hence implicitly far more dangerous) Strange Situation setting, a rejected infant employs an "organized shift of attention" (i.e., active visual, auditory and physical avoidance) to assist with the inhibition of attachment behavior. Main has further proposed that infant avoidance may have historically led a mother to decrease her attention to, and hence decrease her rejection of, the infant.

In contrast to both secure and avoidant infants, ambivalent infants— a small minority of infants, whose mothers' responsiveness has been unpredictable—display attachment behavior even long following their mothers' return to the laboratory room. This is a change in conditions that should normally signal "safety" and hence lead to a return to exploration and play.

In short, neither of these widely observed "insecure" responses to the Strange Situation seen in a substantial minority of infants are in keeping with the general expectation that the attachment behavioral program will inevitably be activated in conditions suggestive of "danger," while the complementary exploratory behavioral program will be activated under "safe" conditions. And, as regards the fourth Strange Situation category mentioned above, we must also ask why some infants unexpectedly show bouts of disorganized behavior.

Because differences in response to the mother in the Strange Situation in low-risk samples are relatively stable across the early years—and even in high-risk samples are found to be predictive of aspects of social behavior many years later in new settings (see Weinfield, Sroufe, Egeland, & Carlson, 1999)—the question of whether these differences should be attributed primarily to *genetic* or rather to *experiential* sources has not infrequently arisen. An example of a "behavior genetics" approach to understanding these differences is the proposal that the *specific, heritable genetic makeup* of a given individual may place him or her within a subset of species members who differ, say, in being *more* (or instead, *less*) fearful than others in new situations. It has thus been suggested by some that heritable or genetically based differences in tendencies to fear new situations could account for the differing response patterns observed. In this view, infants who seek their mothers on the mothers' return to an unfamiliar setting may be carrying genes that create a lower fear threshold for new situations (especially ambivalent infants), and those who fail to approach (avoidant infants) may have a heritably (i.e., genetically based) high fear threshold. This explanation, however, has yet to be supported by the data (see Stevenson-Hinde, Chapter 8, this volume).

In fact, following a series of earlier data-based arguments for an environmental origin to individual differences in attachment patterns (see Main & Weston, 1981; Sroufe, 1985), a recent family genetics study has supported the presence of strong environmental input, and the absence of substantial indices of genetic influence, with respect to all four Strange Situation categories (Bokhorst et al., 2003). Moreover, while two molecular genetics studies involving one particular sample of 70 Hungarian infant–mother dyads seemed to point to particular genetic alleles related to disorganized attachment (Lakatos et al., 2000, 2002), these findings were not replicated in a larger sample (n = 132) in the Netherlands, nor were they replicated when the Dutch and Hungarian samples were combined (Bakermans-Kranenburg & van IJzendoorn, 2004). It therefore appears that despite the species-wide nature of attachment behavior, placing virtually any infant in one of Ainsworth's three rearing contexts (i.e., relatively stably sensitive, rejecting, or unpredictable parental behavior) or in the context elucidated by Main and Hesse (frightening parenting) is likely to produce one of the systematically predictable outcomes (secure, avoidant, ambivalent, or disorganized Strange Situation behavior).

Thus, although we believe that intriguing gene–environment interactions may yet be uncovered, at present it appears that the primary place to look regarding the origin of systematically differing behavioral displays during the Strange Situation is to systematically differing environmental input. Differing environmental input *could* of course lead to differing behavior via the activation of species-wide genes, "turning on" or "activating" differential displays according to the nature of the environment (e.g., certain environments could "turn on" genes controlling a prewired "avoidance behavioral program"). These genes—unlike those for high or low fear thresholds, each available to only some individuals—would then be present in all species members, but "activated" only when, for instance, the attachment figure is rejecting (see Belsky, 1999).

We have suggested instead that there exist species-wide abilities that are not part of the attachment system itself, but can, within limits, manipulate (either inhibit or increase) attachment behavior in response to differing environments. An example taken from Main (e.g., 1979, 1981, 1999) is the proposal that the display of attachment behavior can be inhibited so long as all species members have developed the ability to engage in (1) an organized shift of attention, (2) *together with* the capacity to tie this attentional shift to the inhibition of action.[10]

Review

To review, then, the phenomena of attachment appear in virtually all human infants, and are genetic in the nonheritable sense (i.e., all infants are similarly equipped, no matter what their parentage). At its most basic level, the attachment behavioral program is viewed as leading to (1) the *formation* of an early attachment to caregiving figures, given even minimally consistent social interaction, after which (2) *propensities* to seek that individual are aroused in stressful or dangerous situations. And, again, this behavioral program is presumed to result from an evolved species-wide adaptation to particular dangers faced by ground-living primate infants.

At the same time, once an attachment has been formed, differences in the generation of rules for *if*, *when*, *where*, and *how much* attachment behavior should be exhibited with relation to a specific figure are now largely considered to depend upon the rearing environment. This is consistent with theory and research in fields concerned with other population-wide behavioral programs, which also focus mainly upon environmental rather than genetic sources of variation (Daly, 1996). Thus the capacity to inhibit (or, in contrast, maximize) the display of attachment behavior under certain circumstances can be seen as an indication of the operation of what are currently called "contingent decision rules" or, similarly, "conditional behavioral strategies" available for use in alternate and perhaps somewhat less psychologically "optimal" environments (see Hinde & Stevenson-Hinde, 1990; see also Belsky, 1999; Main, 1979, 1981, 1990; Simpson, 1999; Trivers, 1974). Although in theory these can arise via the environment-specific activation of organized ("prewired") sets of genes available to the species as a whole, to date we have favored the hypothesis that differences in the appearance of attachment behavior simply depend upon the use of very general species-wide abilities (such as alterations of attention). However, even if these general abilities can, for example, inhibit the appearance of attachment behavior in circumstances in which it is expected, it nonetheless remains the case that the species-wide attachment system remains present and potentially ready to be reactivated.

THE BERKELEY LONGITUDINAL STUDY:
SAMPLE, METHODS, AND PERIODS
OF DATA COLLECTION

With the discussion above in mind, we describe the first phases of the Berkeley Longitudinal Study of individual differences in parent–child attachment relationships. As many readers will be aware, by 1985 our laboratory had developed a number of new methods for assessing attachment. Besides Ainsworth's original tripartite analysis of the Strange Situation procedure (described below), in this chapter we emphasize only four: (1) disorganized attachment, devised by us as a new category of infant Strange Situation behavior, together with its equivalents at age 6 and in young adulthood; (2) 6th-year reunion responses to the parents following a 1-hour separation; (3) Kaplan's method of assessing transcripts of 6-year-olds' responses to the Separation Anxiety Test (SAT); and (4) the AAI as administered at age 19. We selected these four measures for the sake of simplicity, and because for each our original findings have been well replicated. Moreover, training in each is now available.[11]

We report all tests run to date, and have yet to examine relations among the remaining measures devised in conjunction with our study. This is the case despite the fact that some of the remaining measures have proven to be promising.[12]

Characteristics of the Sample

Our sample was selected to be "low-risk" and "stable," in the hope that our findings might serve to elucidate exactly those developmental transformations in attachment that occur under relatively consistent life conditions. We believed that only after the sequelae "naturally" arising out of enduring differences in attachment relationships have been delineated can researchers begin to trace—as P. T. Medawar put it in another context—the "variations which depart."

The sample consisted of 189 Bay Area families drawn from birth records, with 84% of those contacted participating. The great majority of participants were middle- to upper-middle-class, and the majority of infants were secure. Sibling order varied; infants were healthy at birth and beyond; and mothers worked no more than 24 hours per week. Families with recent parent–child separations were excluded. Each infant was seen at 12 (or 18) months with the mother (or father), first in the Strange Situation, and a week later in free play and a structured "Clown Session" (Main & Weston, 1981). Each infant visited Berkeley four times over a period of 6 months, and each parent came twice. The sessions in which each parent participated were identical (i.e., one Strange Situation and one play session).

The 6th-Year Follow-Up and the
"Move to the Level of Representation" in Attachment

When the children in the initial wave of the 3-year data collection had reached age 6, we brought a relatively modest subgroup ($n = 40$)[13] back for a follow-up study. Until that time, consideration of the sequelae to individual differences in the infant's attachment to the parent had been almost exclusively confined to behavioral outcomes, with numerous works emerging from Minnesota (as well as other laboratories) showing that children secure with their mothers at age 1 were highly favored in social and emotional development several years following (see Weinfield et al., 1999, for a review of the Minnesota studies).

Reasoning with Bowlby and many others that individual differences in behavior must be guided via differences in attention, thinking, language, and memory, we decided to investigate both children's *representational products* (such as language usage and family drawings) and their *responses to representations* (such as pictured separations and family photographs).

While the children were examined in our playroom, we asked their parents (each in separate offices) for their life histories with respect to attachment (the AAI). Once parents and children were reunited just prior to leaving, their dialogues were recorded (see Main, Kaplan, & Cassidy, 1985).

As we wrote in introducing the rationale for this "move to the level of representation,"

> The aim of this chapter is to discuss individual differences in attachment relationships as they relate to individual differences in mental representation, that is, in the individual's "internal working models" of attachment. . . . We define the internal working model of attachment as a set of conscious and/ or unconscious rules for the organization of information relevant to attachment and for obtaining or limiting access to that information, that is, to information regarding attachment-related experiences, feelings, and ideations. Previous definitions of individual differences in attachment organization, for example, secure, insecure-avoidant, and insecure-ambivalent, have relied on descriptions of the organization of the infant's nonverbal behavior toward a particular parent in a structured separation-and-reunion observation, the Ainsworth Strange Situation. . . .
>
> Our re-conceptualization of individual differences in attachment organization as individual differences in the mental representation of the self in relation to attachment permits the investigation of attachment not only in infants but also in older children and adults and leads to a new focus on representation and language. This conceptualization leads further to the proposal that the secure versus the various types of insecure attachment organizations can best be understood as terms referring to particular types of internal working models of relationships, models that direct not only feelings and behavior but also attention, memory, and cognition insofar as these relate directly or indirectly to attachment. Individual differences in these internal working models will therefore be related not only to individual differences in patterns of nonverbal behavior, but also to patterns of language and structures of mind. . . . (Main et al., 1985, pp. 66–67)

In this 1985 study, we deliberately selected a subsample of 6-year-olds that consisted of approximately one-third disorganized/disoriented with their mothers during infancy, one-third secure, and one-third insecure-avoidant. We were unable to include an exploration of the insecure-ambivalent attachment category, as only two subjects were available. (Following the advent of the disorganized infant attachment category and its AAI equivalent, unresolved/disorganized, the ambivalent category and its adult equivalent, insecure-preoccupied, have become rare. This is because many individuals previously classified as insecure-ambivalent in infancy or preoccupied in adulthood have been found to be disorganized or unresolved. However, the interested reader should refer to Main [2000, pp. 1074–1076, 1086–1088; see also Cassidy & Berlin, 1994] for a description of insecure-ambivalent Strange Situation responses, as well as related child and adult measures.)[14] Eighty-four percent of participants contacted agreed to return, and each measure was found to be strongly related to 1st-year attachment to the mother.

We present here the results of the two 6th-year measures that have most frequently been used to replicate or extend our original findings—namely, Kaplan's (1987, 2003) version of the SAT (see Solomon & George, 1999, for an overview of the success of this measure and its close variants), and Main and Cassidy's (1988) 6th-year reunion procedure (see a meta-analysis by Fraley, 2002, who found this reunion classification to be closely related to the same infants' Strange Situation response in several independent samples).

Follow-Up Study Conducted in Young Adulthood

When the subset of individuals seen in the Social Development Project at age 6 (and a few others seen in these same procedures a few months later) began to reach age 19, we brought them back into the laboratory for a full day's assessments. A surprising 90% of participants seen in this follow-up study contacted returned. As earlier, we divided this sample fairly evenly in terms of the offspring's early attachment classification to their mothers, with 11–15 participants available from each classification (except for ambivalent/resistant, $n = 2$). As 13 years previously, both coders and interviewers were unaware of the participant's response to all other assessments.

Despite the fact that we are testing strong hypotheses, we have erred on the side of caution and used only two-tailed tests, with significance set at $p = .05$. Because a subset of participants were utilized as pilot subjects for the 6th-year measures, the sample available at 6 is sometimes relatively small, with $n = 42$ (25 males) for comparisons between 1st-year and 19th-year procedures, and fewer at 6 years. Early classifications with father failed to predict either 6th-year or 19th-year outcomes, and hence our report focuses upon early attachment to the mother and its sequelae only.

The interviewers for the 19th-year follow-up study were two graduate students in clinical psychology at Berkeley, each trained by Erik Hesse across more than 30 hours in AAI protocol administration. Isabel Bradburn—then at Harvard, and unacquainted with the Bay Area sample—scored and classified the transcripts. Bradburn was regarded as an expert coder, since she had not only been certified in the 30-case reliability test provided by Main and Hesse in conjunction with AAI training, but also established 100% reliability with Hesse to subclass across a set of 14 transcripts. In addition, following Ainsworth's stringent standards, we too required a high level of agreement across 100 Strange Situations for our coders.

Considered together, our standards for training and reliability have no doubt increased the opportunity to find matches between our 1st-year and 19th-year assessments, should these be present.

ASSESSING SECURITY AT 1, 6, AND 19 YEARS: FROM SECURE ATTACHMENT TO THE MOTHER TO OVERALL SECURE-AUTONOMOUS STATES OF MIND

Our chapter began with an overview of primate evolution, and the critical role of the attachment figure in providing protection to young infants. Before moving into a review of our own findings regarding infant security with the mother and its sequelae, we therefore remind the reader that, as primate anthropologist Sarah Hrdy has stated, "Lurking predators, not to mention strange males . . . or the prospect of maternal ambivalence are precisely the threats little primates ought to fear most deeply. What infants yearn for is the reassurance that they will never lose their caretaker's love— that no matter what, [their attachment figures] will keep them safe from any lurking hazard. From an infant's point of view, the desired message is best summed up by an Egyptian incantation from the 16th century B.C., chanted to forestall evil spirits covetous of the child—spirits who might otherwise approach under the cover of dark" (1999, p. 540). The ancient incantation Hrdy cites (p. 541) is, she asserts, the "lullaby" that the infant primate wants to hear and, "in the old mammalian recesses of his brain, emotionally processes to himself as he nestles against his caretaker's breast . . . and falls securely asleep."

> *Hast thou come to kiss this child?*
> *I will not let thee kiss him!*
> *Hast thou come to silence him?*
> *I will not let thee set silence over him!*
> . . . .
> *I will not let thee injure him!*
> *Hast thou come to take him away?*
> *I will not let thee take him away from me!*

Identifying Security of Attachment to the Mother at 1 Year of Age: Procedure, Indices, and Relations to Maternal Sensitivity and Infant Secure-Base Behavior in the Home

Security of attachment in infancy was first explored in Uganda, via Ainsworth's (1967) extensive home observations of 26 infant–mother dyads. Among the dyads Ainsworth considered secure, the infants showed a notable absence of anxiety in their mothers' presence, although they took flight to their mothers as "havens of safety" in times of alarm. Later, in studying her Baltimore sample, Ainsworth additionally identified infants as secure in the home when they were accepting *both* of being picked up and put down; when they showed little distress when the mothers left a room, but greeted them positively upon return; and, most importantly (Waters, Vaughn, Posada, & Kondo-Ikemura, 1995), when they used their mothers as "secure bases" for exploration.

We begin these delineations of security of attachment as inferred from infant home behavior, because—particularly among researchers working outside the field—security has undoubtedly become too closely identified with certain kinds of behavioral responses to the Strange Situation procedure (see Grossmann, 1990; Grossmann & Grossmann, 1990). Although security as assessed in this procedure was found to be strongly *related to* security as identified independently in the home, it is, as Waters informally has put it, "a sign, not a sample" of what goes on in the home. For example, most securely attached infants eventually cry when left alone in the unfamiliar laboratory room—a behavior almost never exhibited when their mothers change rooms at home.

As noted earlier, Ainsworth deliberately structured the Strange Situation procedure to include three of Bowlby's (1969/1982) "natural clues to danger" as he envisioned their appearance within a ground-living primate's "environment of evolutionary adaptedness." Each was expected to arouse *some* propensities to seek proximity to the attachment figure. Moreover, these clues to danger (the "activators" of attachment behavior, such as separation) were intentionally succeeded by what we might now term clues to *safety* (to Bowlby, 1969/1982, "terminators" leading to the reduction or cessation of attachment behavior)—namely, the attachment figure's proximity. The procedure therefore consists of eight episodes, and, following a 1-minute introduction to the room by a research assistant, the succeeding seven are each designed to be 3 minutes in length. However, when an infant is strongly distressed, an episode is terminated in less than 30 seconds. Following introduction to the room, then, the episodes of what Bretherton once called this "miniature drama" are as follows:

- *Episode 2.* The mother (or other primary caregiver) and infant are left alone in a toy-filled environment whose unfamiliarity supplies the first natural clue to danger. However, the mother's presence is expected to provide the infant with security sufficient for interested exploration and/or play.
- *Episode 3.* Providing a second clue to danger, a stranger joins the mother and infant. Since Ainsworth first designed this procedure, new stud-

ies of primate troops have affirmed that strangers do provide a clue to possible danger (see Hrdy, 1999).

• *Episode 4.* The mother leaves the infant with the stranger, providing two combined clues to increased danger. At this time, the infant often cries and begins to search for the mother, who has left her purse or other belongings behind to assure her intention to return.

• *Episode 5.* The mother returns, and the stranger unobtrusively departs. The mother—who throughout this procedure has been otherwise asked to "behave as you normally would," but not to "attempt to direct the infant's activities"—calls from outside, then pauses in the doorway to permit the infant time to mobilize a response. Many infants initially seek proximity but then, reassured of their mothers' nearness, resume play.

• *Episode 6.* The mother leaves, reassuring the infant of her return, and the infant remains entirely alone in the unfamiliar setting. Infant distress can be strong at this point, and this episode is often terminated rapidly. Note that in the environments of evolutionary adaptedness in which humans and other primates evolved, calling and searching immediately upon being left alone would usually be a requirement for survival (see Hinde, 1974; Hrdy, 1999).

• *Episode 7.* The stranger, rather than the mother, enters the room. Here Ainsworth wished to ascertain whether any distress exhibited has resulted simply from being alone without general companionship, or is due specifically to the absence of the attachment figure.

• *Episode 8.* This is the second and final reunion episode. The mother returns as in Episode 5 (again, the stranger leaves unobtrusively), but this time she is instructed to try to pick the infant up. By now, most infants are expected to be crying, and actively and rapidly not only seeking proximity to their mothers, but also perhaps pulling themselves up on the mothers' legs and indicating a strong desire to be held. They may also require a somewhat lengthier period of holding than is typical for Episode 5. Nonetheless, they are expected to settle and renew their interest in exploration and play by the end of this final 3-minute period.

In the Strange Situation as outlined above, the following behaviors encapsulate the form of infant response that Ainsworth ultimately termed "secure." To summarize, an infant who is judged secure in relation to a particular parent does the following:

• Plays happily with the toys and explores the environment prior to separation.
• Shows signs of missing the parent during separation, such as crying or calling.

- Seeks proximity immediately and actively at least by the time of the second separation, often indicating as well a desire to be held.
- And, before the end of each 3-minute reunion episode, returns to exploration and play, "secure" once again in the parent's presence.

Ainsworth found that a "secure" response to the mother in the Strange Situation was associated with the mother's "sensitivity to infant signals and communications" in the home, including (1) perceiving that a signal had occurred, (2) interpreting it accurately, (3) responding promptly, and (4) responding appropriately. In Ainsworth's sample (unequaled to this date in the extensive time given to home observation—i.e., 66 waking hours across the first year), the association between maternal sensitivity and security was very strong (Ainsworth et al., 1978).

Assessing Security at 6 Years at the Behavioral and Representational Levels: Procedures, Indices, and Relations to Early Security with the Mother

Sixth-Year Reunion Responses: Secure

At the conclusion of our assessments of 6-year-olds and their parents as described by Main and colleagues (1985), we included a deliberately casual parent–child reunion. Here, once both parents had completed the AAI in separate offices, one would return to the playroom, followed in 3–5 minutes by the second. Parents were then asked to sign some final consent forms and to prepare the child for leaving. Six-year-olds were termed "secure" when no major changes in affect or behavior appeared on hearing their parents' approach, and when they calmly but affectionately welcomed them, easily incorporating them into their ongoing activities and play. This response was strongly related to early security with the mother (Main & Cassidy, 1988). Children secure in infancy were also less likely than others to have shown distress during the hour-long separation (Cassidy & Main, 1984).

Sixth-Year Responses to Kaplan's Version of the SAT: Secure-Resourceful

In the SAT, the participant is presented with pictures of various kinds of parent–child separations. What is happening during each separation is clearly described by the examiner, and then followed up by questions regarding what the separated child might feel or do. This method was originally devised for use with adolescents (Hansburg, 1972), but was adapted for 6-year-olds by Klagsbrun and Bowlby (1976).

Kaplan (1987) retained the above-described six separation photographs, and as in the Klagsbrun and Bowlby version of the SAT, the examiner asked what the pictured child would *feel*, as well as what the pictured child would *do*. Rather than counting frequencies of precategorized answers, however, Kaplan transcribed the entire conversational exchange, and then analyzed the text via a new system. The SAT text was considered "secure" if the pictured child (1) expressed feelings of sadness, anger, or some other form of distress, *and also* (2) was able to provide a "constructive solution" for the pictured child (e.g., persuading the parents not to leave, or finding something positive to occupy the child during the parents' absence). It is interesting to note that, taken together, these 6-year-old responses indicate both the early development of an open valuing of attachment (as seen in response to the "feel" questions), and an early development of autonomy (as evidenced in the "constructive" answers to the "do" questions). This SAT response was strongly related to early security with the mother in the Strange Situation, and was called "secure-resourceful."

The Adult Attachment Interview:
Assessing Security via Language at Age 19

The AAI is a well-known procedure for assessing "state of mind with respect to attachment" in young adulthood and beyond (see Hesse, 1999a). The AAI protocol (George et al., 1984, 1985, 1996) consists of 18 questions, with set probes. The interview generally takes about 1 hour (ranging from 40 minutes to almost 2 hours), and is transcribed verbatim, including place-holding responses ("um . . . uh"), stammers, and so forth. During the interview, speakers are repeatedly asked to describe their attachment histories. This includes a call for the selection of five adjectives that would, in the speaker's view, best describe the relationship with each parent (first the mother, and then the father). Speakers are then asked for memories or specific incidents to support each adjectival choice. They are asked which parent they were closer to, what happened when they were hurt or ill, whether they experienced threat or abuse from parents, and whether any of their early experiences with parents seemed to them to create a "setback" to their further development. They are also asked to discuss and evaluate the import of any critical loss experience(s) occurring throughout their lifetimes.

Before we report the AAI security findings for our young participants at age 19, it will be helpful to discuss earlier research with the AAI. Ruth Goldwyn and Mary Main initially created a three-category system for scoring and classifying the AAI (Main & Goldwyn, 1984; see Main et al., 2003, for the most recent, five-category version of this system). Using a "development sample" of 44 out of 110 available texts (i.e., 44 texts wherein infant Strange Situation behavior was known), they then attempted to sort out differences in speech among the parents of children who as infants had been placed in one of Ainsworth's three categories of the Strange Situation 5 years earlier. (Note additionally that while Ainsworth had created three major and 8 subclassifications for the Strange Situation, we have ultimately created five major and 12 subclassifications for states of mind seen in the AAI; Main et al., 2003).

From the first, it became clear that it was not the *content* of the parents' apparent history or "experiences" with respect to their own parents, but rather their *mental state with regard to those apparent experiences*, that differentiated AAI texts of individuals whose infants were securely versus insecurely attached to them. Borrowing a term from philosophy, we eventually referred to this as an individual's "overall state of mind with respect to attachment." In fact, what distinguished the AAI texts of the parents of infants who had been judged secure with them in the Strange Situation could be described as "valuing of attachment relationships and experiences, but coherent and apparently objective regarding any particular relationship or experience." These "secure-autonomous" texts underscored a speaker's ability to value relationships, while simultaneously taking an internally consistent or "autonomous" stance toward any individual person (for other explorations of autonomy as related to the AAI, see Allen & Hauser, 1996; Waldinger et al., 2003).

Because coherence was the overall key to secure-autonomous status in adults, not only participants reporting favorable early experiences, but also those describing untoward ones, could be and were found to have secure babies. Speakers who were coherent despite apparently unfavorable backgrounds were termed "earned secure" (alternatively "discontinuous secure").

Having looked "down" on our interview transcripts from the categorical to the subcategorical level by creating taxonomic descriptors, we began to develop *continuous scales* for "probable experiences" with each parent during childhood, as well as scales representing various aspects of a speaker's apparent "state of mind" with respect to particular persons or experiences. These included, for example, "idealization," "preoccupied anger," and "unresolved/disorganized responses to loss or abuse." We also developed scales to represent specific recurring speech usages, such as "vague speech" and "insistence on lack of memory." Some of these scales will be discussed in greater detail later.

Expectable relations between the continuous scores assigned for varying overall classifications or "states of mind" are outlined in a table; this allows the coder to work up from scale score configurations towards the final classification.[15] However, coders also double-check their categorization via a set of generalized descriptors delineating each category and then subcategory.[16] This is why we often refer to classifying an AAI text as a task that combines "bottom-up" (scale-to-category) and "top-down" (category-to-subcategory) approaches.

The central scale ascertaining the extent to which a speaker evidenced a secure-autonomous state during this life history interview was termed "overall coherence of transcript" (this scale was created several years prior to our first reading of Grice). We found that where parental texts were coherent, the child (seen with the same parent) had tended to be secure (Main & Goldwyn, 1984), whereas incoherent texts tended to come from the parents of insecure infants.

Later, as Main began to read the work of the linguistic philosopher Grice and discovered his four "conversational maxims" for cooperative, rational discourse (Grice, 1975, 1989), we began to refer to "coherent" AAI texts as both "consistent" (in keeping with Grice's maxim of "quality" or "truthfulness"—i.e., being internally consistent, or thus most probably "truthful") and "collaborative" (being appropriate in length of conversational turn, or, in Grice's terminology, adhering to the maxims of "quantity," "manner," and "relevance"). However, speakers could also "license" violations of any maxim (e.g., in regard to quantity, opening a conversational turn with "Well, this could be a really long story"; see Mura, 1983).

Following Goldwyn's coding of our remaining 66 AAI transcripts (conducted without knowledge of the infant's Strange Situation behavior), we were able to reconfirm that both mothers and fathers manifesting a secure-autonomous state of mind most frequently had had babies judged secure with them 5 years previously (Main & Goldwyn, 1984; see also Main et al., 1985). These findings have been well replicated, and in van IJzendoorn's (1995) meta-analysis across 18 samples (854 dyads), parents whose AAI texts were classified as secure-autonomous were likely to have had secure babies, while parents whose AAI texts were incoherent during the discussion of their life histories (i.e., were *not* secure-autonomous) were likely to have had insecure offspring. This association (75%) was very strong (effect size $[d] = 1.06$, $r = .49$, biserial $r = .59$), and a statistic utilized by van IJzendoorn led to the conclusion that it would take more than 1,087 further studies with null results to reduce these findings to insignificance. In addition, van IJzendoorn's meta-analysis showed that mothers (and fathers) whose AAI texts were classified as secure-autonomous were more sensitive and responsive than others to their offspring.

AAI classifications assigned to a given speaker have now proven stable across periods extending to 5 years (see Crowell & Waters, Chapter 9, this volume); AAI coherence in the discussion of life history has repeatedly been discriminated from simple intelligence or verbal fluency, and is independent of interviewer (see Bakermans-Kranenburg & van IJzendoorn, 1993; Sagi et al., 1994); and Waters and his colleagues have demonstrated that patterns of discourse discriminating among AAI categories arise specifically when life history with respect to attachment is being discussed, as opposed to the technical aspects of work history (Crowell et al., 1996). Among the pioneering studies involving the AAI (each now well replicated), several included parents whose interviews were conducted before their first infant was born (e.g., initially, Fonagy, Steele, & Steele, 1991); several used high-risk samples (e.g., initially, Ward & Carlson, 1995); several discriminated clinically distressed from control participants (initially, Crowell & Feldman, 1991); and several showed that parental AAIs are predictive of maternal sensitivity (e.g., Grossmann, Fremmer-Bombik, Rudolph, & Grossmann, 1988). Each of these researchers had attended one of the two first AAI institutes, organized by Mary Ainsworth (1985) and then by John Bowlby and John Byng-Hall (1987).

It should be noted in closing this discussion, that, unlike the Strange Situation behaviors of infants (see below), the AAI texts of adults are judged "secure-autonomous" *not* regarding any other particular person or relationship, but rather with respect to the overall state of mind that arises during discussion of an entire series of topics and relationships. In theory, then, an adult with all attachment figures deceased and no close relationships available could still be secure-autonomous and raise secure offspring. In strong contrast, an infant or young child in this same position could not be judged secure, since his or her attachment status is always identified with respect to a particular person (e.g., "securely attached to father").

We now specifically examine the 19th-year AAI responses of our young participants. The first question we address is, of course, whether children securely attached to their mothers on our 6th-year measures or during infancy would become secure-autonomous 13–18 years later on the AAI.

Secure-Autonomous States of Mind in Young Adulthood as Related to Earlier Security

Both secure responses to the mother in the 6th-year reunion procedure, and secure-resourceful status on Kaplan's version of the SAT, significantly predicted a secure-autonomous state of mind on the AAI when the participant had reached age 19. In addition, a significant match was uncovered between infant security (or insecurity) with the mother at age 1 and secure-autonomous (or insecure) status on the AAI 18 years later.

In all analyses, there was an especially low likelihood that a child judged insecure would be judged secure-autonomous on the AAI. Moreover, according to the criteria long established within the AAI manual

(Main & Goldwyn, 1984–1998; Main et al., 2003), not one of our 26 participants insecure in infancy was classified "earned secure" at 19. This finding is understandable, given the age of the sample (cf. Roisman, Padron, Sroufe, & Egeland, 2002, who also found few or no "earned secure" subjects in their poverty sample at age 19, when using the AAI manual criteria).

Similar significant infant Strange-Situation-to-AAI matches in adolescence or young adulthood have been reported in three other U.S. samples—specifically, those of Hamilton at UCLA, and of Waters working with his original Minneapolis middle-class sample (Hamilton, 2000; Waters, Merrick, Trevoux, Crowell, & Albersheim, 2000) and most recently by Sroufe, Egeland, Carlson, and Collins (2005) on predicting AAIs for the Minnesota poverty sample at age 26. Relatedly, even prior to these reports, Benoit and Parker (1994) had found strong matches between mothers' security versus insecurity on the AAI and that of their *adult* daughters. This finding allows us to posit (although it cannot prove) predictability across time on the part of the adult offspring and also, of course, continuity from infancy to adulthood. Finally, Beckwith, Cohen, and Hamilton (1999) found that maternal insensitivity—a substantial correlate of infant insecure Strange Situation behavior—predicted insecure-dismissing adolescent AAIs from 1 month through 24 months of age.

The participants in each of the samples referenced above were Americans or Canadians. Early (19-year as opposed to 26-year) results for the Minnesota poverty sample (Weinfield, Sroufe, & Egeland, 2000) and for two German middle-class samples differed. For example, in the high-stress Minnesota poverty sample, infant security with mother in the Strange Situation failed to predict secure-autonomous status on the AAI at age 19 (n = 125; Weinfield, Whaley, & Egeland, 2004). It is critical to note, however, that in the Minnesota poverty sample, as opposed to the Berkeley (Main & Weston, 1981) and Minnesota (Sroufe & Waters, 1977) middle-class samples, 12- to 18-month stability in Strange Situation behavior to mothers was significant, but low (62% stability; Vaughn, Egeland, Sroufe, & Waters, 1979). One interpretation of the initial 19-year results could be that in a high-stress context, the frequent disruptions and changes occurring in early relationships may fail or else take longer to "stabilize" the offspring's mental organization with respect to attachment sufficiently to predict long-term outcomes.

Furthermore, in presenting the combined results for their two German middle-class samples (Bielefeld and Regensburg), the Grossmanns report only a partial replication of our findings (Grossmann, Grossmann, & Kindler, Chapter 5, this volume). As in our study, below, secure versus insecure responses to the AAI could be predicted forward from middle childhood, but—in contrast to our investigation and to those noted above—were not predictable from infancy. However, D codes were not utilized in the German reports, since D coding was available for the Regensburg but not the Bielefeld sample, and the Grossmanns wished to report pooled findings.[17]

In our Bay Area study, we have gradually begun to place increased emphasis on the continuous scales underlying the taxonomic aspects of both the Strange Situation and the AAI. Among her four 7-point scales assessing aspects of infant reunion response, Ainsworth regarded "proximity seeking" as the most strongly indicative of infant security. We therefore correlated proximity-seeking scores at age 1 with scores assigned to the same participants for our central AAI scale, "coherence of transcript." At the high end of the proximity-seeking scale, the infant immediately, actively, and fully approaches the parent on reunion. At the high end of our 9-point scale for coherence, the speaker is (following Grice, 1975, 1989) reasonably internally consistent and clear, with conversational turns being relevant and appropriate in length. The correlation between these two central continuous scales—proximity seeking in infancy and coherence of transcript on the AAI—was strong over the 18-year period. However, given our paucity of ambivalent-resistant ("C" infants, $n = 2$), our results could be sample-specific and should be tested in samples with higher proportions of C babies. Also, prior to Main and Solomon's (1990) discovery of D, van IJzendoorn and Kroonenberg (1990) had published an algorithm for Strange Situation continuous scales that, like proximity seeking, appears to well represent overall infant security.

AAI Estimates of Mothers' "Loving Behavior during Childhood" as Compared to Early Security

As noted earlier, near the outset of the AAI, speakers are asked to illustrate each of the adjectives they have selected to describe their early relationship to each parent ("support" in the sense of providing specific descriptive incidents), and are then queried regarding parental responses to injury, illness, separation, and so on. The coder's best estimate of parental loving behavior during the speaker's childhood is rated on a 9-point scale (mother and father are scored separately). Again, a coder often assigns a higher or lower rating for overall loving behavior in childhood than would be assigned based on the speaker's choice of adjectives.

To the best of our knowledge, we may be the first researchers to examine AAI coders' "accuracy" in estimating early experiences with the parent. But how could this be done? As was already known, maternal sensitivity scores assigned in infancy relate *prospectively* to infant security in the Strange Situation (Ainsworth et al., 1978; see also De Wolff & van IJzendoorn, 1997). With this in mind, we undertook a *retrospective* examination of whether, as based on Strange Situation responses assessed in infancy, an AAI coder's *estimate* of the mother's loving/"sensitive" behavior in childhood reflected a participant's likely early experience of maternal sensitivity. This undertaking was admittedly somewhat awkward, given that we had no direct measure of maternal sensitivity, and should therefore be attempted again in laboratories with direct access to sensitivity measures. Note also that (a) coder estimates, not specific participant "memories," are being utilized and (b) this correlation will be lowered in any sample having a high proportion of "earned secure" adults (see also footnote 18).

Nonetheless, we did find an impressively significant relation between our AAI coder's estimate of maternal loving behavior in childhood as derived from texts produced by 19-year-olds, and the same speaker's observed overall security with their mothers in the Strange Situation. The AAI coder's estimate of maternal loving behavior during childhood was related even more strongly to secure 6th-year reunion behavior toward the mother, and to Kaplan's security estimates for the SAT.[18]

Consideration of the Role Played by Intervening Trauma

Starting with Waters and colleagues' (2000) study, which linked Strange Situation security with the mother to secure-autonomous status on the AAI, researchers have looked to intervening trauma to explain changes in attachment status. Among the participants in our study, no intervening abuse by parents was reported. However, nine subjects had experienced other forms of trauma—specifically, death of a parent or close parental figure; an ongoing fatal illness in a parent; or a long, potentially fatal illness in the self. We found that intervening trauma had occurred at about three times the rate among participants who were discontinuous in attachment as among those who were continuous, and this result was highly significant. Interestingly and unexpectedly, one participant who had been insecure-disorganized with the mother in infancy had become secure in response to intervening trauma, directly describing the intervening traumatic experience as causal in changing their behavior and feelings toward their family.

When participants with trauma were removed from our analysis, the percentage of secure versus insecure Strange-Situation-to-AAI matches increased, as it had in other laboratories—in ours, to well above 80%. However, because the removal of these nine subjects markedly reduced our sample size, all data reported in the remainder of this presentation include the sample as a whole.

Security: Summary

1. Drawing on Ainsworth's original observations, we can understand secure Strange Situation behavior as a function of earlier experiences of maternal sensitivity and responsiveness (Ainsworth et al., 1978), or, in our more recent terms, as the result of repeated experiences of "fright/distress with (ready) solution" (see Hesse & Main, 1999).

2. Security with the mother at 1 year of age predicted a secure reunion response to her at age 6, as well as a failure to show marked distress or anger during the hour-long separation.

3. Security at 1 year predicted secure-resourceful responses to the SAT.

4. At 6 years, both a calm, secure reunion response, and a secure-resourceful response to the SAT (the pictured child misses the parent, but can act constructively during the separation), predicted a secure-autonomous AAI at 19 years. Each of these 6th-year responses (as well as the failure to show distress on separation seen at 6) is suggestive of a developing sense of autonomy, increasing our understanding of the pathway to secure-autonomous states of mind in young adulthood.

5. Infant security versus insecurity with the mother in the Strange Situation predicted a secure-autonomous versus an insecure AAI. This result has also been reported for two middle-class U.S. samples and for the large Minnesota poverty sample at age 26.

6. Continuous scores for "proximity seeking" during the Strange Situation (Ainsworth's primary continuous index of infant security) predicted continuous scores for "coherence of transcript" on the AAI (the primary continuous scale estimating security in the AAI). This finding may, however, be sample-specific due to our low number of insecure-ambivalent infants.

7. Change in security status between the Strange Situation and the AAI was strongly related to intervening trauma. With cases involving trauma omitted, a substantial as opposed to a slight majority of secure infants were found to have become secure-autonomous, and the secure–insecure match between infancy and the AAI was well above 80%.

8. The scores AAI coders assigned to the participants' mothers for "loving behavior during childhood" were significantly correlated with observed security with the mothers at both 1 and 6 years. Despite the absence of direct measures of maternal sensitivity, this implies a surprising accuracy of coder "experience" estimates, at least in samples with few participants who are "earned secure."

9. Many of the results above can be interpreted in terms of a continuing *flexibility of attention*. This is shown at 1 year in alternating attention between the mother and the toys during the Strange Situation, and at 6 years via the secure-resourceful capacity both to express distress and to find

constructive solutions during the SAT. It is exhibited again at age 19, where the speaker alternates smoothly between attending to the interviewer's queries and coherently responding to them (Hesse, 1996; Main, 1995).

ASSESSING AVOIDANCE OF THE ATTACHMENT FIGURE AT 1 YEAR, AND ITS EQUIVALENTS AT 6 AND 19 YEARS OF AGE

Avoidance is commonly identified by absence of responsiveness when another individual approaches or offers positive overtures. Avoidant behavior includes ignoring, looking away, turning away, moving away, and showing an apparent "lack of recognition." Although the first formal scoring and classification system for avoidance was, to the best of our knowledge, developed by Mary Ainsworth and her collaborators (see Ainsworth et al., 1978), the phenomenon has long been noted in human history. A specific early illustration of the association between avoidance and reunion following long separations is given in *The Odyssey* of Homer (circa 700 B.C.[19]). Here Penelope, 20 years separated from her husband, has just been informed by her son that—having recently triumphed over her many suitors—Odysseus is once more within her halls. She descends to meet him.

Telemachus' voice came to her ears:

> "*Mother,*
> *cruel mother, do you feel nothing,*
> *drawing yourself apart this way from Father?*
> *Will you not sit with him and talk and question him?*
> *What other woman could remain so cold? . . .*
> *Your heart is hard as flint and never changes!*"

Penelope answered:
> "*I am stunned, child.*
> *I cannot speak to him. I cannot question him.*
> *I cannot keep my eyes upon his face.*" (Homer [Fitzgerald, Trans.], 1963, p. 432)

Within the field of attachment, the best-known examples of avoidance following separations are based on the early observations of Robertson and Bowlby (1952) and Heinicke and Westheimer (1966). In both investigations, toddlers subjected to separations lasting weeks to months in which they resided in stressful, unfamiliar environments came to actively avoid and ignore their primary attachment figures. In an important and surprising contrast, secondary figures, together with neighbors and others, were readily greeted and recognized. Heinicke and Westheimer proposed that the initial avoidant response to reunion could be best understood as serving a defensive function, permitting a child to maintain control over an anger (and probably also, distress) that had grown too intense to otherwise permit continued behavioral organization (see also Main, 1981).

Identifying Avoidance of the Mother during Infancy: Indices, and Links to Maternal Rejection and Infant Expressions of Anxiety and Anger in the Home

By the time she undertook her Baltimore study of infant Strange Situation behavior, Mary Ainsworth had already spent several years in London becoming well acquainted with the work of Bowlby, Heinicke, and Robertson, with its focus upon the avoidance of the parent as described above. However, she had no expectation that avoidance could occur (1) following very brief (30-second to 3-minute) separations (2) in home-reared 1-year-olds (3) who had undergone no previous major separation from their parents (M. Ainsworth, personal communication to M. Main, 1979). In the laboratory, she expected to see only proximity seeking following these separations.

An infant who is judged avoidant not only does not cry when left by the mother and fails to greet her on reunion, but also actively avoids looking at her, indicates a wish to be put down if picked up, and explores the toys and room throughout the procedure. This imbalance between exploration and attachment behavior in relation to changes in cues regarding danger and safety suggests the active presence and use of restriction of attention under moderate stress (Main, 1995). Thus, unlike secure infants, who demonstrate flexibility in attention, avoidant infants attend virtually inflexibly to the toys or inanimate environment throughout the procedure.[20]

We can summarize the Strange Situation behavior that leads to placement in the insecure-avoidant attachment classification (Ainsworth et al., 1978) as follows:

- Like secure infants, these infants play or explore prior to separation.
- However, an avoidant infant ignores—or appears, at the least, indifferent to—the parent's leave taking on both the first and second separations.
- When left alone entirely, the infant fails to cry and continues to explore the room.
- On reunion, the infant ignores and avoids the parent. If picked up, the infant indicates a desire to be put down, and if called, will most likely turn away to a toy, or even will move (sometimes sharply) further away from the parent.

Intriguingly, in reviewing her narrative records, Ainsworth found that four of her six avoidant infants had shown strong anxiety regarding mothers' taking leave in the home, so that behavior in the stressful Strange Situation procedure appeared to involve a suppression of their more usual expressions of distress and anxiety. In addition, as Main and Stadtman (1981) discovered, avoidant infants expressed strong anger toward their mothers in the home, but little or none in the Strange Situation.

Ainsworth's records also revealed that avoidance in the Strange Situation was sharply associated with the mother's rejection of attachment behavior in the home (Ainsworth, Bell, & Stayton, 1971; Ainsworth et al., 1978)—a finding replicated by Main and Stadtman (1981) for two further independent U.S. samples. Rejection was exemplified in refusal of tactual contact with and proximity to the infant and, in Ainsworth's sample, in direct statements such as "I wish I had never had this baby."

Assessing Avoidance at 6 Years at the Behavioral and Representational Levels: Indices and Relations to Early Avoidance of the Mother

Sixth-Year Reunion Responses: Avoidant

Main and Cassidy (1988) found that at age 6, previously avoidant infants were distinguished by their continued, but now less overt, avoidance of proximity and conversation. Rather than completely refusing to communicate when addressed, as they often had at age 1, these children allowed a small time lapse prior to taking their conversational turn, and then responded minimally (e.g., "Yeah," "That one," "It's over there," "Nope"). They also edged subtly away from their mothers, and as in infancy, increased attention to the toys and other inanimate objects (or, in a few cases, the examiner). The similarity to their behavior during infancy was obvious, and despite their now more "socially appropriate" demeanor, they were easily identified. The relation to early avoidant status with the mother was strong (this finding was replicated in Regensburg by Wartner, Grossmann, Fremmer-Bombik, & Suess, 1994).

Sixth-Year Responses to Kaplan's Version of the SAT: Insecure-Inactive

Surprising in prospect, children avoidant of the mother during infancy gave responses to the "feel" questions of the SAT virtually indistinguishable from those of the secure children (the separated child was described as feeling sad, crying, or feeling angry). However, in direct opposition to the secure children, who then offered "constructive" solutions as to what a separated 6-year-old could *do* about the situation, previously avoidant children typically responded with "I don't know," "Nothing," or even "Run away." Kaplan termed this response pattern "insecure-inactive," since the child seemed unable to imagine a useful or constructive strategy for acting on his or her self-admitted feelings (Kaplan, 1987; Main et al., 1985).

Dismissing States of Mind in the AAI

From their first examination of their 44 "development" AAI transcripts in the early 1980s, Main and Goldwyn found it relatively straightforward to discriminate the texts of the parents of avoidant infants. This was because—at least during the semistressful task of describing and evaluating early attachment relationships and their influences—these parents (ultimately termed "dismissing of attachment") seemed strongly to resemble their infants (who had behaviorally "dismissed" both separations from and reunions with their mothers under stress). Overall, parents who attempted to avoid the topics of attachment experiences and any untoward effects were termed "dismissing," "devaluing," or "cut off" from attachment relationships and experience.

In most texts judged dismissing, the speakers described their early relationships to their parents as good or normal, and themselves as strong and/ or independent. Thus, just as their infants behaved in the Strange Situation as though nothing untoward was happening, and showed little or no overt distress in the face of what in fact for an infant are highly stressful circumstances, their parents spoke as though their childhoods had included little or no real difficulty, tending to use positive to highly positive adjectives for one or both parents. However, given the positive adjectival constellation usually provided, these texts were considered inconsistent in that the speakers usually then failed to support their adjectival choices ("I said she was loving because she was caring"), or even actively contradicted them (a "very loving" mother may, later in the text, have been described as having gotten so frequently angry with the speaker for hurting himself that he once had hidden a broken arm) either immediately or later within the interview. These inconsistencies lead to a score for "idealization of the mother," and a strong tendency to idealize one or both parents is perhaps the primary index used to place a text in the dismissing AAI category. In sum, then, like an infant who "ignores" the natural clues to danger implicit within the Strange Situation procedure, the dismissing interviewee has attempted to act as though all is/was well (*"tutto bene"*), despite weak or even contradictory evidence.

Another transcript characteristic pointing to this category is a tendency to cut the interview or interview response short via what we have come to call "insistence on lack of memory" for childhood events and relationships. Of course, some thoughtful speakers will worry about whether they are able to remember as much as seems to be called for in the interview, and will say that they do not know whether they remember much, but that they will try. The discourse strategy that we have come to call "insistence on lack of memory" differs from this, in that the speaker indicates not only inability, but perhaps also unwillingness, to proceed with an attempt to respond ("I don't remember. No. I just can't remember anything about that").

We do not know at present whether these speakers in fact cannot remember, or are simply attempting to block discourse, or some combination. Nonetheless, such attempts to dismiss the topic tend to mark the AAI texts of the parents of avoidant infants.

Again, all of the AAI scales dealing with the "organized" categories (e.g., idealization, insistence on lack of memory, coherence) were devised by Main and Goldwyn by 1984, prior to Main's reading of Grice in 1988. Nonetheless, it can be seen here that idealization is a violation of Grice's maxim of quality ("Be truthful, and have evidence for what you say"), while insistence on lack of memory is a violation of Grice's maxim of quantity ("Be succinct, and yet complete"), in that the response is excessively brief. Note that the indices leading to high scale placement are reminiscent of infant avoidance, where the infant seems "not to remember" (i.e., behaviorally indicates that "nothing has happened") either that the parent has left, or that the parent is important at return.

In van IJzendoorn's (1995) meta-analysis of studies comparing parental AAI status and infant Strange Situation response to that same parent, the relation between a mother's or father's dismissing AAI status and the infant's tendency to be classified as avoidant with that parent was very strong, with an effect size of 1.02 (equivalent to $r = .49$).

Dismissing States of Mind in the AAI as Related to Avoidance in Childhood and Infancy

When we looked forward from the 6th-year reunion to the AAI in the Berkeley Longitudinal Study, a strong majority of avoidant children had become dismissing. However, the chi-square for association between a child's 6th-year reunion status as avoidant and dismissing (vs. not-dismissing) status on the AAI was not significant, due to the fact that many children who had not been avoidant on reunion at 6 were also found to be dismissing (the majority of these had been disorganized).

A majority (9 of 11) of children who had been insecure-inactive (avoidant) on the SAT at age 6 were, as expected, judged dismissing on the AAI 13 years later.[21] However, the chi-square test was again not significant, since, as in the case of the 6th-year reunion, many children who were not insecure-inactive at six (largely D-controlling) had also become dismissing by the time of the AAI.

When we moved to an examination of relations between infancy and the AAI, our results were much the same, with 10 of 11 children avoidant of their mothers during infancy being classified as dismissing of attachment on the AAI.[21] As in the case of 6th-year responses, however, dismissing responses also occurred in formerly disorganized infants. Consequently, the overall association with infant avoidance was not significant.

Finally, we examined our continuous Strange Situation scales in conjunction with the appropriate AAI scales. Ainsworth's 7-point scale for avoidance is, like proximity seeking, averaged across the two reunion episodes (refusal to greet the parent immediately upon reunion, and also ignoring her further attempts to attract attention, are scored high, while briefly turning or looking away is scored low). Avoidance of the mother significantly predicted idealization of her 18 years later in the AAI, as well as insistence upon lack of recall for childhood.[22]

As noted above (pp. 254–255), we have proposed that avoidance may represent the early development of a "conditional" or "alternative" behavioral strategy available for surviving in altered or nonoptimal circumstances. Specifically, an avoidant conditional strategy may permit the infant raised by a relatively rejecting (but not frightening) mother to maintain whatever proximity to her is possible (Main, 1981). In other words, our reasoning has been that approach to a mother who normally rejects the infant's proximity seeking would be especially likely to chance increasing danger (infant–mother distance) in unfamiliar settings.

Avoidance of a nonfrightening but rejecting attachment figure is, then, seen by us as a compromised (but optimal in context) response to situations of fright stemming from the external environment (see Belsky, 1999). Furthermore, perhaps precisely because it reduces attention to the withdrawal-prone, rejecting mother, avoidance may simultaneously permit the adaptive maintenance of self-organization, as opposed to dysregulating combinations of tendencies to approach, take flight, or express hostility.[23] In other words, organized avoidance may permit the infant to maintain whatever degree of proximity to the mother seems currently possible.

Avoidance: Summary

1. Avoidance of the mother in the Strange Situation is associated with experiences of rejection of attachment behavior in the home.

2. At age 6, a strong majority of children who had been avoidant of their mothers at age 1 avoided her on reunion.

3. Similarly, a strong majority of children who had been avoidant at 1 were insecure-inactive on the SAT at 6.

4. Both children classified as avoidant on reunion and children classified as insecure-inactive on the SAT at age 6 were very likely to be judged
dismissing on the AAI. However, other children had also become dismissing, and the chi-square was not significant.

5. Children who were avoidant of their mothers at age 1 strongly
tended to be dismissing of attachment on the AAI, although other insecure
children had also become dismissing. Here too, therefore, the chi-square
test was not significant.

6. As expected, continuous scores for proximity avoidance averaged
across the two reunions in the Strange Situation at age 1 predicted the continuous scores for idealization of the mother, as well as insistence on lack of
memory, during the AAI.

7. Inflexibility of attention was seen across all three age periods. That
is, those participants judged avoidant of their mothers in the Strange Situation also tended in varying ways to focus attention *away* from attachment-
related experiences at ages 6 and 19.

ASSESSING DISORGANIZED ATTACHMENT STATUS AT AGE 1: ITS EQUIVALENTS AND SEQUELAE AT 6 AND 19 YEARS OF AGE

The ancient Sumerian epic poem *Gilgamesh*, dating from about 2000 B.C.,
gives perhaps the earliest illustration of one of the causes of the "frightening" behavior of the parents of infants falling in the fourth Strange Situation category, disorganized/disoriented—that is, unresolved grief:

> *Gilgamesh wept bitterly for his friend. . . .*
>
> *He was no more a king*
> *But just a man who had lost his way*
> *Yet had a greater passion to withdraw*
> *Into a deep isolation. Mad,*
> *Perhaps insane, he tried*
> *To bring* [his friend] *Enkidu back to life*
> *To end his bitterness,*
> *His fear of death. . . .*
>
> *And when* [a woman at whose door he knocked] *called: Where are*
>   *you going,*
> *Traveler? And came to see, she saw him as half-crazed.*
> *Perhaps he is a murderer! She thought*
> *And drew away from him in fear.* (Mason [Trans.], 1970, pp. 53–55,
>   62–63)

This Strange Situation category—"disorganized/disoriented" or "D,"—was first recognized on the basis of our work with the Bay Area sample; it was later expanded via Main and Solomon's (1990) analysis of 100 low-risk and 100 high-risk dyads. First noticed due to the anomalous or odd nature of their appearance, D behaviors were systematized only following the earlier discovery of their association with *unclassifiability* in Strange Situation behavior (see Main & Weston, 1981[24]). Some years later, a review of Bay Area Strange Situation videotapes was conducted, and here we reported that "unclassifiable" (as opposed to "classifiable") infants exhibited a diverse array of inexplicable or overtly conflicted behaviors in the parent's presence. One unclassifiable infant, for example, cried loudly while attempting to get into her mother's lap, and then suddenly fell silent and stopped moving for several seconds. Others were seen rocking on hands and knees following an approach; moving *away* from the parent to the wall when frightened by the stranger; screaming for the parent while separated, and then moving silently away upon reunion; raising hand to mouth in a confused or apprehensive gesture immediately on the parent's entrance; and while in an apparently good mood, swiping at the parent's face.

The most striking theme running through these behaviors was "disorganization," or an observed contradiction or lack of explicability in movement pattern. The term "disorientation" was added to describe behaviors that simply indicated a lack of orientation to the present environment (e.g., trance-like expressions). The title of this third form of insecure Strange Situation response therefore became "disorganized/disoriented."

In recent years, infant disorganized/disoriented Strange Situation behavior (Main & Solomon, 1990), together with its 6th-year equivalent, D-controlling behavior (Main & Cassidy, 1988), have become among the most closely pursued topics within developmental and clinical research. This upsurge in interest follows on a meta-analysis of studies of D children (van IJzendoorn, Schuengel, & Bakermans-Kranenburg, 1999), which pointed to an impressive relation between disorganized attachment and increased vulnerability to psychopathology. For example, in a finding the author termed "unprecedented," Carlson (1998) reported that overall psychopathology at age 17 was predictable from the early D classification. Moreover, in keeping with a proposal advanced by Liotti (1992) that infant D attachment would be associated with a vulnerability to dissociation, Carlson also found that children who had been classified as D with their mothers in infancy later showed significantly more dissociative-like behavior as observed by teachers in both elementary and high school, as well as dissociative indices on the Schedule for Affective Disorders and Schizophrenia for School-Age Children. In addition, Lyons-Ruth (1996; see also Lyons-Ruth & Jacobvitz, 1999) discovered that disruptive-aggressive disorders were linked to infant D attachment status with the mother—a finding that has been well replicated.

But why would these anomalous and unpredictable behaviors—most often consisting of very brief interruptions to otherwise "organized" Strange Situation responses—be predictive of an enhanced vulnerability to such dramatic developmental sequelae? As the reader is aware, our proposal has been that these sequelae may emerge out of circumstances for which an infant is not biologically prepared. More specifically, it is a tenet of evolutionary theory that organisms are constrained by the behavioral systems with which they have been phylogenetically (biologically) endowed. Thus it is reasoned that attachment behavior became "universal" within our species as a result of its immediate necessity to survival in our environment(s) of evolutionary adaptedness (for more detailed discussions, see pp. 252–257 as well as Hesse & Main, 1999, 2000, and Hesse, Main, Abrams, & Rifkin, 2003). Therefore, regardless of the nature of any given infant–mother relationship, the mother (or any other primary attachment figure) is the haven of safety that *must* be approached in times of danger. However, when the infant's biologically channeled haven of safety has simultaneously become a source of fright, the infant is placed in an irresolvable and disorganizing approach–flight paradox. We have proposed that when this occurs, anomalies in behavior, attention, and reasoning may arise, and (following Liotti, 1992) may ultimately increase vulnerability to disorders involving dissociative processes.

Identifying Disorganized Attachment with the Mother at Age 1: Relations to Maternal and Infant Behavior in Home and Laboratory

Disorganized/disoriented Strange Situation behavior differs from Ainsworth's two "insecure-organized" attachment categories, in that it represents a breakage or collapse of behavioral patterning, which can occur in conjunction with any of the remaining classifications (including secure). Since by definition no exhaustive list of anomalous (D) behaviors can be created, we delineated seven thematic headings identifying these kinds of Strange Situation responses, each followed by readily fitting behavioral examples. The thematic headings are as follows:

- Sequential display of contradictory behaviors.
- Simultaneous display of contradictory behaviors.
- Undirected, misdirected, incomplete, and interrupted movements and expressions.
- Stereotypies, asymmetrical, or mistimed movements, and anomalous postures.
- Freezing, stilling, and slowed movements and expressions.
- Direct indices of apprehension regarding the parent.
- Direct indices of disorganization, disorientation, and confusion.

Bouts of disorganization sufficient for assignment to the D category can be brief, sometimes lasting just 10–30 seconds. Since these bouts are understood as evidencing a *temporary* "collapse of behavioral and/or attentional strategy" under stress, a best-fitting alternative secondary placement (e.g., "disorganized/avoidant") is always assigned as well.

Disorganized behavior has been found to be associated with a variety of constitutional (e.g., neurological or physiological) as well as experiential origins (see Hesse, 1999b). However, in the meta-analytic overview by van IJzendoorn and colleagues (1999), infants who were seen independently with both parents were almost always D with one parent only, while no overall relation between difficult temperament or even severe health problems and D attachment was found among neurologically normal infants. And finally, despite Main's (1995, 1999) prediction that one would be found, no "family" genetic contribution appears to date in the production of D (or any other) attachment status (Bokhorst et al., 2003).

Because a genetic basis involving infant D attachment status has yet to be substantiated, researchers are continuing to turn to the investigation of potential contributory experiential factors, including any situation in which an infant is frightened *by* the attachment figure(s). Such situations will, of course, include maltreating relationships—and as first established by Cicchetti (Carlson, Cicchetti, Barnett, & Braunwald, 1989), as well as by Lyons-Ruth (see Lyons-Ruth & Jacobvitz, 1999, for an overview), infant D attachment status is reported in a strong majority (an average of 70%) of maltreated subjects (see also Cicchetti & Barnett, 1991).

However, since disorganization also appears in a notable minority of infants in low-risk samples (averaging 15%, but ranging as high as 30%; see Ainsworth & Eichberg, 1991), Main and Hesse (1990) reasoned that other, perhaps subtler forms of frightening parental behavior could also produce disorganization. Eventually, we concluded that for reasons discussed below, some traumatized but nonmaltreating parents of D infants might sporadically enter into dissociative or quasi-dissociative states (Hesse & Main, 1999). While in these fright-associated states, the parent might exhibit any of the "classic" responses to fear—including freezing (cf. trance), attack (as in quasi-predatory movements), and flight (including subtle indications of propensities to increase distance from the infant, suggesting that the infant is experienced as alarming or dangerous). We and a number of colleagues in other laboratories have in fact observed each of these behaviors in parents in low-risk as well as high-risk samples, and it appears that, like maltreatment, they are associated with infant disorganization. Therefore, we developed a coding system for "frightened/frightening/dissociated" (termed "FR") parental behavior (Main & Hesse, 1991–1998; see note 11), which has now been utilized in several samples. In each, the "FR system" has predicted infant D attachment (e.g., Abrams, Rifkin, & Hesse, in press; Schuengel, van IJzendoorn, & Bakermans-Kranenburg,

1999; True, Pisani, & Oumar, 2001). It may be important to add here that aspects of D behavior (especially perhaps as it develops into D-Controlling behavior [see below]), may, like the other forms of insecure infant attachment, ultimately have sequelae that enhance the likelihood of survival in the face of nonoptimal parenting.

Assessing Disorganization and Its Correlates at 6 Years at the Behavioral and Representational Levels: Indices, and Relations to Early Disorganization with the Mother

Sixth-Year Reunion Responses: D-Controlling

In Main and Cassidy's (1988) Bay Area study of 6-year-olds reunited with their parents following a 1-hour separation, the great majority of former D infants exhibited role-inverting or "D-Controlling" behavior. Some, described as "D-Controlling-punitive," ordered the parent about ("Sit down and shut up, and keep your eyes closed! I said, keep them closed!"); others, described as "D-Controlling-caregiving," were excessively and inappropriately solicitous (e.g., "Are you tired, Mommy? Would you like to sit down and I'll bring you some [pretend] tea?"). A few actively "clowned" in an apparent effort to entertain and regulate their parents' state (a behavior pattern seen in repeated clips of the child protagonist clowning and turning cartwheels in an attempt to cheer his depressed mother in Lasse Hallström's film *My Life as a Dog*). D-Controlling behavior at age 6 was predicted from disorganized infant Strange Situation behavior in our sample—a finding replicated in three further laboratories (van IJzendoorn et al., 1999).

Note that at 6 an unanticipated behavioral transformation had occurred, in that these children were *organized* in structuring the reunion with their mothers.

Sixth-Year Responses to Kaplan's Version of the SAT: D-Fearful

Overall, Kaplan (1987) described the previously disorganized 6-year-olds seen in her version of the SAT as seeming "inexplicably afraid and unable to do anything about it" (p. 109). These children were therefore termed "D-Fearful," a category placement that was found to be strongly linked to early disorganized attachment to the mother (Main et al., 1985). Indices of fear included silence and whispering, inexplicable linguistic disorganization ("yes–no–yes–no–yes–no"), and catastrophic fantasies in which the parents or child died.

The association between D-Fearful responses to the SAT and early disorganized attachment to the mother led Kaplan (1987) to speculate that because many D infants had parents who were still experiencing frightening ideation with respect to their own loss experiences (see below), queries regarding parent–child separations might have had a particularly disorganizing effect on their offspring. In essence, Kaplan was proposing that the children's fearful fantasies, silences, and disorganized language or behavior in response to queries regarding parent–child separations might have resulted from repeated interactions with parents who were still fearful and confused (in AAI terms, below, "unresolved/disorganized") regarding an important loss.

The AAI Categories Most Equivalent to Infant Disorganization: Unresolved/Disorganized and Cannot Classify

From the beginning of our AAI research in general, we had noted that among the parents of disorganized infants, speech surrounding important loss experiences in the AAI had anomalous qualities not found during similar discussions held with the parents of infants falling into Ainsworth's three original Strange Situation categories. By the late 1980s, Main, DeMoss, and Hesse (cited in Main & Goldwyn, 1984) were able to delineate two central ways of speaking about loss (and later, abuse) experiences, which identified what we came to term "unresolved/disorganized" or "U" AAI texts (see Hesse, 1999a, 1999b):

1. Speech usages that seemed to violate a "normal" monitoring of the interview context, as manifested by apparent "absorption" into extreme detail and lengthy and/or inappropriate description. For example, the speaker might discuss the exact position and clothing of each person in a car traveling to a funeral, and then the specific streets taken. Or the speaker might suddenly shift into inappropriate, eulogistic, or "funereal" speech (e.g., "She was young, she was lovely, and she was torn from us by that most dreaded of diseases, tuberculosis").

2. Speech usages indicating beliefs inconsonant with ordinary conceptions of time–space relations and physical causality. For example, a speaker might state that he or she had "killed" a deceased loved one by failing to think of the person at the moment of death, or describe a deceased individual as both dead and alive in the physical sense (see Hesse et al., 2003; Main et al., 2003).

These speech acts (together with a third U indicator, termed "extreme behavioral response" and rare in low-risk samples[25]) were associated *specifically with discussions of potentially traumatic events*. They were not uncommon in the texts of speakers who were otherwise readily classifiable as secure-autonomous, dismissing, or preoccupied.

Language usages such as those described above seemed likely to us to originate in anomalous mental states involving dissociated negative emotions or memories. These states of mind might then be indicative of a temporary collapse of mental, attentional, or linguistic strategy (perhaps associated with a fright-induced lapse in working memory; see Main, 1999). We have therefore speculated that such mental states may account for the occurrence of frightened, frightening, or dissociated (FR) behavior in the parents of disorganized infants.

The kinds of discourse "lapses" described above (see also note 25) now lead to placement in the *unresolved/disorganized* (U) AAI category and are predictive of infant D attachment status. As is the case with infant D attachment, the U classification is always assigned together with a best-fitting secondary category (e.g., U/secure-autonomous, or U/dismissing). In van IJzendoorn's (1995) meta-analysis of the relations between U parental status on the AAI and infant D status in the Strange Situation with the same parent, the overall effect size was moderate (d = .65, equivalent to a correlation of r = .31). However, even this moderate relation is surprising, given that assignment to the U (adult) and D (infant) classifications often depends upon only a very few sentences during the AAI, or a few seconds of Strange Situation behavior, respectively.

U placement on the AAI is now considered to be the direct equivalent of infant D attachment status. However, a more recently developed AAI category, "cannot classify" ("CC"; see Hesse, 1996; Minde & Hesse, 1996) may also be expected to predict infant disorganization (as found by Ammaniti & Speranza, 1994). CC status is assigned to an AAI text when, for example, the discussion of a given parent is first dismissed and then becomes an object of preoccupied anger. Hesse has suggested that whereas U status is indicative of the presence of brief and circumscribed bouts of disorganization in speech or reasoning, CC status implies a global disorganization or collapse of a singular or consistent discourse strategy that runs throughout the interview. Thus we anticipated that some former D infants would not "organize" over time, but in the absence of intervening trauma might instead become unclassifiable or CC with respect to the AAI.

In the Berkeley longitudinal study, we therefore predicted that children disorganized with their mothers during infancy would not infrequently be placed in the U category (and occasionally the CC category) of the AAI at age 19. At this point in time, U and CC categories are combined in data reports by most investigators, and hence we collapsed U status with CC status as representing our predicted AAI "outcome variable."

Unresolved and/or Cannot Classify States of Mind in the AAI as Related to Disorganized Attachment Status at 6 Years of Age and in Infancy

Being classified as D-Controlling on reunion at age 6 approached a trend level (p = .12, two-tailed test) in its association with U and/or CC, while being D-Fearful in the SAT related significantly to U/CC on the AAI. Having been D in the Strange Situation with the mother in infancy was related at a trend level to being judged U/CC at age 19.

However, when we converted our AAI measure to a 3-point scale for U/CC (so that primary U or CC status was assigned a value of 3, alternative placements a 2, and texts insufficient for alternative U or CC placement a 1), the increase in available "range" yielded the following results. First, D-Fearful status on Kaplan's version of the SAT at age 6 was significantly related to U/CC status on the AAI, while D-Controlling behavior was related at a trend level to U/CC placement (p = .06, two-tailed). Finally, being D in the Strange Situation now significantly predicted U/CC status on the AAI (see also Main, 2001).

Because disorganization with the mother is currently considered the strongest index of infant insecurity in terms of attachment, we also ran a simple chi-square testing D versus non-D status with the mother during infancy against adult status on the AAI. Of 15 D infants, 14 were insecure on the AAI, and the relation between simply being disorganized versus "organized" with the mother during infancy and secure-autonomous versus insecure AAI status approached significance (p = .06, chi-square, two-tailed). With these results in mind, we also found that 9 out of 10 (90%) of children judged D-Controlling during the 6th-year reunion were insecure on the AAI, as were all 9 (100%) judged D-Fearful on Kaplan's version of the SAT.

Other Sequelae to Early D Attachment Status

Finally, examination of the 15 AAIs of participants who were D with their mothers at age 1 showed that over half had been judged dismissing, although several were judged U/CC, and one text was now judged secure. This explained the low chi-square results for the sequelae to avoidant attachment status at ages 1 and 6, since while a very strong majority of avoidant children became dismissing, so had many who had initially been disorganized. These latter individuals, then, may have shifted attention inflexibly away from their disorganizing early attachment experiences.

We also compared outcomes for the seven infants judged disorganized/secure with the mother during infancy to outcomes for the eight judged disorganized/insecure. All seven disorganized/secure babies were insecure at 19, and the only disorganized baby judged secure at 19 had in fact been disorganized/insecure at age 1. This result is worth contemplating, given that one might assume a greater resiliency underlying a secondary placement of security in infancy. However, perhaps once fear intervenes to disrupt any organized system, whether the disrupted system was optimal or not becomes of little import. More specifically, if attachment and fear become intertwined, fear may override all else. In closing this brief section, we should additionally note that without D coding (often based on just a few seconds), we would in many cases have incorrectly predicted security on the AAI.

As this book goes to press, we have learned that using the high-risk Minnesota poverty sample (*n* = 125), Weinfield and her colleagues (2004) have also found that disorganized versus "organized" (both secure and insecure) status with mother in infancy predicts security versus insecurity on the AAI at age 19 (*p* = .03), a result that has replicated at stronger levels in this same sample at age 26, *p* = .001 (Sroufe et al., 2005). Surprisingly, our proportions are similar, with 86% of disorganized children in the Minnesota poverty sample being insecure 18 years later on the AAI, compared to 93% of former D babies in the Bay Area. Again as in our sample, most former D infants in Minnesota also became dismissing on the AAI, with the remaining participants most likely to be classified as U (or, in our sample, U or CC). Finally, in Minnesota as in Berkeley, disorganized/secure infants were no more likely than those who had been judged disorganized/insecure to be secure-autonomous at age 19.

Disorganized/Disoriented Attachment Status: Summary

1. Disorganized (D) attachment has been found to be related to frightening parental behavior, which—because the parent is the infant's biologically based haven of safety—leads to disorganizing experiences of "fright without solution" (Hesse et al., 2003; Main & Hesse, 1990).

2. Across multiple studies, infant D attachment status has been found to be predictive of psychopathology from middle childhood to young adulthood, including especially dissociative and externalizing disorders (see meta-analysis by van IJzendoorn et al., 1999).

3. D attachment status with the mother strongly predicted D-Controlling behavior on reunion following an hour-long separation at age 6, as well as being classified D-Fearful on the SAT.

4. Almost all D-Controlling and D-Fearful 6-year-olds were insecure on the AAI at age 19.

5. When U/CC status was converted to a 3-point scale, infant D status and both of its 6th-year equivalents (D-Fearful and D-Controlling) predicted their "adult" parallel (U/CC status on the AAI).

6. D versus non-D status in infancy *in itself* predicted being insecure versus secure-autonomous on the AAI.

7. D infants who were alternatively secure were no more likely than D infants who were alternatively insecure to become secure-autonomous on the AAI. Both this and the preceding result (6) also held for the Minnesota poverty sample (Weinfield et al., 2004).

8. As in Weinfield and colleagues' (2004) study, we found a significant tendency for D infants to become U or CC on the AAI at age 19. This result was replicated again in the Minnesota poverty sample at age 26 (Sroufe et al., 2005).

9. Again as in Weinfield and colleagues' (2004), study we found that more than half of our D infants were insecure-dismissing in their AAI transcripts.

10. Rather than indicating either flexibility or inflexibility in attention, infant D behavior and its adult U and CC equivalents represent local (U) or global (CC) collapses of behavioral, attentional, or linguistic strategy.

CONCLUDING REMARKS

Considered in sequence, we have presented, in addition to Ainsworth's Strange Situation procedure and her three "organized" categories of infant response, four of the methodologies for the assessment of attachment devised in our laboratory. These have included (1) the development of a fourth, "disorganized" infant Strange Situation category; systems for examining (2) real-life and (3) representational processes related to separation at age 6; and finally (4) a life history interview for adults focusing upon attachment. We have summarized the data for each of the three "developmental pathways" that the distribution of infant categories in our sample permitted us to examine—that is, those taken by secure, avoidant, and disorganized infants.

Since this chapter has been constructed so that each attachment category is traced and summarized within its own section, rather than providing a review, we now turn to a few salient topics that have not yet been either directly or fully addressed to this point in the text.

Interpreting Our Long-Term Outcomes:
Stability, Functional Equivalence, and Predictability

We selected a low-risk, relatively stable sample for our longitudinal study in order to maximize opportunities for tracing lawful sequelae to differing infant "categories of attachment," should these exist—that is, as part of a search for *lawful outcomes in stable circumstances.* More specifically, it was our hope to capture and articulate the natural development of individual differences in mind, language, and behavior as a function of childhood attachment relationships.

Prediction, however, may be considered in three ways: "stability" (an outcome almost identical to its precedent, and within the same modality); "functional equivalence" (an outcome mirroring or strongly reflecting its precedent, but within a different modality); and "pure" predictability per se (an outcome that does not reflect or resemble its precedents, whether or not within the same modality). In other words, simple stability is observing the same thing twice inside a given modality; functional equivalence, more interesting than simple stability, shows the mirroring of a thing across modalities; and "pure" predictability is perhaps the most interesting of all, because there is a presumably replicable transformation in both the form and the modality of the phenomenon. With all this in mind, then, consider that between ages 1 and 6, only two of the six infant response patterns (secure and avoidant reunion behavior) "mirrored" the participant's earlier behavior (i.e., represented simple stability). However, regarding lawful transformations in the absence of simple stability—that is, functional equivalence and pure predictability—consider the following:

1. The reunion behavior of disorganized infants had become organized (D-controlling) by age 6. This exemplifies pure predictability, being a transformation in both modality and form that has been replicated in further samples (van IJzendoorn et al., 1999).

2. Consider next Kaplan's (1987, 2003) finding that insecure-avoidant infants who were "affectless" and explored the laboratory room during the separation episodes 5 years later described a pictured child as feeling distress on separation from the parent, but were unable to think what the child could do while separated. Here our observations moved from the nonverbal to the verbal modality. If these children had, as anticipated, lawfully tended to reply that the pictured child would "feel" nothing, but would constructively play or explore, we would have seen an instance of prediction via functional equivalence. However, our previously avoidant infants unexpectedly said that the child would feel distress, but could not think of anything that the separated child could do. This was a *reversal* of Strange Situation behavior, and hence represents "pure" prediction in the absence of functional equivalence.

In general, whether working with Kaplan's version of the SAT or with the AAI, what we uncovered as we moved from nonverbal to linguistic processes only sometimes represented functional equivalence. At 19, for example, we did see functional equivalence across time with respect to early disorganization, since brief early episodes of disorganization in nonverbal behavior predicted disorganization in discourse or reasoning within the AAI. However, we also found that internal consistency and collaboration within the text was predicted by secure nonverbal responses to reunion with the mother in infancy—an instance of "pure" predictability, replicating Waters and colleagues (2000) as well as Hamilton (2000).

Despite the impressive predictability in our sample, our study cannot address the question of whether there is a "sensitive period" influencing long-term outcomes, or, in contrast, whether these outcomes are guided by interactions ongoing into adolescence. Questions of this kind can only be investigated in studies that include a substantial proportion of individuals whose life circumstances have been relatively unstable, as in the Minnesota poverty sample. In fact, early versus later influences on functioning in the Minnesota sample showed that when early attachment to the mother was compared to social functioning in middle childhood, early attachment provided the better predictor of long-term social functioning (Sroufe, Egeland, & Kreutzer, 1990).

Let us now consider, however, the *absence* of long-term predictability specific to attachment in the Minnesota sample when secure versus insecure Strange Situation behavior (as opposed to D vs. non-D behavior, discussed above) was initially used to predict security on the AAI at age 19 (Weinfield et al., 2004). Here, we note that whereas in our study attachment to the mother was stable from 1 to 6 years of age, the Minnesota group found only low, albeit significant, stability in infant attachment to the mother even across a far shorter period (12–18 months; Egeland & Farber, 1984; Vaughn et al., 1979). If, as we assume, (1) when exploring the issue of sensitive periods we are implicitly considering the effects of early experience upon later brain organization with respect to attachment, then (2) *we should not expect predictability in any individual whose early attachment-related experiences were markedly unstable.* Thus, where no "single" strategy representing any particular attachment-related brain organization is stably evident across the first 18 months, marked predictability to adolescence would hardly be expectable. However, the most recent report from the Minnesota group does show significant stability between security versus insecurity in the Strange Situation at age 18 months and secure-autonomous versus insecure AAI status at age 26 (Sroufe et al., 2005).

Why Are There Marked Resemblances between Strange Situation Behavior and Linguistic Responses to the AAI?: Accounts via Procedural Memory, Attention, and Emotion

When participants with intervening trauma were excluded in the Bay Area study, infants' systematically differing responses to separation from and reunion with their mothers in the unfamiliar laboratory setting often predicted the discourse characteristics of their later discussion of life history. Earlier, we offered the simple interpretation that these similarities emerged out of parent–child interactions that had systematically differed in kind.

We now consider some of the differences in "procedural" memories, attentional processes, and affects that may have helped to account for these

outcomes. More specifically, we explore the possibility that repeated interactions may act to predict discourse during the AAI via the patterning of
early actions, affects (see Amini et al., 1996), and attentional processes.

One reason why insecure individuals in particular might "return" to
early procedures, routines, attentional processes, or affective states when
undertaking the AAI is that its central questions and probes force attention
toward early experience and require a rapid succession of speech acts, giving speakers little time to prepare a response. This will enhance the necessity for making rapid action (speech) choices, and will encourage the kind
of inflexible, relatively routinized responses seen in previously avoidant
infants (and also in ambivalent infants, not studied here). For example, in
our study, previously avoidant infants almost from the start of the interview used restriction of attention (and sometimes also response refusal) to
"avoid" the topic of early relationships and experiences. In addition, as
mentioned above, a significant proportion of infants who had experienced
a procedural collapse (disorganization) in the stressful Strange Situation
manifested a similar procedural collapse in response to the trauma-related
questions in the AAI. In contrast, for previously secure infants, discourse
appeared less routinized—a finding consonant with the possibility that
most of these participants were able to explore the interview topics in
a flexible and relatively relaxed manner, not unlike that observed by
Ainsworth regarding a secure infant's "secure-base" explorations in the
home (see Waters et al., 1995). "Earned secure" or "discontinuous secure"
texts suggest that, following Amini and colleages (1996), these speakers
somehow have in contrast learned new procedures related to attachment
(new action patterns that have become implicit and now guide thinking).

Finally, an "emotional" analysis of the consistencies observed can be
considered. With respect to individuals continuous for security, we can
infer an underlying confidence and calm. For example, briefly returning to
infancy, note that Spangler and Grossmann (1993), who assessed cortisol
output following the Strange Situation (cortisol is indicative of preparation
for long-term stress), found that even though secure infants often cried during the procedure, their pre- to post-Strange-Situation cortisol rise was
exceptionally low. Spangler and Grossmann interpreted this finding as
indicative of a (calm) confidence that a well-working "strategy" (i.e., crying
and calling) was available for regaining the mother's presence. Indices that
security is also associated with relatively calm emotional states in young
adulthood can be taken from the psychophysiological studies conducted by
Dozier and Kobak (1992) and from personality Q-sorts obtained from the
friends and acquaintances of secure-autonomous college students by Kobak
and Sceery (1988). With respect to the association between early avoidance
of the mother and the dismissing AAI classification, we have simply to look
to the suppression of (overt) expression of negative experience or emotion

in attachment-related contexts (but see Kobak & Sceery, 1988, for descriptions of hostility observed in dismissing adolescent speakers in other contexts). And, as regards disorganization and its prediction of U/CC status, early behavioral and later linguistic collapses may both involve experiences of temporarily overwhelming fright.

Emotion, attention, and procedural memories are, of course, not mutually exclusive (see Amini et al.'s [1996] emphasis upon affect as well as memory). All three must be mutually influential, all effect narrative, and all three have no doubt contributed to the continuities observed.

Is Stability Enhanced through Attempts by Parents in Insecure-Organized States of Mind to Maintain a State of "Felt Security" with Respect to Their Own Primary Attachment Figures?

In papers first circulated at the University of Virginia in 1985 (see also Main, 1995), we suggested that many parents whose AAI texts are placed in insecure-organized categories may (1) implicitly act to encourage their infants to assist them in maintaining their present (insecure) states of mind, either by (2) specifically discouraging attachment behavior, a form of behavior that may raise anxiety for insecure-dismissing parents, or else by (3) discouraging autonomous/exploratory behavior, which may raise anxiety for insecure-preoccupied parents.

In other words, *both infant "attachment" behaviors and infant "independent" exploratory behaviors may threaten to lead dismissing or preoccupied parents away from the state of mind that had seemed optimal for maintenance of the relationship to their own parents during childhood, and hence may still create feelings of anxiety.* As one example, being faced with infants' crying and proximity seeking could create feelings of anxiety in parents who had "learned" that inhibiting attachment behavior (minimizing relatedness under stress) was the best strategy for maintaining relationships with their own parents. Thus, insofar as it serves to minimize attachment displays, the rejection of infant attachment behavior may help parents who produce dismissing AAI texts to maintain their historically desired, and currently "working," state of mind. The same argument could hold for parents who produce preoccupied texts, for whom independent exploration as well as autonomous gestures they had displayed as young children may have led to anxiety for their own parents, and produce anxiety if exhibited by their own infants.

Thus, a sense of *"false* but *felt* security" may be preserved via maintenance of any mental state that originally allowed some continued proximity to the parents' parents, and be threatened[26] by any infant behaviors so inconsonant with that mental state as to potentially alter it. At another level, of course, insofar as the infant begins to respond by behaving like the parents' parents, both "rejecting" and unpredictable, "autonomy-discouraging" parents may find the repetition of their own parents' behavior by their offspring distressing.

Finally, we may speculate that various kinds of "insensitive" behavior, at least for some insecure parents, act to preserve the original tie to their own parents, and that—because their state of mind has yet to become autonomous—this may in fact remain their primary tie.

"Looking Backward" from Late Adolescence to Infancy and Early Childhood: What Can We Learn from a Longitudinal Study?

The value of prospective studies in attachment—first suggested by John Bowlby—is now well recognized, and in the present chapter we have for the most part presented our data via this prospective path. Here, we look briefly at our data from a retrospective vantage point.

Expected Findings and Their Implications

A majority of secure-autonomous AAI texts in our study came from individuals with apparently secure backgrounds, while the majority of insecure texts were produced by individuals whose childhoods appeared to have been insecure. These were both expected findings. If sufficient replications of our study are forthcoming, researchers who need to employ the AAI in the absence of earlier attachment measures may have some confidence that for a majority of AAI participants without intervening trauma, they are assessing a stable phenomenon. The likelihood of replication will of course be increased where sample selection is similar to ours, and where coders are trained to comparable levels of expertise.

Another expected finding was that CC status on the AAI had some association with infant disorganization, as well as the mothers' unexplained fears for the death of the (child) participant. These findings appear to support the notion that such texts do come—as Hesse (1996) has proposed—from frightening interactions with a primary attachment figure.[27]

Unexpected Findings and Their Implications

Most researchers are inclined to expect that when trauma changes security status, it will "move" a secure individual into insecurity. A first unexpected finding, then, is the case mentioned earlier, in which a traumatic event in fact appeared to lead an adolescent who had been insecure in infancy and at 6 to secure-autonomous AAI status.

Another informative and unanticipated finding comes from an additional single case—a child who appeared to us to be exceptionally robust, self-confident, and high-spirited in free-play observations made in infancy and at age 6, and had been coded as secure with both parents at both time periods. However, at 19, following an intervening trauma, this participant's text was coded as unresolved/preoccupied—meaning that the adolescent not only "lapsed" while discussing a frightening event, *but also* discussed the parents with whom there had been security for the first 6 years in a manner indicative of strong insecurity. This outcome was especially surprising, because the form of speech usage leading to this particular preoccupied category placement ("passive/vague discourse") is very rare. We had presumed that speech of this kind would stem from a background of extreme early insecurity, probably including neglect.

These are, of course, only single cases. In addition, we found that quite a few 19-year-olds producing dismissing texts came from disorganized (hence probably frightening) backgrounds, as opposed to rejecting backgrounds (as imagined). This has been discussed in detail earlier in the text. Nevertheless, it is important to remember that it was an entirely unexpected yet systematic outcome, and is virtually identical to Weinfield and colleagues' Minnesota outcomes.

The assumption that individuals sharing the same present attachment classification are "now" the same (or at least highly similar), whatever their differences in history, is widespread. Of course, an individual's AAI text, insofar as it leads to a particular classification, does imply certain important similarities with others in that same classification. We would argue, however, that this "retrospective" examination of our data has not only emphasized that individuals with the same AAI classification can differ sharply in earlier experience, but also that those alike in AAI classification but differing in early experience may soon be found to differ as well in neurophysiological and brain organization (see also Main, 1999). Moreover, note that our discontinuous unresolved/preoccupied text came from a speaker who may later reveal unexpected resiliency, while some dismissing texts may come from individuals with continuing but as yet unrevealed vulnerabilities to trauma.

Among the many current investigations utilizing the AAI, some now involve psychophysiology and neuroimaging. In these and other similarly complex and intensive investigations, it will be particularly important to bear in mind that those assigned to the same adult attachment classification may well differ in lawful ways, depending on whether this classification is or is not consonant with early attachment organization and early attachment-related states of mind.

ACKNOWLEDGMENTS

This chapter is dedicated to the memory of Fariboz Amini, MD (1930–2004), whose 1996 article influenced our thinking regarding the mediators of the long-term effects of early attachment relationships. For support of the studies described here, we are grateful to several foundations and fellowships. First, following the kind intervention of Klaus and Karin Grossmann, Lotte Kohler and the Kohler-Stiftung Foundation of Munich provided the initial funds for the 19th-year follow-up study, as did the American Psychoanalytic Foundation. A Guggenheim Fellowship to Mary Main assisted with the development of our methods, and the study was further supported by the William B. Harris Foundation of Chicago, the William T. Grant Foundation, and the Amini Foundation for the Study of Affects. We are grateful to Jude Cassidy, Carol George, Ruth Goldwyn, Judith Solomon, Ellen Richardson, and Donna Weston for their assistance with early phases of this project. Jennifer Ablow and Daniel Silver conducted the Adult Attachment Interviews for the most recent follow-up study; Isabel Bradburn analyzed them; Kazuko Behrens assisted with data analysis; and Wanda Bronson, Pehr Granqvist, Siegfried Hesse, Sarah Hrdy, Deborah Jacobvitz, Joan Stevenson-Hinde, and Marinus Van IJzendoorn provided conceptual, technical, and terminological improvements to this manuscript. We thank the then-11-year-old David van IJzendoorn for the extraordinary technological expertise and assistance he and his parents provided in Leiden prior to our trip to Regensburg, and Marinus van IJzendoorn for acting as our discussant.

NOTES

1. Only two "insecure-ambivalent/resistant" infants were available; hence their trajectories could not be traced.
2. Recently, attention has been drawn to the positive role played by the attachment figure's "mind-mindedness" in the development of infant security. However, it should be noted that from its inception Ainsworth's sensitivity scale had included the mother's capacity to reflect upon and acknowledge the infant's mind (see Main, 1999).
3. For readers who are less familiar with idiomatic U.S. English, the term "being a pill" is a light term of nonendorsement of the behavior patterns currently shown by another person, often a child.
4. Again for readers who may need clarification, this is a contraction for the very young of the more adult usage, "an expression."
5. Mary Ainsworth would not think of or countenance asking mothers to visit her laboratory without a full and friendly visit and description of the procedures in the comfort of their homes.
6. Not all outcomes of conflict appear anomalous; for example, grooming behavior can be a normal-appearing form of "displacement."
7. As used here, "heritable" refers to variations in genetic makeup originating in the parents of some, but not other, individuals within a given species. Attachment is not considered "heritable" in this sense, because all individuals and their ancestors in the same species are born equipped with this same "behavioral program."
8. Even less than an hour of social interaction with a consistent caregiver per day may facilitate the formation of an attachment. Moreover, attachments are as readily formed to abu-

sive caregivers as to others. Thus the nature of the interaction is not as critical as that it originates consistently from a particular person.

9. Note, however, that studies of infants raised without any consistent caregivers indicate that the ability to form attachments may decrease by the end of the third year of life.

10. Humans evidently have these associated inhibitory capacities, whereas, for example, in rhesus monkeys, "organized" avoidance (as opposed to simple flight) appears yet to be observed.

11. Training in assessing disorganized attachment from videotapes is available each summer at the Institute of Child Development at the University of Minnesota (contact Elizabeth Carlson at 612-626-8668). Training in the Adult Attachment Interview is available in six or more institutes per year worldwide (contact Mary Main or Erik Hesse at the Department of Psychology, University of California, Berkeley, CA, 94720, or else fax 510-642-5293 for a list of certified trainers and their contact numbers). Use this fax number also for inquiries regarding training in the 6th-year system held at Berkeley, Main and Hesse's "FB" coding system and Kaplan's training in her version of the SAT. Inquiries regarding the latter trainings can be addressed to us at the Department of Psychology, or else, again, faxed to us at 510-642-5293.

12. For example, our method for estimating a child's attachment status in infancy from family drawings with the mother (developed by Kaplan & Main, 1986) has been replicated in the Minnesota poverty sample (Fury, Carlson, & Sroufe, 1997), in Regensburg (Grossmann & Grossmann, 1991), and at the University of Maryland (J. Cassidy, personal communication, 1987).

13. The size of this group ($n = 40$), selected at random beyond the relatively even groups representing infant attachment to the mother, obviously contrasts sharply with the numbers of families actually available to us. This was due to Mary Ainsworth's recommendation to Mary Main to select for any intensive and pioneering study a group of persons no larger than could be comprehended, remembered, and thought through, both at the time of data collection and over succeeding years. With respect to her own selection of 26 infant–mother dyads for intensive study (in both Uganda and Baltimore), she had said that this was just about the size of most hunter–gatherer troops, and hence probably represented the number of other people that a person could naturally come to understand.

14. Fewer secure children than would have been representative of the sample were returned to the laboratory, because of our special interest in the sequelae to early insecurity, especially early disorganization.

15. Continuous score configurations are usually sufficient for singular category placement, but when scores indicate directly contradictory category placements, Hesse's (1996) "cannot classify" category is considered.

16. However, as is the case with the algorithm for category assignment from our continuous scales developed by Waters (Waters, Treboux, Fyffe, & Crowell, 2001), this "bottom-up" approach is insufficient to move beyond the five major categories of the AAI to the 12 subcategories, which are also of special interest. Here the top-down approach remains necessary.

17. The Grossmanns' AAI report, however, rested not on the method of AAI analysis developed in our laboratory, but rather upon Roger Kobak's Q-sort analysis (Kobak, 1993), a system derived from but by no means identical to ours. However, as we understand it (K. E. Grossmann, personal communication, 2002), the Main and Goldwyn (1984–1998) method fared no better in predicting AAI responses from infancy.

18. Our sample was young and, as noted above, contained no "earned secure" transcripts. Therefore, coherence was of course strongly associated with scores for maternal loving. In samples containing a high proportion of "earned secure" texts, the relation between maternal loving and early security would ideally be recomputed, controlling for relations between security and coherence.

19. *Columbia Encyclopedia* (1993, p. 1260).
20. Some avoidant infants do, however, attend to and appear to enjoy the presence of the stranger.
21. For AAI matches to 1st-year and 6th-year avoidance here, we were using a three-way analysis. When we used a five-way analysis, two adolescents received "cannot classify" designations, with dismissing as the first alternative.
22. These are the only two continuous AAI scores that could be linked to early avoidance of the mother in this sample, since "fear of loss of the child" (associated with dismissing placement in parents) could not be used with adolescent college students, and "deroga- tion" (also associated with the dismissing category) is rare in low-risk samples.
23. Maintenance of self-organization as an adaptive or biological function of avoidance had been suggested for the nonhuman context both by Michael Chance (1962) and—albeit less directly—by Niko Tinbergen (Tinbergen & Moynihan, 1952).
24. During her year in Bielefeld, Main (1977) was already assigning some of the Grossmanns' middle-class infants to a new code ("N.T.C." or "not to classify").
25. Lapses in the monitoring of (1) discourse or (2) reasoning are by far the most frequent indices of unresolved/disorganized states of mind as seen in the AAI. A third, very rare response (which also leads to unresolved/disorganized category placement) is seen in reports of "extreme behavioral reactions," including especially suicidal attempts and/or psychiatric hospitalization following a loss.
26. It would go beyond the bounds of this chapter to present this theory at its fullest. How- ever, it is most likely (as Ainsworth suggested in a letter to Main) that dismissing parents not only attempt to obtain their infants' cooperation in maintaining their own "safest" state of mind via rejection, thus creating avoidance, but also are simultaneously dismayed by it, since avoidance mimics the rejection they may have earlier experienced.
27. However, others came from secure backgrounds (and were coded unresolved/secure), and two coded as CC had been avoidant as infants but had mothers who had feared their deaths without being able to trace this fear to any source. Insofar as we are aware, the infant–mother interaction pattern for this rare dismissing subcategory (Ds4, "fear of loss from an unknown source") has yet to be ascertained, but may well be frightening.

REFERENCES

Abrams, K. Y., Rifkin, A., & Hesse, E. (in press). Examining the role of parental fright- ened/frightening (FR) subtypes in predicting disorganized attachment within a brief laboratory session. *Development and Psychopathology.*

Ainsworth, M. D. S. (1967). *Infancy in Uganda: Infant care and the growth of love.* Baltimore: Johns Hopkins University Press.

Ainsworth, M. D. S., Bell, S. M., & Stayton, D. J. (1971). Individual differences in strange situation of one-year-olds. In H. R. Shaffer (Ed.), *The origins of human social relations* (pp. 17–57). London: Academic Press.

Ainsworth, M. D. S., Blehar, M., Waters, E., & Wall, S. (1978). *Patterns of attach- ment.* Hillsdale, NJ: Erlbaum.

Ainsworth, M. D. S., & Eichberg, C. G. (1991). Effects on infant–mother attachment of mother's unresolved loss of an attachment figure or other traumatic experi- ence. In C. M. Parkes, J. Stevenson-Hinde, & P. Marris (Eds.), *Attachment across the life cycle* (pp. 160–183). London: Routledge.

Allen, J. P., & Hauser, S. T. (1996). Autonomy and relatedness in adolescent–family interactions as predictors of young adults' states of mind regarding attachment. *Development and Psychopathology, 8,* 793–809.

Amini, F., Lewis, T., Lannon, R., & Louie, A. (1996). Affect, attachment, memory: Contributions towards psychobiologic integration. *Psychiatry: Interpersonal and Biological Processes, 59*, 213–239.

Ammaniti, M., & Speranza, A. M. (1994). *Maternal attachment patterns and disorganized patterns of attachment in children.* Poster presented at the International Conference on Infant Studies, Paris.

Bakermans-Kranenburg, M. J., & van IJzendoorn, M. H. (1993). A psychometric study of the Adult Attachment Interview: Reliability and discriminant validity. *Developmental Psychology, 29*, 870–879.

Bakermans-Kranenburg, M. J., & van IJzendoorn, M. H. (2004). No association of the dopamine D4 receptor (DRD4) and –521C/T promoter polymorphisms with infant attachment disorganization. *Attachment and Human Deveopment, 6*, 211–218.

Beckwith, L., Cohen, S. E., & Hamilton, C. (1999). Maternal sensitivity during infancy and subsequent life-events relate to attachment representations in early adulthood. *Developmental Psychology, 35*(3), 693–700.

Belsky, J. (1999). Modern evolutionary theory and patterns of attachment. In J. Cassidy & P. R. Shaver (Eds.), *Handbook of attachment: Theory, research, and clinical applications* (pp. 141–161). New York: Guilford Press.

Benoit, D., & Parker, K. (1994). Stability and transmission of attachment across three generations. *Child Development, 63*, 1444–1456.

Bokhorst, C. L., Bakermans-Kranenburg, M. J. Fearon, P. M. van IJzendoorn, M. H., Fonagy, P., & Schuengel, C. (2003). The importance of shared environment in mother–infant attachment security: A behavioral genetic study. *Child Development, 74*, 1769–1782.

Bowlby, J. (1969/1982). *Attachment and loss: Vol. 1. Attachment.* New York: Basic Books.

Bowlby, J. (1988). A secure base: Parent–child attachment and healthy human development. New York: Basic Books.

Bretherton, I. (1985). Attachment theory: Retrospect and prospect. In I. Bretherton & E. Waters (Eds.), Growing points of attachment theory and research. *Monographs of the Society for Research in Child Development, 50*(1–2, Serial No. 209), 3–38.

Bretherton, I. (1992). The origins of attachment theory: John Bowlby and Mary Ainsworth. *Developmental Psychology, 28*, 759–775.

Carlson, E. A. (1998). A prospective longitudinal study of disorganized/disoriented attachment. *Child Development, 69*, 1107–1128.

Carlson, V., Cicchetti, D., Barnett, D., & Braunwald, K. (1989). Disorganized/disoriented attachment relationships in maltreated infants. *Developmental Psychology, 25*, 525–531.

Cassidy, J., & Berlin, L. (1994). The insecure-ambivalent pattern of attachment: Theory and research. *Child Development, 65*, 971–981.

Cassidy, J. & Main, M. (1984). Secure attachment in infancy as a precursor of the ability to tolerate a brief laboratory separation at five years. In J. D. Call, E. Galenson, & R. L. Tyson (Eds.), *Frontiers of infant psychiatry* (Vol. 2, pp. 132–136). New York: Basic Books.

Chance, M. R. A. (1962). An intrerpretation of some agonistic postures: The role of "cut-off" acts and postures. *Symposium of the Zoological Society of London, 8,* 71–89.

Cicchetti, D., & Barnett, D. (1991). Attachment organization in maltreated pre-schoolers. *Development and Psychopathology, 3,* 397–411.

Columbia Encyclopedia (5th ed., B. A. Chernow & G.A. Valasi, Eds.). (1993). New York: Columbia University Press.

Crook, J. H., & Gartlan, J. S. (1966). Evolution of primate societies. *Nature, 210,* 1200–1203.

Crowell, J. A., & Feldman, S. S. (1988). Mothers' internal models of relationships and children's behavioral and developmental status: A study of mother–child interaction. *Child Development, 59,* 1273–1285.

Crowell, J., Waters, E., Treboux, D., O'Connor, E., Colon-Downs, C., Feider, O., Golby, B., & Posada, G. (1996). Discriminant validity of the Adult Attachment Interview. *Child Development, 67,* 2584–2599.

Daly, M. (1996). Evolutionary adaptationism: Another biological approach to criminal and antisocial behaviour. In G. R. Bock & J. A. Goode (Eds.), *Genetics of criminal and antisocial behaviour* (Ciba Foundation Symposium, London, 14–16 February, 1995). Chichester, UK: Wiley.

Dawkins, R. (1976/1989). *The selfish gene.* Oxford: Oxford University Press.

De Wolff, M., & van IJzendoorn, M. (1997). Sensitivity and attachment: A meta-analysis on parental antecedents of infant attachment. *Child Development, 68*(4), 571–591.

Dozier, M., & Kobak, R. R. (1992). Psychophysiology in Adult Attachment Interviews: Converging evidence for de-activating strategies. *Child Development, 63,* 1473–1480.

Egeland, B., & Farber, E. (1984). Infant–mother attachment: Factors related to its development and changes over time. *Child Development, 55,* 753–751.

Fonagy, P., Steele, H., & Steele, M. (1991). Maternal representations of attachment during pregnancy predict the organization of infant–mother attachment at one year of age. *Child Development, 62,* 891–905.

Fraley, R. C. (2002). Attachment stability from infancy to adulthood: Meta-analysis and dynamic modeling of developmental mechanisms. *Personality and Social Psychology Review, 6,* 123–151.

Fury, G., Carlson, E., & Sroufe, L. A. (1997). Children's representations of attachment relationships in family drawings. *Child Development, 68,* 1154–1164.

George, C., Kaplan, N., & Main, M. (1984, 1985, 1996). *Adult Attachment Interview.* Unpublished protocols, University of California, Berkeley.

Grice, H.P. (1975). Logic and conversation. In P. Cole & J. L. Moran (Eds.), *Syntax and semantics III: Speech acts* (pp. 41–58). New York: Academic Press.

Grice, H. P. (1989). Studies in the way of words. Cambridge, MA: Harvard University Press.

Grossmann, K., Fremmer-Bombik, E., Rudolph, J., & Grossmann, K. E. (1988). Maternal attachment representations as related to patterns of infant–mother attachment and maternal care during the first year. In R. A. Hinde & J. Stevenson-Hinde (Eds.), *Relationships within families: Mutual influences* (pp. 241–260). Oxford: Clarendon Press.

Grossmann, K. E. (1990). The wider concept of attachment in cross-cultural research. *Human Development, 33*, 31–47.

Grossmann, K. E. (1995). The evolution and history of attachment research and theory. In S. Goldberg, R. Muir, & J. Kerr (Eds.), *Attachment theory: Social, developmental, and clinical perspectives,* (pp. 85–122). Hillsdale, NJ: Analytic Press.

Grossmann, K. E., & Grossmann, K. (1990). The wider concept of attachment in cross-cultural research. *Human Development, 33*, 31–47.

Grossmann, K. E., & Grossmann, K. (1991). Attachment quality as an organizer of emotional and behavioral responses in a longitudinal perspective. In C. M. Parkes, J. Stevenson-Hinde, & P. Marris (Eds.), *Attachment across the life cycle* (pp. 93–114). London: Routledge.

Grossmann, K. E., Grossmann, K., & Zimmermann, P. (1999). A wider view of attachment and exploration: Stability and change during the years of immaturity. In J. Cassidy & P. R. Shaver (Eds.), *Handbook of attachment: Theory, research, and clinical applications* (pp. 760–786). New York: Guilford Press.

Hamilton, C. E. (2000). Continuity and discontinuity of attachment from infancy through adolescence. *Child Development, 71*, 690–694.

Hansburg, H. G. (1972). *Adolescent separation anxiety: A method for the study of adolescent separation problems.* Springfield, IL: Thomas.

Heinicke, C., & Westheimer, I. (1966). *Brief separations.* New York: International Universities Press.

Hesse, E. (1996). Discourse, memory and the Adult Attachment Interview: A note with emphasis on the emerging cannot classify category. *Infant Mental Health, 17*, 4–11.

Hesse, E. (1999a). The Adult Attachment Interview: Historical and current perspectives. In J. Cassidy & P. R. Shaver (Eds.), *Handbook of attachment: Theory, research, and clinical applications* (pp. 395–433). New York: Guilford Press.

Hesse, E. (1999b). *Unclassifiable and disorganized responses in the Adult Attachment Interview and in the infant strange situation procedure: Theoretical proposals and Empirical findings.* Unpublished doctoral dissertation, Leiden University, Leiden, The Netherlands.

Hesse, E., & Main, M. (1999). Second-generation effects of unresolved trauma in non-maltreating parents: Dissociative, frightened, and threatening parental behavior. *Psychoanalytic Inquiry, 19*(4), 481–540.

Hesse, E., & Main, M. (2000). Disorganization in infant and adult attachment: Description, correlates, and implications for developmental psychopathology. *Journal of the American Psychoanalytic Association, 48*(4), 1097–1127.

Hesse, E., Main, M., Abrams, K., & Rifkin, A. (2003). Unresolved states regarding loss or abuse can have "second-generation" effects. In M. F. Solomon & D. J. Siegel (Eds.), *Healing trauma: Attachment, mind, body, and brain* (pp. 57–106). New York: Norton.

Hinde, R. A. (1966). *Animal behaviour: A synthesis of ethology and comparative psychology.* New York: McGraw-Hill.

Hinde, R. A. (1974). *Biological bases of human social behavior.* New York: McGraw-Hill.

Hinde, R. A. (1983). The study of interpersonal relationships: Dialogue with Robert Hinde. In J. Miller (Ed.), *States of mind.* New York: Random House.

Hinde, R. A., & Stevenson-Hinde, J. (1990). Attachment: Biological, cultural and individual desiderata. *Human Development, 33*, 62–72.

Homer. (1963). *The odyssey* (R. Fitzgerald Trans.). Garden City, NY: Anchor Books.

Hrdy, S. (1999). *Mother nature: A history of mothers, infants and natural selection.* New York: Pantheon.

Kaplan, N. (1987). *Individual differences in six-year-olds' thoughts about separation: Predicted to actual experiences of separation.* Unpublished doctoral dissertation, University of California, Berkeley.

Kaplan, N. (2003, April). *The development of attachment in the Bay Area study: One year, six years, nineteen years of age.* Paper presented at the biennial meeting of the Society for Research in Child Development, Tampa, FL.

Kaplan, N., & Main, M. (1986). *Assessment of attachment organization through children's family drawings.* Unpublished manuscript, University of California, Berkeley.

Klagsbrun, M., & Bowlby, J. (1976). Responses to separation from parents: A clinical test for children. *British Journal of Projective Psychology, 21,* 7–21.

Kobak, R. R. (1993). *The attachment Q-sort.* Unpublished manuscript, University of Delaware.

Kobak, R. R., & Sceery, A. (1988). Attachment in late adolescence: Working models, affect regulation, and representation of self and others. *Child Development 59,* 135–146.

Lakatos, K., Toth, I., Nemoda, Z., Ney, K., Sasvari-Szekely, M., & Gervai, J. (2000). Dopamine D4 receptor (DRD4) gene polymorphism is associated with attachment disorganization in infants. *Molecular Psychiatry, 5,* 633–637.

Lakatos, K., Nemoda, Z., Toth, I., Ronai, Z., Ney, K., Sasvari-Szekely, M., & Gervai, J. (2002). Further evidence for the role of the dopamine D4 receptor (DRD4) gene in attachment disorganization: Interaction of the exon III 48-bp repeat and the −521 C/T promoter polymorphism. *Molecular Psychiatry, 7*(1), 27–31.

Liotti, G. (1992). Disorganized/disoriented attachment in the etiology of the dissociative disorders. *Dissociation, 5,* 196–204.

Lyons-Ruth, K. (1996). Attachment relationships among children with aggressive behavior problems: The role of disorganized early attachment patterns. *Journal of Consulting and Clinical Psychology, 64* (1), 64–73.

Lyons-Ruth, K., & Jacobvitz, D. (1999). Attachment disorganization: Unresolved loss, relational violence, and lapses in behavioral and attentional strategies. In J. Cassidy & P. R. Shaver (Eds.), *Handbook of attachment: Theory, research, and clinical applications* (pp. 520–554). New York: Guilford Press.

Main, M. (1973). *Exploration, play, and cognitive functioning as related to child–mother attachment.* Unpublished doctoral dissertation, Johns Hopkins University.

Main, M. (1977). Sicherheit und Wissen [Security and knowledge]. In K. E. Grossmann (Ed.), *Entwicklung der Lernfahigheit in der sozialen Umwel [Development of learning competence in the social world]* (pp. 47–95) München, Germany: Kindler.

Main, M. (1979). The ultimate causation of some infant attachment phenomena: Further answers, further phenomena and further questions. *Behavioral and Brain Sciences, 2,* 640–643.

Main, M. (1981). Avoidance in the service of attachment: A working paper. In K. Immelmann, G. Barlow, L. Petrinovitch, & M. Main (Eds.), *Behavioral develop-*

ment: The Bielefeld interdisciplinary project (pp. 651–693). New York: Cambridge University Press.

Main, M. (1990). Cross-cultural studies of attachment organization: Recent studies, changing methodologies and the concept of conditional strategies. *Human Development, 33,* 48–61.

Main, M. (1995). Recent studies in attachment: Overview, with implications for clinical work. In S. Goldberg, R. Muir, & J. Kerr (Eds.), *Attachment theory: Social, developmental, and clinical perspectives* (pp. 407–474) Hillsdale, NJ: Analytic Press.

Main, M. (1999). Epilogue. Attachment theory: Eighteen points with suggestions for future studies. In J. Cassidy & P. R. Shaver (Eds.), *Handbook of attachment: Theory, research, and clinical applications* (pp. 845–888). New York: Guilford Press.

Main, M. (2000). The Adult Attachment Interview: Fear, attention, safety and discourse processes. *Journal of the American Psychoanalytic Association, 48*(4), 1055–1096.

Main, M. (2001, April 21). *Attachment to mother and father in infancy, as related to the Adult Attachment Interview and a self-visualization task at age 19.* Poster presented at the biennial meeting of the Society for Research in Child Development, Minneapolis, MN.

Main, M., & Cassidy, J. (1988). Categories of response to reunion with the parent at age 6: Predicted from infant attachment classifications and stable over a 1-month period. *Developmental Psychology, 24,* 415–426.

Main, M., & Goldwyn, R. (1984). *Adult attachment scoring and classification system.* Unpublished manuscripts, University of California, Berkeley.

Main, M., Goldwyn, R., & Hesse, E. (2003). *Adult attachment scoring and classification system.* Unpublished manuscript, University of California, Berkeley.

Main, M., & Hesse, E. (1990). Parents' unresolved traumatic experiences are related to infant disorganized/disoriented attachment status: Is frightened and/or frightening parental behavior the linking mechanism? In M. T. Greenberg, D. Cicchetti, & E. M. Cummings (Eds.), *Attachment in the preschool years: Theory, research, and intervention* (pp. 161–182). Chicago: University of Chicago Press.

Main, M., & Hesse, E. (1991–1998). *Frightening, frightened, dissociated, deferential, sexualized and disorganized parental behavior: A coding system for frightening parent–infant interactions.* Unpublished manuscript, University of California, Berkeley.

Main, M., Kaplan, N., & Cassidy, J. (1985). Security in infancy, childhood and adulthood: A move to the level of representation. In I. Bretherton & E. Waters (Eds.), Growing points of attachment theory and research. *Monographs of the Society for Research in Child Development, 50*(1–2, Serial No. 209), 66–104.

Main, M., & Solomon, J. (1990). Procedures for identifying infants as disorganized/disoriented during the Ainsworth Strange Situation. In M. T. Greenberg, D. Cicchetti, & E. M. Cummings (Eds.), *Attachment in the preschool years: Theory, research, and intervention* (pp. 121–160). Chicago: University of Chicago Press.

Main, M., & Stadtman, J. (1981). Infant response to rejection of physical contact by the mother: Aggression, avoidance and conflict. *Journal of the American Academy of Child Psychiatry, 20,* 2992–3007.

Main, M., & Weston, D. R. (1981). The quality of the toddler's relationship to mother and to father: Related to conflict behavior and the readiness to establish new relationships. *Child Development, 52*, 932–940.

Mason, J. H. (Trans.). (1970). *Gilgamesh: A verse narrative.* New York: New American Library.

Minde, K., & Hesse, E. (1996). The role of the Adult Attachment Interview in parent–infant psychotherapy: A case presentation. *Infant Mental Health Journal, 17*, 115–126.

Mura, S. S. (1983). Licensing violations: Legitimate violations of Grice's conversational principle. In R. T. Craig & K. Tracy (Eds.), *Conversational coherence: Form, structure and strategy.* Beverly Hills, CA: Sage.

Plato (1959). *Samliche Werke [Collected works]: Vol. 6. Nomoi.* Hamburg: Rowohlt.

Robertson, J., & Bowlby, J. (1952). Responses of young children to separation from their mothers. *Courrier Centre Internationale Enfance, 2*, 131–142.

Roisman, G. L., Padron, E., Sroufe, L. A., & Egeland, B. (2002). Earned-secure attachment status in retrospect and prospect. *Child Development, 73*(4), 1204–1219.

Sagi, A., van IJzendoorn, M. H., Scharf, M. H., Koren-Karie, N., Joels, T., & Mayseless, O. (1994). Stability and discriminant validity of the Adult Attachment Interview: A psychometric study in young Israeli adults. *Developmental Psychology, 30*, 771–777.

Schuengel, C., van IJzendoorn, M. H., & Bakermans-Kranenburg, M. (1999). Frightening maternal behavior linking unresolved loss and disorganized infant attachment. *Journal of Consulting and Clinical Psychology, 67*, 54–63.

Simpson, J. A. (1999). Attachment theory in modern evolutionary perspective. In J. Cassidy & P. R. Shaver (Eds.), *Handbook of attachment: Theory, research, and clinical applications* (pp. 115–140). New York: Guilford Press.

Solomon, J., & George, C. (1999). The measurement of attachment security in infancy and childhood. In J. Cassidy & P. R. Shaver (Eds.), *Handbook of attachment: Theory, research, and clinical applications* (pp. 287–316). New York: Guilford Press.

Spangler, G., & Grossmann, K. E. (1993). Biobehavioral organization in securely and insecurely attached infants. *Child Development, 64*, 1439–1450.

Sroufe, L. A. (1985). Attachment classification from the perspective of infant–caregiver relationships and infant attachment. *Child Development, 2*, 1–14.

Sroufe, L. A., Egeland, B., Carlson, E., & Collins, W. A. (2005). *The development of the person: The Minnesota study of risk and adaptation from birth to adulthood.* New York: Guilford Press.

Sroufe, L. A., Egeland, B., & Kreutzer, T. (1990). The fate of early experience following developmental change: Longitudinal approaches to individual adaptation in childhood. *Child Development, 61*, 1363–1373.

Sroufe, L. A., & Waters, E. (1977). Attachment as an organizational construct. *Child Development, 48*, 1184–1199.

Stern, D. (1985). *The interpersonal world of the infant: A view from psychoanalysis and developmental psychology.* New York: Basic Books.

Tinbergen, N., & Moynihan, M. (1952). Head flagging in the black-headed gull: Its function and origin. *British Birds, 45*, 19–22.

Trivers, R. L. (1974). Parent–offspring conflict. *American Zoologist, 14*, 249–264.

True, M., Pisani, L., & Oumar, F. (2001). Infant–mother attachment among the Dogon in Mali. *Child Development, 75*(5), 1451–1466.

Underwood, B. (1966). *Experimental psychology* (2nd ed.). New York: Appleton-Century-Crofts.

van IJzendoorn, M. H. (1995). Adult attachment representations, parental responsiveness, and infant attachment: A meta-analysis on the predictive validity of the Adult Attachment Interview. *Psychological Bulletin, 117,* 387–403.

van IJzendoorn, M. H., & Kroonenburg, P. M. (1990). Cross-cultural consistency of coding the Strange Situation. *Infant Behavior and Development, 13,* 469–485.

van IJzendoorn, M. H., Schuengel, C., & Bakermans-Kranenburg, M. J. (1999). Disorganized attachment in early childhood: Meta-analysis of precursors, concomitants, and sequelae. *Development and Psychopathology, 11,* 225–249.

Vaughn, B. E., Egeland, B., Sroufe, L.A., & Waters, E. (1979). Individual differences in infant–mother attachment at twelve and eighteen months: Stability and change in families under stress. *Child Development, 50,* 971–975.

Waldinger, R. J., Seidman, E. L., Gerber, A. J., Liem, J. H., Allen, J. P., & Hauser, S. H. (2003). Attachment and core relational themes: Wishes for autonomy and closeness in the narratives of securely and insecurely attached adults. *Psychotherapy Research, 13*(1), 77–98.

Ward, M. J., & Carlson, E. A. (1995). The predictive validity of the Adult Attachment Interview for adolescent mothers. *Child Development, 66,* 69–79.

Wartner, U. G., Grossmann, K., Fremmer-Bombik, E., & Suess, G. (1994). Attachment patterns at age six in south Germany: Predictability from infancy and implications for preschool behavior. *Child Development, 65*(4), 1014–1027.

Waters, E., Merrick, S. K., Treboux, D., Crowell, J., & Albersheim, L. (2000). Attachment security from infancy to early adulthood: A twenty-year longitudinal study. *Child Development, 71*(3), 684–689.

Waters, E., Treboux, D., Fyffe, C., & Crowell, J. (2001). *Scoring secure versus insecure and dismissing versus preoccupied attachment as continuous variables: discriminant analysis using AAI state of mind scales.* Manuscript submitted for publication.

Waters, E., Vaughn, B. E., Posada, G., & Kondo-Ikemura, K. (Eds.). (1995). Caregiving, cultural and cognitive perspectives on secure-base behavior and working models: New growing points of attachment theory and research. *Monographs of the Society for Research in Child Development, 60*(2–3, Serial No. 244).

Weinfield, N. S., Sroufe, L. A., & Egeland, B. (2000). Attachment from infancy to adulthood in a high-risk sample: Continuity, discontinuity, and their correlates. *Child Development, 71,* 695–702.

Weinfield, N. S., Sroufe, L. A., Egeland, B., & Carlson, E. A. (1999). The nature of individual differences in infant–caregiver attachment. In J. Cassidy & P. R. Shaver (Eds.), *Handbook of attachment: Theory, research, and clinical applications* (pp. 68–88). New York: Guilford Press.

Weinfield, N. S., Whaley, G., & Egeland, B. (2004). Continuity, discontinuity and coherence in attachment from infancy to late adolescence: Sequelae of organization and disorganization. *Attachment and Human Development, 6*(1), 73–97.

CHAPTER 11

Lessons from the Longitudinal Studies of Attachment

MARY DOZIER
MELISSA MANNI
OLIVER LINDHIEM

We first take this opportunity to thank the authors of the chapters in this volume for their critical contributions to the field. As we and others began our longitudinal studies in the 1990s and 2000s, we were informed by what these individuals had already accomplished in the way of developing and refining attachment theory, and developing and refining methodologies for studying it. As a result of these investigators' longitudinal studies, we now have an understanding of developmental trajectories under a range of circumstances that inform our questions, our methodologies, and the range of possibilities open to us. In this chapter, we highlight some of their many contributions and point to issues with which we continue to struggle.

Our research program has focused on children who experience disruptions in care as the result of their placement in foster care. Recently, we have also begun to focus on children who have not experienced disruptions in care, but rather have remained in their parents' care following maltreatment. Although children who experienced early attachment disruptions were of interest to Bowlby, such children have received relatively little attention from attachment researchers more recently, with several exceptions (e.g., Hodges & Tizard, 1989a, 1989b). As a result of this lack of attention, there are a number of issues that the study of these children has raised that we discuss in this chapter. We consider such issues vital and informative not just for the study of foster children, but for furthering our understanding of attachment more generally. We also consider the contributions of others and the challenges for the next generation of researchers in the context of the questions that we are asking.

CHALLENGES FOR CHILDREN IN FOSTER CARE

One night as I watched the news in the early 1990s, I saw a toddler being taken away from her foster parents who had raised her since birth. The couple wanted to adopt her, but a judge determined that the child should be with parents of her own ethnicity (she was Hispanic and her foster parents were non-Hispanic). I remember so well the child's anguished cries as social workers took her from her foster parents. At the time I was studying how attachment state of mind affected use of treatment among adults with serious psychiatric disorders. But within several hours of seeing this child's reaction to being taken from her foster parents, I began to think about changing the focus of my research.

According to Bowlby (1969/1982), the attachment behavior system evolved because it served to protect the infant, and thus enhanced reproductive fitness. In the evolutionary history of humans (and of many other primate species), survival was enhanced if infants were in proximity to their parents under conditions of threat. In Bowlby's view, when infants were sick, hurt, in the company of strangers, or under other threatening conditions, it was advantageous for them to be close to the parent. Infants who showed such behaviors were more likely to survive and to pass on their genes than other infants, and this characteristic was thus favored. As Bowlby pointed out, the attachment behavioral system was not secondary to other systems in terms of its evolutionary significance. Whereas the infant could go for hours without food, he or she would not survive without a caretaker under conditions of threat for very long at all. Hence, the immediacy, the strength of the system, is apparent. Separations thus represent the ultimate threat. For example, Levine and colleagues (Coe, Glass, Wiener, & Levine, 1983; Levine, Johnson, & Gonzalez, 1985) found that, regardless of the number of times that infant squirrel monkeys were separated from their mothers, they never habituated in terms of neuroendocrine response.

As I thought about this foster child who was taken away from her attachment figures, what struck me was how difficult were the challenges for her and for others like her. Even if the previous attachment figure had been insensitive or had maltreated the child, this disruption would not be easy. It was immaterial to the child whether the parents were foster parents or birth parents—in either case, the child would need to form an attachment to a new caregiver after having lost the parents to whom he or she had become attached.

Developing Attachments in a New Relationship

The Grossmanns' work (see K. Grossmann, K. E. Grossmann, & Kindler, Chapter 5, this volume, for a summary) has highlighted how critical multiple assessments of the child and parents can be to understanding the relationship fully. When considering a developing relationship between a foster mother and a foster infant, it was apparent that we needed to assess attachment behaviors frequently, even daily. Clearly, the Strange Situation was not the instrument that would allow us to look at a developing attachment on a daily basis. After he or she had one or two encounters with the Strange Situation, he or she would no longer experience the same impact from the experimental condition. Although Waters and Deane's (1985) Attachment Q-sort was a somewhat more plausible alternative, it was nonetheless untenable because of the time involved and its high stability. We were not aware of other existing measures that could be collected frequently (i.e., daily) that were highly sensitive to change. Therefore, we developed a diary measure of children's attachment behaviors. Given Bowlby's (1969/1982) suggestion that attachment behaviors should be seen when children are frightened, hurt, and separated from caregivers, we asked parents to generate examples of their children's behaviors under these conditions in our daily inventory. Each day, parents were asked to provide a brief narrative of an incident that had occurred that day in which their child had been hurt (and a second in which their child had been frightened, and a third in which the child had been separated from the caregiver). Parents also completed a checklist corresponding to the narrative of the child's initial behaviors, the parent's response, and the child's response to the parent. We attempted to make the measure as objective as possible by asking parents to describe *specific* events that happened *that day*. Daily inventories of these behaviors have a number of advantages to more global, retrospective reports of child behavior. Daily report minimizes parent bias and error, measures factual events rather than parents' subjective attitudes, and provides specific time frames for parents to recount events (Furey & Forehand, 1983). Using this methodology, we followed the development of children's attachment behaviors over a 2-month period (see Stovall & Dozier, 2000).

The answer to our question regarding how long it takes for an infant to form a new attachment was complicated. To our surprise, infants younger than a year of age tended to show stable attachment behaviors very, very quickly (Stovall & Dozier, 2000; Stovall-McClough & Dozier, 2004). Certainly, within 2 weeks, attachments behaviors had become stable for nearly all infants. For many young infants, attachment behaviors were stable within the first week. However surprising this may seem, it is important to keep in mind our evolutionary history: an infant without an attachment figure would not have survived in the wild for long. Therefore, a several-day period is not a short time in the life of an infant. Nonetheless, differences between younger infants (younger than about 10 months of age) and older infants (older than about 1 year of age) were striking. Older infants did not show stable attachment behaviors for an extended period of time following placement. For most, stability was not seen for at least several weeks, and for some, attachment behaviors were still not stable 2 months after placement. We have posited that stability reflects, to some extent, the consolidation of the attachment for the child (Stovall-McClough & Dozier, 2004). Certainly, on the basis of these behavioral data, the process of consolidating a new attachment appears more difficult for the older infant than for the younger infant. Nonetheless, we are aware that converging methods are critical to make strong claims with regard to this thesis. For example, even young infants show evidence that they are dysregulated at the neuroendocrine level although their behavior may appear well regulated (Dozier et al., 2004), so we do not want to suggest that the process is easy for younger infants.

Parental State of Mind and Infant Attachment

As overviewed in this volume (Sroufe, Egeland, Carlson, & Collins, Chapter 4; H. Steele & M. Steele, Chapter 6; and Main, Hesse, & Kaplan, Chapter 10), Main and colleagues developed the parental measure that best predicts infant attachment quality. Amazingly, even before an infant is born, the parents' state of mind predicts the child's attachment (Fonagy, Steele, & Steele, 1991; Steele, Steele, & Fonagy, 1996). Nonetheless, there were a number of reasons to think that such associations might not hold for foster parent–infant dyads. First, given that the foster mother and the infant were unrelated genetically, any temperamental aspects that were important to the transmission would not play a part. Second, the child's earlier experiences might interfere with taking advantage of the foster mother's contribution to the interaction, as suggested by our diary findings. However, we found that the association between foster mother state of mind and child attachment was nearly as high as that reported in van IJzendoorn's (1995) meta-analysis. In particular, we found a two-way correspondence of 72% between foster mother state of mind and foster infant attachment, as contrasted with van IJzendoorn's 75%. These findings, particularly among older infants, surprised us. The findings suggested that, after some period in the relationship, the foster mother was able to lead the dance (using Daniel Stern's [1977] metaphor). Furthermore, along with other studies (e.g., O'Connor & Croft, 2001), this study suggests that the primary mechanism of transmission is not genetic.

Internal Working Models and Other Developmental Outcomes

Bowlby (1969/1982) proposed that, on the basis of attachment experiences, the child develops internal working models of relationships. One can think of the internal working model as a roadmap, providing predictability for an otherwise uncertain journey. Just as there are costs to an inaccurate map (e.g., it will provide the wrong direction at times), an inconsistent map (e.g., it will be confusing at times), or a map that cannot be updated and revised (e.g., it will not allow for new roads, changes in roads, etc.), there are costs to an inaccurate, inconsistent, or rigid internal working model. Bretherton develops these issues elegantly in her chapter in this volume (see Chapter 2).

K. Grossmann, K. E. Grossmann, and Kindler (Chapter 5, this volume) emphasize that these models are formed on the basis of attachment experiences with both parents. In their work, both mothers' and fathers' interactions with children powerfully predict later representations of relationships, some assessed 15–20 years later when these children have become young adults. Fathers' early and ongoing support of exploration appears to be especially critical to developing feelings about the self. We consider this finding especially important because fathers' contributions as attachment figures have been neglected in many investigations, including our own.

As Avi Sagi-Schwartz and Ora Aviezer emphasize (Chapter 7, this volume), the question of how attachments to different caregivers affect the development of internal working models is a thorny one. As hierarchies become more complex (e.g., mother, father, grandmother, foster mother) and as conditions become more unstable (as elaborated by Belsky, Chapter 4, this volume), it becomes increasingly difficult to predict effects on developmental outcomes (Sroufe, Egeland, Carlson, & Collins, Chapter 3, this volume). On the other hand, with greater complexity and instability, large sample sizes will allow assessment of the relative role of early attachments. Sagi-Schwartz and Aviezer have asked the important question, What is the "special" place for early attachments? If we see lawful discontinuity (Weinfield, Sroufe, & Egeland, 2000), can we nonetheless see the residual of the early attachment later? For example, consider a child who has a secure attachment to a mother who dies when the child is age 3. The child's subsequent caregiving is unstable, and he shows behavioral problems in adolescence. Nonetheless, can we see the effects of his early attachment when he forms a marital relationship or is a parent to his own children? The work of Grossmann and Grossmann (detailed in this volume) has been critical to understanding the complexities of relationship influences over time. Our work with foster children (who may have secure attachments to caregivers they never see again or secure relationships with caregivers following very unstable early care) provides an extreme test of the importance of early attachments. These and other conditions (as overviewed below) can allow us to gradually unpack effects.

Associations between infant attachment quality and later developmental outcomes have been seen in a number of studies. Sroufe and colleagues (Chapter 4, this volume) found that attachment quality was associated with many salient developmental outcomes. Although Grossmann and Grossmann (K. Grossmann, K. E. Grossmann, & Kindler, Chapter 5, this volume) did not find that attachment quality predicted later outcomes, parent and child relationship indices were important predictors of later outcomes.

Among foster children, we do not find that attachment quality predicts later behavioral outcomes, such as performance in the tool task (e.g., Bates & Dozier, 2002) or representations of attachment figures (e.g., Ackerman & Dozier, 2004). Given the complexities of these children's attachment hierarchies and the lack of stability in their lives, perhaps this is not surprising. Indeed, a host of findings suggest that the more unstable a child's environment is, the less predictability is allowed with regard to later outcomes (see K. Grossmann, K. E. Grossmann, & Kindler, Chapter 5, this volume; Sroufe, Egeland, Carlson, & Collins, Chapter 3, this volume).

On the other hand, whereas attachment quality (measured in the Strange Situation) is not associated with developmental outcomes, foster parents' commitment to their children has predicted a number of such outcomes. For example, foster parents who indicated that they were more highly committed to their children were rated as more supportive in the problem-solving task and their children were more enthusiastic in problem solving (Bates & Dozier, 2002). Greater commitment was also associated with children showing more adequate resolutions on the Separation Anxiety Test (Ackerman & Dozier, 2004). We consider it plausible that having a *committed* caregiver is a more fundamental need than having a *responsive* caregiver. There may be relatively little variability along this dimension among most intact parent–child dyads, but quite a lot of variability when surrogate caregivers are involved.

Children's Ability to Adapt to Various Conditions

Typically, children's ability to function in a range of environments cannot be tested experimentally. Whereas nonhuman primate work allows experimental manipulation of such things as the duration of mother–infant separations, human research is usually limited to natural experiments. The types of natural experiments range from daycare (e.g., National Institute of Child Health and Human Development [NICHD] Early Child Care Research Network, 1997) to parents who stress early independence (e.g., Bielefeld sample of K. Grossmann, K. E. Grossmann, Spangler, Suess, & Unzner, 1985) to kibbutz-rearing (e.g., Sagi-Schwartz & Aviezer, Chapter 7, this volume) to foster care (e.g., Dozier, Stovall, Albus, & Bates, 2001) to orphanage placements (e.g., Chisholm, 1998). These natural experiments are critical in suggesting what conditions are optimal to development, what conditions are nonoptimal but for which children can typically develop an organized response, and what conditions may leave children with limited adaptive coping strategies. There are many opportunities for counterintuitive findings in these studies, such as the nontransmission of unresolved states of mind among Holocaust survivors (Sagi-Schwartz et al., 2003). Such counterintuitive findings lead to a refinement and qualifying of theory.

From an evolutionary perspective, placing children in child care for much of the day could represent a failure to provide protection, although there is some evidence for "baby-sitting" among nonhuman primates. This issue was therefore of great interest to a number of researchers in attachment and child care. It was plausible that children were not able to cope with not having a primary attachment figure available for long periods of the day. The effects of child care on attachment have been mixed and complex. For example (see Belsky, Chapter 4, this volume), the NICHD Early Child Care Research Network (1997) found that child care, in and of itself, had no significant effect on attachment security among infants and their caregivers. Under specific conditions, however (e.g., poor quality of care, more than 10 hours of care per week, or more than one child-care setting within the first 15 months of life), infants were more likely to form insecure attachments to caregivers, but only if their caregiver was low in sensitivity. Other child-care evidence suggests that center-based care, in and of itself, does indeed have a negative effect on the development of secure attachment relationships (e.g., Sagi, Koren-Karie, Gini, Ziv, & Joels, 2002). In any event, there is consistent evidence that child care is stressful for children, as shown in increasing levels of cortisol over the course of the day in center-based child-care settings (e.g., Dettling, Gunnar, & Donzella, 1999; Tout, de Haan, Campbell, & Gunnar, 1998; Watamura, Donzella, Alwin, & Gunnar, 2003).

Routine nighttime separations may be even more difficult than daytime separations for young children. Sagi-Schwartz and Aviezer (Chapter 7, this volume) found that children who slept away from their parents in kibbutzim showed low levels of security to parents. Children whose parents are routinely absent when they go to bed may become less able to trust in their parents' availability. Plausibly, these findings suggest that parents' physical presence when children go to bed may be crucial to a developing sense of security.

Nonetheless, it seems that, whereas conditions of regular, routine separations may not be optimal, children can develop strategies for coping with these separations. The variation is typically considered in terms of individual differences in attachment quality. Rarely has the question been *whether* a child is attached to his or her caregiver under these differing conditions.

When young children experience severe deprivation or privation for an extended period of time, they typically thrive physically when given stimulation and care (see Gunnar, 2003). For some, though, or perhaps even for many, there is a point after which it seems to become difficult to establish meaningful relationships with others. O'Connor and colleagues (O'Connor, Marvin, Rutter, Olrick, & Britner, 2003) studied children who had spent their early months in Romanian orphanages as they adjusted to new adoptive homes in the United Kingdom. They found a dose–response association between length of time in orphanage care and disturbed attachment behaviors. About half of the children who had been in orphanages between 6 and 24 months showed anomalous behaviors in the Strange Situation. Some showed disinhibited attachment, similar to the indiscriminate friendliness described by Chisholm (1998). Others showed an odd inconsistent pattern of behaviors with the stranger (e.g., friendliness followed by wariness). Bowlby (1946) described similar behaviors among his "affectionless thieves." What these children shared was a period of extreme privation and/or deprivation with regard to primary attachment relationships. Although we occasionally see such behavior among children who are placed in foster care (Albus & Dozier, 1999), at least at the anecdotal level, it appears to be a rarer phenomenon than seen among children who have experienced more serious privation.

Conditions for Change

Whether mind-minded relationships (i.e., those involving reflection on oneself, one's partner, and one's relationship) can lead to revision of working models is a question elaborated in Crowell and Waters (Chapter 9, this volume) consideration of couples' relationships with one another and with their children. Mind-minded relationships could include psychotherapy, relationships with partners, and relationships with children, among others. In the assessment of change, we expect that studying quantitative shifts (e.g., changes in dimensional score for autonomy) will be more fruitful than studying categorical shifts (e.g., changes from dismissing to autonomous states of mind). The measure of reflective functioning developed by Howard and Miriam Steele, in collaboration with Peter Fonagy (see H. Steele & M. Steele, Chapter 6, this volume), is an example of a variable that should be more amenable to change than state of mind more generally.

In our work with foster parents, we have not attempted to directly change working models. One of our intervention components with foster parents involves helping foster parents to provide more nurturing care than they would otherwise. To achieve this goal, we ask foster parents to consider their reactions to their children's bids for reassurance, and the impact on parenting of having their own needs met as children. Rather than attempt to modify parents' state of mind, we help them "override" their propensities. By becoming aware of their own reactions, parents can respond to children in a less automatic fashion, providing nurturance even if that is not what is elicited for them. It is possible that we are helping parents to become more "mindful" (Slade, in press) of their children, and, in so doing, may indirectly affect parents' state of mind. Our primary intention, though, is to affect parental behaviors, and thus eventually the internal working models of the children.

HOW CAN THE FIELD OF ATTACHMENT RESEARCH BECOME MORE OPEN?

The field of attachment research is considered by some researchers to be relatively closed. This is probably partially the result of the time involved in becoming trained and reliable in the use of most measures. Furthermore, there is the perception, whether true or not, that the field is not very open to modifications in constructs and/or methodology, and that discrepant findings or theories are not welcomed. All of this has led to the perception that attachment researchers represent a "guild." This is a serious concern. To the extent that this perception is true, it needs to be countered. We discuss the complexities of some of these issues below.

Open to Disconfirmation

A threat (but also a strength) inherent in most longitudinal studies is that we include measurements of nearly everything, including assessments of cognitive development, social development, neuroendocrine functioning, and so on. It is indeed useful to have information regarding children's functioning across domains. What is critical is that we develop hypotheses about expected associations that are precise and "risky" (Popper, 1963). Karl Popper, a philosopher of science, emphasized that a theory can only be confirmed when risky predictions are supported. Risky predictions are those that would not be made in the absence of the theory. For attachment research, our predictions ought to be sufficiently risky that researchers with different theoretical orientations would make different predictions. In particular, hypotheses should be more specific than those predicted by parental warmth or good parenting more generally. Furthermore, if *any* results could be interpreted as supportive of the theory, then the theory is not falsifiable. On the other hand, it is also critical that we study a wide range of factors that we do not expect to be directly associated with attachment and specify hypothesized associations (or lack of associations) a priori.

Open to Other Operationalizations

The methods relied on most heavily in attachment research are not amenable to easy dissemination. The Strange Situation and the Adult Attachment Interview (AAI), as well as most other measures, require extensive training and are time-consuming to use. Attempts to develop shortcuts for the methods have not been entirely satisfying, so for now we may be reliant upon expensive measures that will not be accessible to all. Self-report measures of attachment style have yielded very interesting findings, but these measures are unrelated or only modestly related to attachment state of mind as assessed using the AAI (e.g., see Crowell & Waters, Chapter 9, this volume). Nonetheless, we encourage attempts to go beyond current methodologies in assessing constructs of interest. The Strange Situation and the AAI are proxies for variables of interest, and we should not be conservative as a field in considering alternative methodologies or conceptualizations.

The Strange Situation (Ainsworth, Blehar, Waters, & Wall, 1978) has proven to be a powerful procedure, as demonstrated in the longitudinal studies presented in this volume. Although the procedure is only about 21-minutes-long and involves observing "strange behavior in a strange environment" (Belsky, Chapter 4, this volume), it appears to capture a critical feature of the infant–parent relationship. Nonetheless, Karin and Klaus Grossmannn remind us in this volume (see K. Grossmann, K. E. Grossmann, & Kindler, Chapter 5) of Bowlby's warning that we not reify the Strange Situation as the sole operationalization of attachment quality. Even though at a concrete level the Strange Situation provides videotaped data regarding the parent–child relationship, the procedure provides only a snapshot of the parent–child relationship. Bowlby (1969/1982) worried that too much stock was being placed in a single assessment when the child was 12 months old. The Grossmanns' data show us the importance of using other measures as well as the Strange Situation. Had they only included the Strange Situation in their assessments, they might well have come to the erroneous conclusion that the parent–child interaction was not critical to the adolescent's and adult's representations of self and others.

Mary Main is an excellent observer of behaviors who has not been constrained by existing methodologies or coding schemes. Some 15 years ago, she recognized that some of the most important variations in attachment were not being captured by Ainsworth's system. As she reports in Chapter 10 (Main, Heese, & Kaplan) in this volume, she first noticed the disorientation of a child who ran away from her mother and toward Main when thunder struck nearby. This observation served as the source of her development of a system for coding disorganized behavior. Using observational skills à la Ainsworth, she developed a coding scheme for disorganized attachment that captured these odd and anomalous behaviors that had been neglected in the prior system.

Elizabeth Carlson's work provides another example in the tradition of Mary Ainsworth, Mary Main, and the Grossmanns. She noted that many children who had spent their early years in orphanages showed anomalous behaviors in the Strange Situation, behaviors that were not well characterized by the existing categorization system. Rather than use a system that did not adequately characterize the sample, Carlson developed a system for rating the extent to which children showed behaviors that are seen typically among orphanage-reared children (see Zeanah, Smyke, Koga, Carlson, & the BEIP Core Group. 2004). Had she simply used the usual coding system, she could have coded these children's behaviors, but would have missed much. Similarly, she has noticed anomalous behaviors among our foster children in coding the tool task. Whereas it is possible to rate children's performance using the same system that has been used for other samples, much is lost in the process.

Karlen Lyons-Ruth's coding of the hostile/helpless state of mind provides an excellent example of a critical innovation with regard to the AAI. Having found that the existing system of classification yielded too many false negatives for parents of disorganized attachment, Lyons-Ruth carefully studied which parents were missed (Lyons-Ruth, Yellin, Melnick, & Atwood, in press). Following Mary Main's lead in analyzing discourse carefully and systematically, she found that mothers with a hostile/helpless state of mind, who had not necessarily been coded as unresolved, typically had infants with disorganized attachments. She argued that the mother and the child share a hostile/helpless approach to interactions, whereby either total control is executed (the hostile orientation) or control is completely given over to the other (the helpless orientation). As Lyons-Ruth points out, this model accounts for the very different outcomes (e.g., controlling vs. passive) for children who had been disorganized in infancy. This is an exciting contribution to the field.

FINAL COMMENTS

One of the reasons that this volume's authors have made such crucial contributions is that most entered the area from a "nonattachment" perspective. Like Bowlby, many of these individuals originally had primary interests and/or expertise in development that were outside of attachment relationships. Klaus Grossmann and Karin Grossmann, Robert Hinde, and Joan Stevenson-Hinde were ethologists who also had experience in experimental animal behavior. Everett Waters was a chemistry major when he met Mary Ainsworth as an undergraduate. Jay Belsky was trained in the "ecology of human development" by scientists who were critical of attachment theory. Howard Steele and Miriam Steele came from a psychoanalytic tradition. Mary Main was primarily interested in language development when she started graduate school. L. Alan Sroufe started his career as a psychophysiologist, and Byron Egeland was interested in child maltreatment. When one considers the richness of these backgrounds, it makes sense that questions were asked and the theory developed in ways that would not have happened otherwise. For example, Sroufe and Waters (1977) were able to provide compelling evidence that avoidant children are not just unperturbed by the separation from their mothers by monitoring their heart rates, an approach unlikely to have been employed if Sroufe did not have expertise in psychophysiological measures. Main's background in language development and linguistics was critical to her ability to develop measures that assess narrative coherence.

As a field, we need to embrace Joan Stevenson-Hinde's suggestion (Chapter 8, this volume) that we become more eclectic. We have trained a generation of attachment researchers, something that most of these pioneers were not. Although that has been useful in developing the foundation of attachment theory, we now need to train students who look more like these pioneers in terms of background and expertise. The National Institutes of Health have recognized the need for researchers who apply knowledge from one area of study to another in funding translational research efforts. Just as these pioneers were translational researchers, we need to train our students to become translational researchers. Such training could involve developing expertise in areas such as neuroscience, cognitive development, and primatology, for example. Rather than working with other attachment researchers, we need to be challenged by working with a group such as that convened by Bowlby in the 1960s (described by Robert A. Hinde, Chapter 1, this volume) that included an ethologist, a primatologist, and a learning theorist, among others. This broadening of expertise, and asking questions that cut across areas, will strengthen and enrich the field of attachment.

ACKNOWLEDGMENTS

We acknowledge the support of Grant Nos. K02 MH01782 and R01 MH52135 from the National Institute of Mental Health to Mary Dozier. We greatly appreciate the helpful feedback of Karin Grossmann, Klaus Grossmann, Abraham Sagi-Schwartz, Inge Bretherton, and Robert Hinde on an earlier version of this chapter.

REFERENCES

Ackerman, J., & Dozier, M. (2004). *Foster parent commitment and children's representations of self and others.* Unpublished manuscript, University of Delaware.

Ainsworth, M. D. S., Blehar, M. C., Waters, E., & Wall, S. (1978). *Patterns of attachment: A psychological study of the Strange Situation.* Hillsdale, NJ: Erlbaum.

Albus, K. E., & Dozier, M. (1999). Indiscriminate friendliness and terror of strangers in infancy: Contributions from the study of infants in foster care. *Infant Mental Health Journal, 20,* 30–41.

Bates, B., & Dozier, M. (2002). The importance of maternal state of mind regarding attachment and infant age at placement to foster mothers' representations of their foster infants. *Infant Mental Health Journal, 23,* 417–431.

Bowlby, J. (1946). *Fourty-four juvenile thieves: Their characters and home life.* London: Tindall & Cox.

Bowlby, J. (1969/1982). *Attachment and loss: Vol. 1. Attachment.* New York: Basic Books.

Chisholm, K. (1998). A three year follow-up of attachment and indiscriminate friendliness in children adopted from Romanian orphanages. *Child Development, 69,* 1092–1106.

Coe, C. L., Glass, J. C., Wiener, S. G., & Levine, S. (1983). Behavioral, but not physiological, adaptation to repeated separation in mother and infant primates. *Psychoneuroendocrinology, 8,* 401–409.

Dettling, A. C., Gunnar, M.R., & Donzella, B. (1999). Cortisol levels of young children in full-day childcare centers: Relations with age and temperament. *Psychoneuroendocrinology, 24,* 519–536.

Dozier, M., Manni, M., Gordon, K., Stovall-McClough, K. C., Gunnar, M. R., Fisher, P. A., & Levine, S. (2004). *Foster children's diurnal production of cortisol.* Manuscript submitted for publication.

Dozier, M., Stovall, K. C., Albus, K. E., & Bates, B. (2001). Attachment for infants in foster care: The role of caregiver state of mind. *Child Development, 72,* 1467–1477.

Fonagy, P., Steele, H., & Steele, M. (1991). Maternal representations of attachment during pregnancy predict the organization of infant–mother attachment at one year of age. *Child Development, 62*(5), 891–905.

Furey, W. & Forehand, R. (1983). The Daily Child Behavior Checklist. *Journal of Behavioral Assessment, 5*(2), 83–95.

Grossmann, K., Grossmann, K.E., Spangler, G., Suess, G., & Unzner, L. (1985). Maternal sensitivity and newborns' orientation responses as related to quality of attachment in northern Germany. In I. Bretherton & E. Waters (Eds.), Growing points in attachment theory and research. *Monographs of the Society for Research in Child Development, 50* (1–2, Serial No. 209), 233–256.

Gunnar, M. R. (2003). Integrating neuroscience and psychological approaches in the study of early experiences. *Annals of the New York Academy of Sciences, 1008,* 238–247.

Hodges, J., & Tizard, B. (1989a). IQ and behavioural adjustment of ex-institutional adolescents. *Journal of Child Psychology and Psychiatry and Allied Disciplines, 30*(1), 53–75.

Hodges, J., & Tizard, B. (1989b). Social and family relationships of ex-institutional adolescents. *Journal of Child Psychology and Psychiatry and Allied Disciplines*, *30*(1), 77–97.

Levine, S., Johnson, D. F., & Gonzalez, C. A. (1985). Behavioral and hormonal responses to separation in infant rhesus monkeys and mothers. *Behavioral Neuroscience*, *99*, 399–410.

Lyons-Ruth, K., Yellin, C., Melnick, S., & Atwood, G. (2003). Childhood experiences of trauma and loss have different relations to maternal unresolved and hostile-helpless states of mind on the AAI. *Attachment and Human Development*, *5*, 330–352.

Lyons-Ruth, K., Yellin, C., Melnick, S., & Atwood, G. (in press). Expanding the concept of unresolved mental states: Hostile/helpless states of mind on the adult attachment interview are associated with atypical maternal behavior and infant disorganization. *Development and Psychopathology*.

Melnick, S., Lyons-Ruth, K., Hobson, P., & Patrick, M. (2003, April). *Discriminating borderline states of mind regarding attachment: Operationalizing the concepts of affective splitting and hostile-helpless states of mind on the Adult Attachment Interview*. Poster presented at the biennial meeting of the Society for Research in Child Development, Tampa, FL.

National Institute of Child Health and Human Development Early Child Care Research Network. (1997). The effects of infant child care on infant–mother attachment security: Results of the NICHD study of early child care. *Child Development*, *68*, 860–879.

O'Connor, T. G., & Croft, C. M. (2001). A twin study of attachment in preschool children. *Child Development*, *72*(5), 1501–1511.

O'Connor, T. G., Marvin, R. S., Rutter, M., Olrick, J. T., & Britner, P. A. (2003). Attachment following early institutional deprivation. *Development and Psychopathology*, *15*, 19–38.

Popper, K. (1963). *Conjectures and refutations: The growth of scientific knowledge*. London: Routledge & Kegan Paul.

Sagi, A., Koren-Karie, N., Gini, M., Ziv, Y., & Joels, T. (2002). Shedding further light on the effects of various types and quality of early child care on infant–mother attachment relationship: The Haifa Study of Early Child Care. *Child Development*, *73*(4), 1166–1186.

Sagi-Schwartz, A., van IJzendoorn, M., Grossmann, K., Joels, T., Grossmann, K., Scharf, M., Koren-Karie, N., & Alkalay, S. (2003). Attachment and traumatic stress in female Holocaust child survivors and their daughters. *American Journal of Psychiatry*, *160*, 1086–1092.

Slade, A. (in press). Parental reflective functioning: An introduction. *Attachment and Human Development*.

Sroufe, L. A., & Waters, E. (1977). Heart rate as a convergent measure in clinical and developmental research. *Merrill-Palmer Quarterly*, *21*, 3–27.

Steele, H., Steele, M., & Fonagy, P. (1996). Associations among attachment classifications of mothers, fathers, and their infants. *Child Development*, *67*(2), 541–555.

Stern, D. (1997). *The first relationship*. Cambridge, MA: Harvard University Press.

Stovall, K. C., & Dozier, M. (2000). The development of attachment in new relationships: Single subject analyses for 10 foster infants. *Development and Psychopathology*, *12*(2), 133–156.

Stovall-McClough, K. C., & Dozier, M. (2004). Forming attachments in foster care: Infant attachment behaviors during the first 2 months of placement. *Development and Psychopathology, 16,* 253–271.

Tout, K., de Haan, M., Campbell, E. K., & Gunnar, M. R. (1998). Social behavior correlates of cortisol activity in child care: Gender differences and time of day effects. *Child Development, 69,* 1247–1262.

van IJzendoorn, M. H. (1995). Adult attachment representations, parental responsiveness, and infant attachment: A meta-analysis of the predictive validity of the Adult Attachment Interview. *Psychological Bulletin, 117,* 387–403.

Watamura, S., Donzella, B., Alwin, J., & Gunnar, M. (2003). Morning to afternoon increases in cortisol concentrations for infants and toddlers at child care: Age differences and behavioral correlates. *Child Development, 74,* 1006–1020.

Waters, E., & Deane, K. E. (1985). Defining and assessing individual differences in attachment relationships: Q-methodology and the organization of behavior in infancy and early childhood. In I. Bretherton & E. Waters (Eds.), Growing points in attachment theory and research. *Monographs of the Society for Research in Child Development, 50* (1–2, Serial No. 209), 41–65.

Weinfield, N. S., Sroufe, L. A., & Egeland, B. (2000). Attachment from infancy to early adulthood in a high-risk sample: Continuity, discontinuity, and their correlates. *Child Development, 71,* 695–702.

Zeanah, C. H., Smyke, A. T., Koga, S., Carlson, E. A., & the BEIP Core Group. (2004). *Attachment in institutionalized and community children in Romania.* Unpublished manuscript.

Index

Page numbers followed by an *f* indicate figure, *t* indicate table

321

LaVergne, TN USA
01 June 2010
184608LV00002B/20/A